Handbook of 3D Printing in Pharmaceutics

Three-dimensional (3D) printing has evolved as an emerging tool for the design of customized or personalized medication that provides the maximum therapeutic benefits to patients. The manufacturing of medicines in small batches customized with tailored dosages, sizes, shapes, and drug release properties is the key prospect of using 3D printing in pharmaceutics.

Handbook of 3D Printing in Pharmaceutics: Innovations and Applications provides a detailed and in-depth technical discussion on the various additive manufacturing processes for the development of pharmaceutical products with experimental justification. It details the characterization, optimization, and numerical modeling of the processes involved and outlines the industrial implications of the resulting products as well as offering solutions for patient-tailored drugs processed by additive manufacturing. The handbook goes on to focus on the various post-processing technologies available to fortify the mechanical, chemical, biological, geometrical, and other characteristics of additively manufactured components and also discusses future directions and possible research gaps that need to be filled.

The buyers of this cutting-edge handbook will learn the complete information and methodology for manufacturing drug delivery systems and customized medicine for biomedical applications. It is also an ideal read for undergraduates, graduates, and postgraduate research scholars. Industrial and academic professionals working and studying industrial, manufacturing, and production engineering, along with those studying mechanical engineering, pharmaceutical sciences, material science, chemical engineering, biomedical engineering, automobile/aerospace engineering, and other relevant domains will want this handbook at their fingertips.

Innovations in Smart Manufacturing for Long-Term Development and Growth

Series Editors: Atul Babbar, Gursel Alici, Yu Dong, Ankit Sharma

Fabrication Techniques and Machining Methods of Advanced Composite Materials
Vikas Dhawan, Atul Babbar, Inderdeep Singh and Jonathan M. Weaver

Advances in Pre- and Post-Additive Manufacturing Processes
Innovations and Applications
Naveen Mani Tripathi and Ankit Sharma

Handbook of 3D Printing in Pharmaceutics
Innovations and Applications
Prakash Katakam, Ranvijay Kumar, Nishant Ranjan and Atul Babbar

For more information about this series, please visit: www.routledge.com/Innovations-in-Smart-Manufacturing-for-Long-Term-Development-and-Growth/book-series/CRCISMLDG

Handbook of 3D Printing in Pharmaceutics

Innovations and Applications

Edited by
Prakash Katakam, Ranvijay Kumar,
Nishant Ranjan, and Atul Babbar

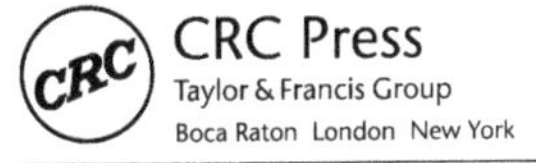

CRC Press
Taylor & Francis Group
Boca Raton London New York

CRC Press is an imprint of the
Taylor & Francis Group, an **informa** business

Designed cover image: Shutterstock - asharkyu

First edition published 2025
by CRC Press
2385 NW Executive Center Drive, Suite 320, Boca Raton FL 33431

and by CRC Press
4 Park Square, Milton Park, Abingdon, Oxon, OX14 4RN

CRC Press is an imprint of Taylor & Francis Group, LLC

ISBN: 978-1-032-57278-9 (hbk)
ISBN: 978-1-032-57466-0 (pbk)
ISBN: 978-1-003-43950-9 (ebk)

DOI: 10.1201/9781003439509

Typeset in Times
by Newgen Publishing UK

Contents

SECTION I 3D Printing, Drug Delivery Systems, and Application Domain Overview

Bhavaraju Lakshmi Ratna Madhavi, J Joysa Ruby,
Prakash Katakam, Ravi Shankar Ayyanar, and
Shanta Kumari Adiki

Popat Mohite, Sudarshan Kakad, and Anil Pawar

SECTION II Quality Characteristics' Challenge in 3D Printing of Pharmaceutical Products

Kanaka Durga Devi Nelluri, Sk. Abdul Rahaman,
Vijaya Lakshmi Marella, Kakani Anil Kumar, and
Kondabrolu Naga Bhargavi

SECTION III Extrusion-Based 3D Printing in Pharmaceutics

Aastha Singh, Mohit Agrawal, Vijay Kumar Sharma,
Hema Chaudhary, Aakriti Patel, Shivendra Kumar,
Sunam Saha, and Md. Sadique Hussain

SECTION IV Binder Jetting-Based 3D Printing in Pharmaceutics

SECTION V SLS and SLA-Based 3D Printing in Pharmaceutics

SECTION VI Hybrid 3D Printing Techniques in Pharmaceutical Applications

SECTION VII Social, Economic, Environmental, Quality, and Regulatory Aspects

Preface

The book entitled *3D Printing in Pharmaceutics: Innovations and Applications* aims to present various experimental outbreaks on the novel methodologies to develop pharmaceutical products by 3D printing, especially for the drug delivery process. The purpose of this book is to emphasize the various types of 3D printing techniques, such as materials extrusion, vat polymerization, binder jetting, inkjet, and associated hybrid processes for customized drugs, medicine, and biomedical utilities, formation of shape, size, and dosage tailored medicines, etc. This book is designed to cover the significant contribution of the research fraternity, across the world, to different classes of pharmaceutical products by 3D printing and end applications. This book is a key source for gathering knowledge about drug delivery processes, 3D printing processes, and mechanisms for the sustainable development of drug delivery systems. This book also provides broad coverage of the theory behind this emerging technology, material development, functional characterization, and the technical details required for readers to investigate the novel applications of the involved methods for themselves.

Dr. Prakash Katakam
Dr. Ranvijay Kumar
Dr. Nishant Ranjan
Dr. Atul Babbar

About the Editors

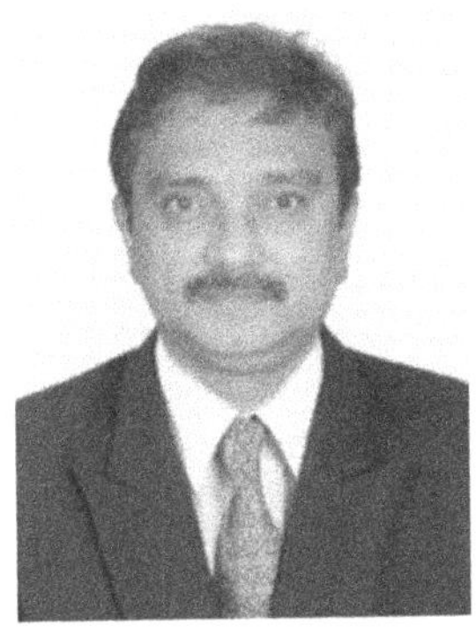

Prakash Katakam is a pharmaceutical scientist working as professor and principal at Indira College of Pharmacy, Nanded, India. He has more than 27 years of professional experience as a teacher and researcher. He published over 150 research articles in indexed journals and guided 14 PhD students. His research areas are 3D printing for personalized drug delivery, pulmonary delivery of vaccines, micro/nanoparticles, phyto-formulations and drug discovery. He is the founder of a research laboratory on 3D printing, RxPrints Lab, 3DFying Inc., Hyderabad, India and Awarded for his invention, "Indigenous 3D Printer Customized Medicine and Pharmaceutics of the Year 2023", by IIT Bombay, India. His major research focus is on identifying applications of various polymers for 3D printing for patient-specific dosage forms. He has been co-principal investigator for a sponsored research project of National Tea Research Foundation, India. Recently he contributed a publication on "Navigating the Challenges of 3D Printing Personalized Medicine in Space Explorations: A Comprehensive Review" in *Critical Reviews in Therapeutic Drug Carrier Systems* Journal and a book chapter "Recent Advancements of Additive Manufacturing for Patient-Specific Drug Delivery" in the book, "Additive Manufacturing Processes in Biomedical Engineering", published by CRC Press (Taylor & Francis Group). Dr. Katakam also published a highly cited review article, "Top-Down and Bottom-Up Approaches in 3D Printing Technologies for Drug Delivery Challenges" in the journal *Critical Reviews in Therapeutic Drug Carrier Systems*.

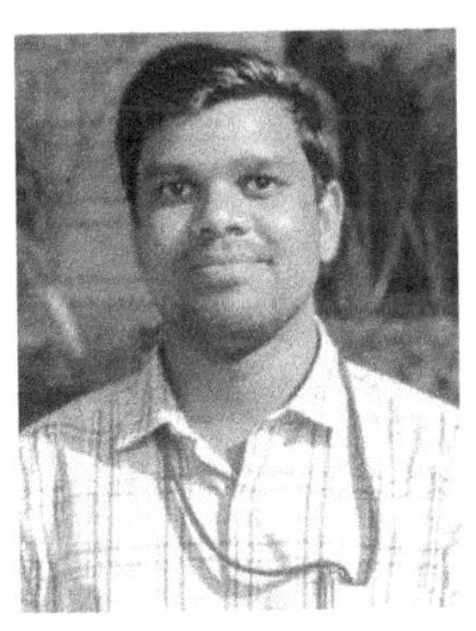

Ranvijay Kumar is an assistant professor at the Marwadi University Research Center, Marwadi University, Rajkot, India. He received a PhD in Mechanical Engineering from Punjabi University, Patiala. Additive manufacturing, shape memory polymers, smart materials, friction-based welding techniques, advanced materials processing, polymer matrix composite preparations, reinforced polymer composites for 3D printing, plastic solid waste management, thermosetting recycling, and destructive testing of materials are Dr. Kumar's expertise. Dr. Kumar has won the prestigious CII MILCA award in 2020. He has co-authored more than 43 research papers in science citation indexed journals, and 38 book chapters, and has presented 20 research papers at various national/international-level conferences. He has contributed extensively to the additive manufacturing literature with publications appearing in *Journal of Manufacturing Processes, Composite Part: B, Rapid Prototyping Journal, Journal of Thermoplastic Composite Materials, Measurement, Proceedings of the Institution of Mechanical Engineers, Part C (iMeche Part C), Proceedings of the Institution of Mechanical Engineers, Part H: Journal of Engineering in Medicine, Journal of Thermoplastic Composite Materials, Materials Research Express, Proceedings of the National Academy of Sciences, India Section A: Physical Sciences, Journal of*

Central South University, Journal of the Brazilian Society of Mechanical Sciences and Engineering, Composite Structures, and CIRP Journal of Manufacturing Science and Technology. He is the editor of the book "Additive Manufacturing for Plastic Recycling: Efforts in Boosting A Circular Economy" publishing by CRC Press (Taylor & Francis Group).

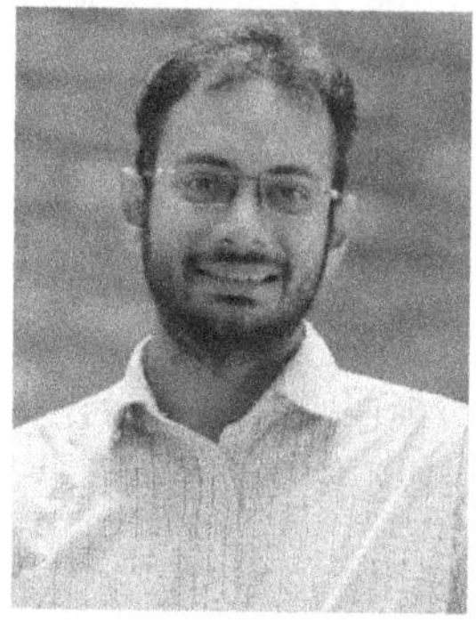

Nishant Ranjan is an assistant professor at the Marwadi University Research Center, Marwadi University, Rajkot, India. Dr. Ranjan has won the prestigious CII MILCA award in 2022. Fused deposition-modeling, extrusion, thermoplastic polymers, Polymer Composites, natural and synthetic biopolymers, scaffolds printing, 3D printing technology, thermal, mechanical, morphological, and chemical properties of thermoplastic polymers, biocompatible and biodegradable fillers, and reinforcement of materials are the main areas of focus for Dr. Ranjan. He has co-authored more than 40 research papers in science citation index journals, 35 book chapters, 2 books and presented more than 10 research papers at various national/international conferences.

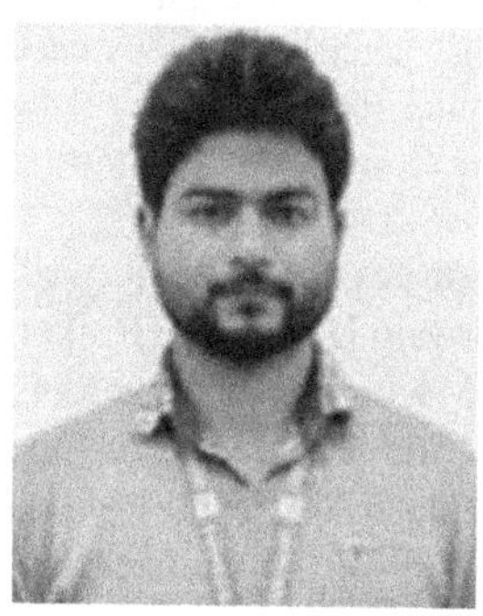

Atul Babbar is an assistant professor at the Mechanical Engineering Department of SGT University, Gurugram. He has taught students in academics and research fields. He is a a level 2 non-destructive testing engineer certified by the American Society of Non-Destructive Testing (ASNT). His research interests include biomedicals, 3D and 4D printing, conventional/non-conventional machining and not limited to that. He has authored several research articles and book chapters in various international/national SCI and Scopus journals. He has reviewed research articles of various peer-reviewed SCI and Scopus indexed journals.

Contributors

Shanta Kumari Adiki
Rajarshi Shahu College of Pharmacy
　　Markhel
Maharashtra, India

Mohit Agrawal
School of Medical & Allied Sciences
　　K.R. Mangalam University
Gurugram, India

Swamita Arora
Department of Pharmacy
　　R.V. Northland Institute
Greater Noida, India

Swati Arya
SGT College of Pharmacy,
　　SGT University
Haryana, India

Ravi Shankar Ayyanar
Commissioner of Police
　　Commissioner of Police Bungalow
Andhra Pradesh, India

Kondabrolu Naga Bhargavi
KVSR Siddhartha College of
　　Pharmaceutical Sciences
Andhra Pradesh, India

P. Sunil Kumar Chaitanya
St. Pauls College of Pharmacy
Telangana, India

Hema Chaudhary
School of Medical & Allied Sciences
　　K.R. Mangalam University
Gurugram, India

Somnath De
St. Pauls College of Pharmacy
Telangana, India

Bhoopathi Deepika
St. Pauls College of Pharmacy
Telangana, India

Tulja Rani Gampa
Department of Pharmaceutical Analysis
　　Malla Reddy Pharmacy College
Telangana, India

Md. Sadique Hussain
School of Pharmaceutical Sciences
　　Jaipur National University
Jaipur, India

J Joysa Ruby
Acharya & BM Reddy College of
　　Pharmacy
Karnataka, India

Keerthi Kadimcharla
National Institute of
　　Pharmaceutical Education and
　　Research (NIPER)
Telangana, India

Sudarshan Kakad
AETs St. John Institute of Pharmacy
　　and Research
Maharashtra, India

Raja Rajeswari Kamisetti
Vardhaman College of Pharmacy
Maharashtra, India

Naga Raju Kandukoori
St. Pauls College of Pharmacy
Telangana, India

Prakash Katakam
Indira College of Pharmacy
Maharashtra, India
and
RxPrints Lab, 3DFying, Inc.
Hyderabad, India

Venu Madhav Katla
St. Pauls College of Pharmacy
Telangana, India

Adarsh Keshari
Department of Pharmacy
 Practice Teerthanker Mahaveer
 College of Pharmacy
 Teerthanker Mahaveer University
Moradabad, India

Kakani Anil Kumar
Assistant Professor, Department of
 Pharmaceutics and Biotechnology
 KVSR Siddhartha College of
 Pharmaceutical Sciences
Andhra Pradesh, India

Shivendra Kumar
Department of Pharmacy
 Rajiv Academy for Pharmacy
Mathura, India

**Bhavaraju Lakshmi Ratna
 Madhavi**
Acharya & BM Reddy College of
 Pharmacy
Karnataka, India

Kiranmai Mandava
Department of Pharmaceutical
 Chemistry
 St. Paul's College of Pharmacy
Telangana, India

Vijaya Lakshmi Marella
Associate Professor, Department of
 Pharmaceutical Analysis
 KVSR Siddhartha College of
 Pharmaceutical Sciences
Andhra Pradesh, India

Popat Mohite
AETs St. John Institute of Pharmacy
 and Research
Maharashtra, India

Kanaka Durga Devi Nelluri
Associate Professor, Department of
 Pharmaceutics and Biotechnology
 KVSR Siddhartha College of
 Pharmaceutical Sciences
Andhra Pradesh, India

Naga Haritha Pamujula
St. Pauls College of Pharmacy
Telangana, India

Aakriti Patel
Bengal college of Pharmaceutical
 Sciences and Research
West Bengal, India

Neha Pathak
Department of Pharmacy
 Practice, Teerthanker Mahaveer
 College of Pharmacy
 Teerthanker Mahaveer University
Moradabad, India

Rashmi Pathak
Department of Pharmacy, Invertis
 University
Bareilly, India

Anil Pawar
MES's College of Pharmacy
Maharashtra, India

Bhupendra Prajapati
Shree S. K. Patel College of
Pharmaceutical Education and
Research
Ganpat University
Kherva, India

Sk. Abdul Rahaman
School of Pharmacy
Galgotias University
Uttar Pradesh, India

Ajmeer Ramkishan
Deputy Drugs Controller-India
CDSCO, Hyderabad Zonal Office
Hyderabad, India

Sameer Rastogi
School of Pharmacy
Noida International University
Greater Noida, India

Nensi Raytthatha
Gujarat Technological University
Gujarat, India

Sunam Saha
Department of Pharmacy
Rajiv Academy for Pharmacy
Mathura, India

Subhas Sahoo
Pulla Reddy Institute of Pharmacy
Telangana, India

Sowmyaranjan Satapathy
DFE Pharma India Pvt. ltd.
Telangana, India

Manoj Shahare
Novartis Health Care Pvt. Ltd.
Telangana, India

Himanshu Sharma
Department of Pharmacology
Teerthanker Mahaveer College of
Pharmacy
Teerthanker Mahaveer University
Moradabad, India

Vijay Kumar Sharma
Dr. K.N. Modi Institute of
Pharmaceutical Education &
Research
Uttar Pradesh, India

Aastha Singh
Dreams College of Pharmacy
Uttar Pradesh, India

Kuldeep Singh
Department of Pharmacy
Rajiv Academy for Pharmacy
Mathura, India

Sudarshan Singh
Faculty of Pharmacy and Office of
Research Administration
Chiang Mai University
Chiang Mai, Thailand

Nagarajan Sriram
Florence College of Pharmacy, Ranchi
Jharkhand, India

Sneha Thakur
Department of Pharmacognosy
St. Pauls College of Pharmacy
Telangana, India

Siddhant Jai Tyagi
Department of Pharmacology
Teerthanker Mahveer College of
Pharmacy
Teerhanker Mahaveer University
Moradabad, India

Prakhar Varshney
Department of Pharmacology
 Teerthanker Mahaveer
 College of Pharmacy
 Teerthanker Mahaveer University
Moradabad, India

Jigar Vyas
Faculty of Pharmacy
 Sigma University
Gujarat, India

Section I

3D Printing, Drug Delivery Systems, and Application Domain Overview

1 Advancements in Tailoring Medication Using 3D Printing

Bhavaraju Lakshmi Ratna Madhavi, J Joysa Ruby, Prakash Katakam, Ravi Shankar Ayyanar, and Shanta Kumari Adiki

1.1 INTRODUCTION

In the realm of modern medicine, a groundbreaking convergence of technology and healthcare is redefining the way we approach diagnosis, treatment, and patient care. At the forefront of this revolution stands three-dimensional printing (3DP), a cutting-edge manufacturing technique that has transcended its industrial roots to become an invaluable asset in the field of personalized medicine (Vaz and Kumar, 2021; Mathew *et al.*, 2020). 3DP, with its ability to create intricate three-dimensional objects layer by layer from digital designs, is offering tailored solutions to individual patients. Medical treatment, once characterized by a one-size-fits-all approach, is now being driven by the recognition of individual uniqueness. Patients vary not only in their medical conditions but also in their anatomical structures, genetic compositions, and treatment responses. Traditional standardized treatments often fall short in addressing the intricacies of each patient's condition, leading to suboptimal outcomes and prolonged recovery times. 3DP technology promises an unprecedented level of personalization into medical care.

Conventional/traditional medicine refers to the mainstream healthcare practices that have been in use for centuries, often based on empirical knowledge, population pharmacokinetics and standardized treatment approaches. The fundamental premise of personalized medicine is simple yet profound: no two individuals are alike. Every patient carries a unique genetic makeup, medical history, and set of circumstances that influence their health journey. Yet, for decades, medical interventions have largely adhered to standardized protocols, treating patients as statistical averages rather than singular entities. The emergence of 3DP, introduces a paradigm shift that aligns seamlessly with the ethos of personalized medicine. Personalized medicine is an approach to improve therapy or prophylaxis designed specifically for each patient. It uses a person's genetic and epigenetic details and takes special care about their preferred choices, faith, attitudes, knowledge and societal influences. Precision medicine is a deeper extent of personalized medicine, the basis of which relies on data from many sources like genomics, biological information, transcriptomics and

DOI: 10.1201/9781003439509-2

proteomics, which are vital to predict diagnoses precisely and accurately, define disease subtypes and suggest treatment. It is an advanced medical strategy with a higher resolution towards understanding a disease condition to facilitate better targeting of disease subtypes with newer therapeutic approach, for example, cystic fibrosis and cancer (Strianese *et al.*, 2020). 3DP operates on the principle of additive manufacturing (AM). It involves building up layers of material, one upon another, guided by digital blueprints. Originally adopted in sectors like manufacturing and design prototyping, the technology has swiftly found its way into healthcare, where its precision and adaptability are revolutionizing patient-specific interventions (Eshkalak *et al.*, 2020; Cox *et al.*, 2016).

3DP has emerged as a promising tool in personalized medicine due to its ability to create highly customized and patient-specific drug delivery systems, medical devices, implants, and even tissues thus aid to greatly improve treatment outcomes and patient experiences. Against the "one-size-fits-all" approach, which may not always be optimal for every patient, 3DP allows for the design and development of implantable systems and other medical devices to suit the individuals as per their anatomy, precisely. This is particularly important in cases of complex surgeries or implantations where the fit and functionality of the device play a critical role in the patient's recovery and overall well-being (Pieters *et al.*, 2022). The other applicative aspect of 3DP towards personalized healthcare is in the area of surgery where 3DP facilitates planning for surgical procedures, offering training and education for surgeons. Intricate surgical procedures may be planned by printing a replica as per the anatomy of the patient. These models allow for better visualization of the patient's unique anatomy, which can help surgeons strategize and practice before the actual procedure. This technology also aids in explaining procedures to patients, improving their understanding and reducing anxiety (Ganguli *et al.*, 2018; Calvo-Haro *et al.*, 2021). Cardiovascular healthcare benefits from 3DP technology. Educationists may utilize patient-specific 3D models to impart knowledge, explore the physiology and functionality of valve and vessel function, plan for catheter-based surgical procedures, design and refine the latest innovations in percutaneous structural devices (Vukicevic *et al.*, 2017)

3DP technology has aided diagnosis for over two decades where abstract medical data like computed tomography (CT) scans, magnetic resonance imaging (MRI) images, and other diagnostic records could be transformed into tactile models, allowing medical professionals to examine intricate details and anticipate potential challenges. This immersive approach to preoperative planning expedites procedures, minimizes complications, and ultimately enhances patient outcomes. By providing surgeons with an accurate physical representation of a patient's unique anatomy, 3DP empowered them to navigate complex surgical landscapes with heightened confidence (Rengier, 2010; Baylon *et al.*, 2017). The versatility of 3DP extends to providing point-of-care manufacturing. In remote or underserved areas, 3DP could bring medical solutions closer to patients. Point-of-care 3DP enables the on-site production of medical devices, reducing the need for extensive supply chains and transportation (Point-of-Care 3D Solutions 3dsystems.com). Integrating 3DP technology into hospitals led to production models, such as point-of-care manufacturing (Calvo-Haro *et al.*, 2021; Biglino *et al.*, 2023).

Biofabrication is another prominent contribution of 3DP for personalizing healthcare by printing biological materials to develop functional tissues and organs that meet specific patient needs. This breakthrough could potentially alleviate the organ shortage crisis and provide patients with life-changing treatments that were previously considered unattainable (Lewis, 2017). Biofabrication using a patient's own cells has the potential to transform the field of transplantation by avoiding the necessity for organ donation as well as minimizing the possibility of its rejection, as the printed tissues would closely match the patient (Agarwal *et al.*, 2020). Biofabrication in tissue engineering and regenerative medicine employs nanobiomaterials. In the bioprinted model, cells will be seeded and grown. These biofabrication techniques may be segregated as bioprinting and bioassembly. An example of biofabrication was the use of polyether urethane-based nanostructured poly lactic glycolic acid (PLGA) biofilm for facilitating adhesion and proper functioning of the bladder smooth muscle cells; use of silver nanoparticles in catheters for lowering the possibility of infection (Di Marzio *et al.*, 2020; Barazanchi *et al.*, 2017).

1.2 ADVANCEMENTS IN 3DP OF PATIENT-SPECIFIC MEDICAL DEVICES

Medical devices are therapeutic solutions to certain kinds of health issues, e.g., orthopedics. The variety of medical devices employed in healthcare is enormous. 3DP sustained-release implants, stents, medical devices and contact lens find use in joint replacement treatment, medical prostheses, ophthalmic or cardiovascular indications. 3DP technology has facilitated the development and production of devices like prosthetics, implants and scaffolds, which are designed to align as per the individual's body. As we look deeper into the intersections of 3DP and personalized medicine, it becomes evident that this synergy has the potential to redefine healthcare paradigms. For hip and knee arthroplasty, traditionally, the surgeon would choose from a limited range of implant sizes that might not perfectly fit the patient's anatomy resulting in discomfort, reduced mobility, and the need for follow-up surgeries. 3DP obliterates these limitations by enabling the creation of implants customized to the finest detail. By translating a patient's medical scans into digital designs and then physically fabricating implants layer by layer, 3DP ensures a precise fit, enhancing not only the implant's functionality but also the patient's overall quality of life (Kumar *et al.*, 2020). Prosthetics, such as limb replacements or orthopedic braces, can be designed to fit unique body shape and requirements of the patient. 3DP enables faster and more cost-effective production of these devices, making them more accessible to a broader range of patients.

Stents that are coated with scaffolds composed of biocompatible and biodegradable materials, and incorporate pharmaceuticals, have the potential to function as drug delivery systems, particularly for antimicrobial agents. Recently, considerable research was carried out on the development of customized patient-specific biocompatible scaffolds that are loaded with antimicrobials. These scaffolds are specifically designed to promote bone regeneration and prevent infections (Elsayed *et al.*, 2019). Surgical meshes were fabricated as interwoven structures, resulting in sheet-like formations composed of biocompatible and sometimes biodegradable materials

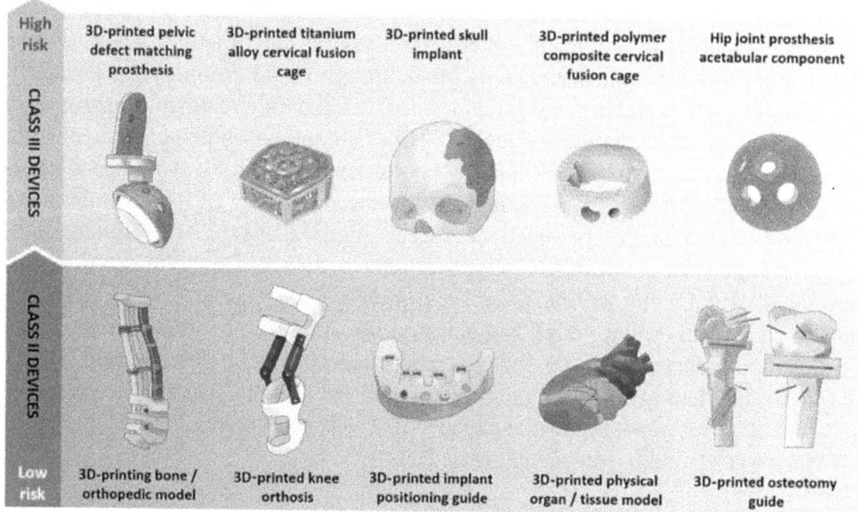

FIGURE 1.1   3D-printed medical devices for various healthcare applications (Jin *et al.*, 2022).

of inorganic origin. Researchers are currently engaged in the development of novel surgical meshes (Baylon *et al.*, 2017). 3DP or AM techniques were employed to produce implants composed of titanium that were capable of eluting antibiotics (Cox *et al.*, 2016). Selective laser-melting (SLM) technique was used to fabricate titanium drug-delivery implants that facilitate drug release via micro-channels (Hassanin *et al.*, 2018). Drug-coated implants, scaffolds and meshes were manufactured utilizing AM technology in order to incorporate clinical functionality aimed at the prevention or treatment of infections, as well as the mitigation of pain (Mohanty *et al.*, 2015). Figure 1.1 presents some examples of 3D-printed medical devices in various applications of healthcare (Jin *et al.*, 2022).

1.3   DENTAL APPLICATIONS OF 3DP TECHNOLOGY FOR PERSONALIZED THERAPY

Dentistry has benefited greatly from 3D printing. Dentists can produce highly accurate crowns, bridges, and even entire sets of dentures tailored to each patient's oral structure. The digital scanning of a patient's mouth combined with 3DP allows for more comfortable and efficient dental procedures (Turkyilmaz and Wilkins, 2021). Research in dentistry has undergone a significant transformation with the advent of 3DP technologies. This transformation has been characterized by a shift towards the production of dental prosthesis, artificial teeth and shattered bone structures that are constructed as per the requirement of the patient (Barazanchi *et al.*, 2017; Patel *et al.*, 2017). AM is now being investigated as a potential method for producing tissue scaffolds used in bone-graft surgeries. In the field of periodontology, 3DP is employed for the production of patient-specific bio-absorbable fiber-guided scaffolds. These scaffolds are utilized for various purposes, such as sinus and bone

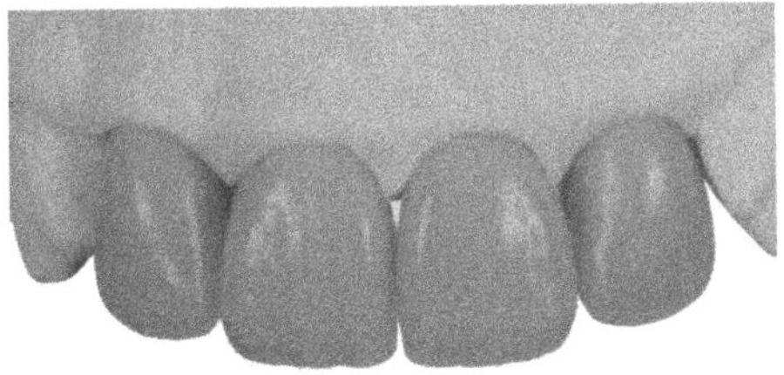

FIGURE 1.2 Crowns of upper jaw incisors produced by 3DP Technology (Schweiger *et al.*, 2021).

augmentation, socket preservation, as well as implant placement and maintenance in cases of periodontal abnormalities (Gul *et al.*, 2019). A guided tissue regeneration membrane using platelet-rich fibrin for the treatment of severe bone deformities could be developed by 3DP (Lei *et al.*, 2019). Bio-resorbable scaffolds specifically designed for periodontal healing purposes were printed. PLGA was identified as a promising polymer employed in scaffold creation in the context of guided bone regeneration (Rasperini *et al.*, 2015). Figure 1.2 shows one of the applications of 3DP in dentistry where crowns of the teeth have been printed (Schweiger *et al.*, 2021).

1.4 3D-PRINTED DRUG DELIVERY SYSTEMS FOR INDIVIDUALIZED THERAPEUTIC APPROACHES

Personalized medicine often involves delivering drugs in specific dosages and formulations tailored to an individual's genetic makeup and health condition. 3DP can create intricate drug delivery systems, such as pills with multiple compartments releasing different medications at various rates, enhancing treatment efficacy and reducing side effects (Mathew *et al.*, 2020; Bacskay *et al.*, 2022). Topical products like dressings for wounds, micro-needle-based delivery systems, and medicated contact lens systems, were created by 3DP techniques. 3D nanoprinting for biologics and nanotech-based drugs offers printed personalized nanomedicines in the years to come. 3DP technology could be facilitated for continuous manufacturing via 3D-printed microfluidic chips and thus enable personalization to reach clinical practice (Serrano *et al.*, 2023). The delivery of drugs through the rectum or vagina has been a longstanding practice, particularly suggested for youngsters, geriatrics, comatose patients, and those with difficulty swallowing, to address a range of etiologies. A recent study conducted research on the production of various patient-specific rectal and vaginal rectal devices using AM. These devices were designed with diverse geometries and incorporated customized drug-eluting mechanisms (Fu *et al.*, 2018). Fused deposition modeling (FDM), stereolithography (SLA), binder jetting, powder-bed, ink-jet printing (IJP) and semisolid extrusion are some 3DP/AM methods employed in pharmaceutical product development. Among such AM technologies, the powder extrusion method led to successful formulation of amorphous solid printlets of itraconazole, which overcame the lapses of FDM technology. AM has a possibility for flexible dosage form development by virtue of the flexibility of materials selection leading to personalized therapeutics (Katakam *et al.*, 2022).

Current studies are mostly centered on achieving high drug loading and developing patient-specific treatments. Researchers are also exploring alternative drug delivery systems, including buccal patches, transdermal patches, biodegradable implants and oral-delivery systems. These alternative approaches are particularly valuable in cases where conventional commercial methods are unable to offer the desired level of pharmaceutical customization. One such advancement is in the development AM technology for lipid-based drug delivery systems for lipophilic pharmaceutical compounds (Vithani *et al.*, 2018). The utilization of 3DP has several advantages, particularly in terms of the flexibility it provides in selecting materials. This attribute enhances its applicability in the field of multi-drug therapies. A poly-pill consisting of four distinct cardiovascular medications was developed by 3DP (Pereira *et al.*, 2019). Similarly, 3D-printed mini-printlets incorporating paracetamol and ibuprofen as separate components were developed (Awad *et al.*, 2019).

1.4.1 ORAL DOSAGE FORMS

Oral solid dosage forms are widely recognized as the oldest and most well-established pharmacological formulations due to their affordability, non-invasiveness, and patient-friendly administration. There are various types of dosage forms available, including pills, tablets, capsules, lozenges, pellets, and films. The fixed-dose combination therapy (FDCT) involves the administration of two medications in a single tablet. This may not provide dosing flexibility tailored to individual patients. Secondly, the utilization of poly-therapy has the potential to exacerbate issues related to drug adherence, hence leading to a subsequent decline in the overall health status of patients. Thus the integration of many medications into a personalized formulation tailored to individual patients suffering from chronic illnesses has the potential to significantly enhance treatment adherence and patient compliance. AM technologies offer the capability to give numerous medications in a formulation with customized shape, size, and desired drug-release patterns, hence circumventing the limitations of conventional approaches (Norman *et al.*, 2017; Alhnan *et al.*, 2016; Angeliki *et al.*, 2020; Goyanes *et al.*, 2019). The utilization of 3DP facilitates dosage form design with customised geometry, design and shape. This capability has been challenging to obtain through traditional manufacturing methods. 3DP methods have several limitations, such as the production of porous materials and uneven shapes in dosage forms (Pravin and Sudhir, 2018). To date, the utilization of FDM method is limited to the printing of products exclusively for thermostable pharmaceuticals, employing a restricted range of appropriate excipients. The utilization of SLA carries the risk of drug degradation upon exposure to ultraviolet (UV) radiation, which serves as the catalyst for the polymerization reaction (Prasad and Smyth, 2016). AM demonstrated efficacy in developing sublingual, orodispersible, fast-disintegrating/dissolving, and immediate-release dosage forms (Jamróz *et al.*, 2017; Musazzi *et al.*, 2018; Kempin *et al.*, 2018; Solanki *et al.*, 2018). Researchers have shown interest in flexible therapeutic dosage forms that provide customized combinations of medicines, dosages and desired release kinetics. For example, impact of varied tablet shapes on drug-release kinetics, enabled the development of innovative dosage forms that possess specific pharmacokinetic properties tailored to particular absorption locations within the gastrointestinal tract (Goyanes *et al.*, 2015).

1.4.2 PARENTERAL SYSTEMS

Parenteral devices are utilized for the administration of medications through the intravenous (IV) route, employing either a catheter or a needle. The primary focus of previous research in the field of intravenous (IV) devices pertained to the development of personalized catheters designed for the targeted administration of pharmaceutical agents. The production of catheters coated with drugs is being undertaken with the aim of mitigating the occurrence of infections. The efficacy of antimicrobial coatings in inhibiting bacterial adhesion to catheter surfaces has been demonstrated (Mathew *et al.*, 2019). In traditional coating procedures, the incorporation of an antimicrobial agent at a concentration of 2% w/w was often employed to prevent bacterial attack. However, the 3D-printed catheter tips exhibited antimicrobial properties at lower concentrations of 1% w/w, thereby demonstrating the technological superiority of AM (Weisman *et al.*, 2019). According to published statistics, the FDM technique has emerged as a prominent method in the fabrication of catheters, showing potential for future advancements (Weisman *et al.*, 2015). The utilization of hot melt extrusion (HME) is widely preferred in various applications due to its inherent benefits, such as the significant reduction in organic solvent wastage and its environmentally sustainable characteristics (Keating *et al.*, 2018). The capabilities of HME utilizing an FDM printer for the development of modified drug-release systems composed of polymer blends consisting of eudragits and polyvinly alcohol (PVA), along with the incorporation of polyethylene oxide (PEO), Polyethylene glycol (PEG), and Tween 80 were investigated (Alhijjaj *et al.*, 2016). A separate investigation was conducted wherein wound dressings with patient-specific antibacterial metal ions were developed, demonstrating the potential of HME technology (Muwaffak *et al.*, 2017). Successful extrusion of filaments composed of PEO, ethyl cellulose (EC), Eudragit RL100, and PVA was performed. These filaments were later utilized to produce discs through the utilization of an FDM printer (Melocchi *et al.*, 2016). The hot melt extrusion (HME) technique can be utilized across a range of polymers in order to produce filaments that possess diverse physical characteristics, hence rendering them appropriate for various medicinal applications (Tappa *et al.*, 2018). A comprehensive examination of patient-specific drug administration in relation to the design of 3D-printed dosage forms was carried out highlighting many novel applications in this field (Dumpa *et al.*, 2021).

1.4.3 TRANSDERMAL APPLICATIONS

Transdermal patches are employed for the purpose of administering medications in a systemic manner via the skin. The conventional manufacturing techniques employed to produce a high rate of production are in direct competition with the need of tailoring medication doses to individual patients (Adamo *et al.*, 2016). In alternative terms, the production of transdermal dosage forms can be expedited and uninterrupted, hence accommodating individualized patient dosages concurrently. Transdermal

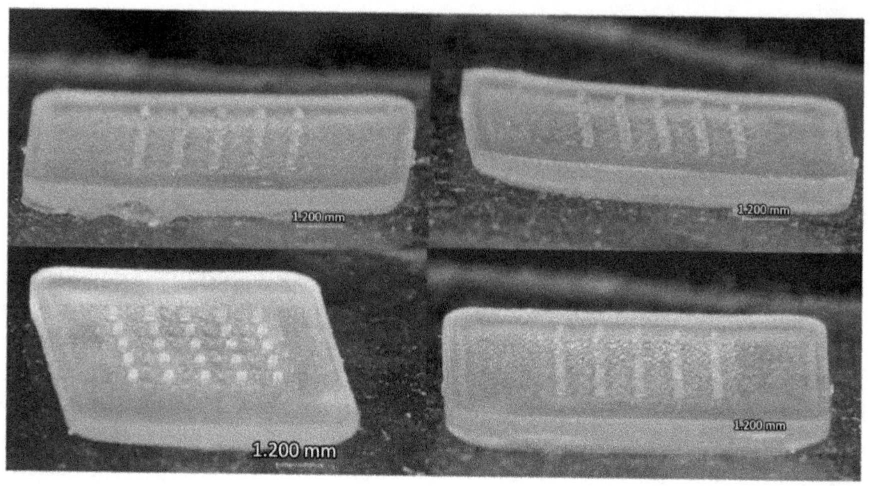

FIGURE 1.3 Transdermal drug-delivery employing microneedle patches made by 3DP (Villota *et al.*, 2022).

thin-film patches and micro-needles are employed for the systemic administration of medications (Ita, 2015). Microneedle patches have emerged as promising formulations for the transdermal delivery of medicines. The utilization of the SLA microfabrication approach has been employed in the production of microneedle patches with a notable level of precision, ranging from 1 to 25 μm (Iliescu *et al.*, 2017). The process of selective laser sintering (SLS) necessitates multiple production phases and the utilization of specialized equipment in order to produce miniature items. Drug-coated and drug-eluting microneedles were manufactured by 3DP, which presents numerous benefits in comparison to traditional microfabrication approaches (Caudil *et al.*, 2018). Figure 1.3 is an image of 3D-printed microneedle patches (Villota *et al.*, 2022).

1.4.4 Films

3DP has been used to design and develop mucoadhesive, orodisperisble or ophthalmic films. Mucoadhesive films are made using a variety of processes, including as hot-melt extrusion, solvent casting, compression and 3D printing. Although the technique most frequently employed in research is solvent casting (Elkanayati *et al.*, 2022). The developed 3D-printed orodispersible films of aripiprazole by FDM, which works on the basis of hot melt extrusion as a suitable method in the formation of film with reproducible shape and drug content (Jamróz *et al.*, 2017). Catechin loaded mucoadhesive oral film was 3D printed employing hydroxypropyl methylcellulose using the semi-solid extrusion-type 3D printer. This study provides useful information on a model pharmaceutical for personalized therapy (Tagami *et al.*, 2019). The Hyrel 30M 3D printer was used to create PLGA films to evaluate drug-release behavior *in vitro* using simulations and molecular models that elucidate drug–polymer interactions (Serris *et al.*, 2020). The mouth dissolving printed film was produced by pneumatic-based

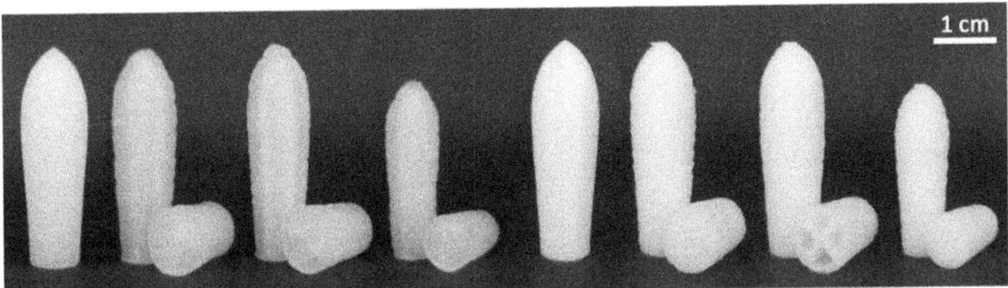

FIGURE 1.4 Photographic images of molded and 3D-printed suppositories containing 10% (*w/w*) paracetamol in the frontal view and internal view of partially printed suppositories. From left to right: PEG mold, PEG "standard", PEG "hollow", PEG "small", HF mold, HF "standard", HF "hollow", HF "small" (Domsta *et al.*, 2022).

microextrusion printing technology with ketorolac (a high potent low-dose and heat-sensitive API) and was found feasible for highly flexible small-scale printing, i.e., for personalized medicine (Khan *et al.*, 2022). Levofloxacin-loaded hydrogel-based ophthalmic patches have been 3D printed to facilitate specified drug release in the eye (Greymi *et al.*, 2022).

1.4.5 SUPPOSITORIES

Drug administration via oral and IV routes is difficult in acute severe ulcerative colitis, which could lead to systemic adverse effects and limited dose availability at the illness site. This would restrict the therapeutic effectiveness of the medication (Hua *et al.*, 2020). Oral medications intended for the colon have to pass through the entire alimentary canal in order to reach the target site, which delays the therapeutic response (Awad *et al.*, 2022; McCoubrey *et al.*, 2023). A rectal formulation, on the other hand, provides a substitute to improve therapeutic efficacy by optimizing medication concentrations at the illness site and reducing systemic side effects (Hua *et al.*, 2019). Suppositories can also be self-administered by the patient unlike parenteral formulations. 3DP has facilitated development of suppository dosage forms. Figure 1.4 shows 3DP paracetamol suppository employing PEG and hard fat (HF) (Domsta *et al.*, 2022).

Extensive work has been done on drug delivery systems employing 3DP, which find use in tailoring medication delivery for personalized treatment. Such reported work has been compiled in Table 1.1.

1.5 CONCLUSION

The utilization of 3DP as an innovative technology across diverse domains in healthcare favors the delivery of personalized treatment because it allows for the creation of patient-specific medical solutions. Such tailor-made interventions enhance treatment outcomes, reduce complications, and improve overall patient satisfaction. The first 3D-printed Spritam (Levitiracetam) tablet has paved the way for the promising use of 3DP technology in developing drug delivery systems. Numerous

TABLE 1.1
Work Done on 3D-printed Drug Delivery Systems

S.No	Drug	Technology	Formulation	Excipients	Parameters Studied
1.	Paracetamol or caffeine (Goyanes*et al.*, 2016)	FDM	Caplets	PVA filament (1.75 mm diameter, print temperature 190–220 °C) – USP grade	Porosity, dissolution test conditions
2.	Budesonide (Goyanes *et al.*, 2015)	FDM	Caplets	PVA (1.75 mm diameter, print temperature 190–220 °C)	Drug loading of filaments and caplets, scanning electron microscopy (SEM), x-ray powder diffraction (XRPD) thermal analysis, dynamic dissolution
3.	4-aminosalicylic acid (ASA) or 5- ASA (Goyanes *et al.*, 2015)	FDM	Tablets	PVA- (1.75 mm diameter, print temperature 190–220 °C)	Tablet morphology, strength, friability, drug loading, dissolution
4.	Hydrochlorothiazide (Gioumouxouzis *et al.*, 2017)	FDM	Tablets	PLA filament (1.75 mm diameter, print temperature 180–220 °C, density 1.24 g/mL)	Drug loading in the filament
5.	Theophylline (Pietrzak *et al.*, 2015)	FDM	Tablets	Eudragit RL100 and RS100 Hydroxypropyl cellulose (HPC) (SSL grade) Triethyl citrate (TEC) and triacetin	Drug content uniformity, drug-release kinetics
6.	Prednisolone (Skowyra *et al.*, 2015)	FDM	Tablets	PVA filaments (melting point 160–170 °C, specific heat 0.4 Cal/g °C, density 1.25–1.35 g/cm^3)	Drug content, SEM
7.	Aripiprazole (Jamróz *et al.*, 2017)	FDM	Oral films	PVA (Poval 4–88), Glycerol (85%), Sodium Acetate Anhydrous, Hydranal®-Water Standard 10.0	Drug content, thickness, mass, tensile strength disintegration time, F_{max}, Young's modulus

No.	Drug (references)	Technology	Dosage form	Materials	Properties evaluated
8.	Methylene blue and alizarin yellow (dyes) (Prasad *et al.*, 2016)	Binder jet printing	Tabular device	Polycaprolactone (PCL), MCC and PEO	Mechanical strength and durability, print accuracy and precision, dissolution testing
9.	Paracetamol and alizarin yellow (dye) (Choi *et al.*, 2009)	Binder jet printing	Tablets	Kollicoat IR and Eudragit L100e55	Print resolution, drug content uniformity, layer adhesion, dissolution rate
10.	Pseudoephedrine (Alhnan *et al.*, 2016)	Binder jet printing	Cubic tabular devices	Kollidon SR, hydroxyl propyl methylcellulose (HPMC)	Print accuracy and precision, print resolution, powder bed uniformity, dissolution rate
11.	Chlorphenamine maleate and fluorescein (Ursan *et al.*, 2013)	Binder jet printing	Tablets	Avicel PH301, Eudragit E-100, RLPO in ethanol or acetone, or PVP and Tween 20 in deionized water.	Binder compatibility, drug content uniformity, dissolution rate
12.	Levetiracetam (Alhnan *et al.*, 2016)	Binder jet printing	Orodispersible tablets	Microcrystalline cellulose (MCC), glycerine, Tween 80, povidone, sucralose	Disintegration time, disintegration and erosion profile, drug content uniformity, dissolution rate
13.	Guaifenesin (Ameeduzzafar *et al.*, 2018)	SSE	Bi-layered tablets (polypill)	Polyacrylic acid (PAA), MCC and sodium starch glycolate	Mechanical properties, drug-release profile
14.	Nifedipine, glipizide, and captopril (Ameeduzzafar *et al.*, 2018)	SSE	Multiactive tablets (polypill)	HPMC K15M (Methocel K15M)	Drug content uniformity, drug release profiles print accuracy and precision, physical integrity and mechanical strength
15.	Hydrochlorothiazide, aspirin, pravastatin, atenolol and Ramipril (Patel *et al.*, 2012)	SSE	Multiactive tablets (polypill)	PEG 600, D-mannitol, cellulose acetate	Hardness, friability, in-process monitoring dissolution
16.	Paracetamol (Jamróz *et al.*, 2018)	SLS	Tablets	Kollicoat® IR or Eudragit® L100–55. Additionally, Candurin® gold sheen was added to aid the sintering process	Dissolution rates (geometry matters)

(continued)

TABLE 1.1 (Continued)
Work Done on 3D-printed Drug Delivery Systems

S.No	Drug	Technology	Formulation	Excipients	Parameters Studied
17.	Progesterone (Salmoria *et al.*, 2012)	SLS	Drug-delivery device	PCL (Molar mass around 70,000–90,000 g/mol, the melting temperature of 60 °C and melt flow rate 1.00 g/10 min). The particles size was 150–212µm)	Drug loading efficiency, mass loss of the reservoirs of PCL, functional drug delivery for gradient reservoirs of the PCL with progesterone
18.	Paracetamol or 4-ASA (Alruwaili *et al.*, 2018)	SLA	Tablets	Polyethylene glycol diacrylate (PEGDA), PEG 300 and diphenyl (2,4,6-trimethyl benzoyl)phosphine oxide	Drug release
19.	Ibuprofen (Martinez *et al.*, 2017)	SLA	Hydrogels	PEGDA, PEG 300, diphenyl (2,4,6-trimethyl benzoyl)phosphine oxide or riboflavin and triethanolamine	Drug content, swelling ratio, and water content, dissolution study
20.	Salicylic acid (Goyanes *et al.*, 2016)	SLA, FDM	Nose mask Patches	PEGDA, PEG 300, diphenyl (2,4,6-trimethyl benzoyl)phosphine oxide	Drug-loading diffusion test
21.	Guaifenesin (Khaled *et al.*, 2014)	Desktop 3D printer	Tablet	HPMC 2910, SSG type A, MCC PH 102	Weight uniformity, hardness, friability
22.	Pseudoephedrine (Jassim-Jaboori and Oyewumi, 2015)	A laboratory-scale 3DP machine	Capsule	Eudragit® E-100 (Rohm Pharma. Average molecular weight of 150,000 and is soluble below pH 5 and permeable above pH 5) and ethanol	Hardness, friability
23.	Nifedipine, captopril, and Glipizide (Khaled *et al.*, 2015)	3D extrusion printing	Tablet	PEG 6000, (HPMC 2910) (hypromellose®), sodium chloride 99 %, and tromethamine USP grade. D-mannitol 99 %, Croscarmellose sodium (CCS) (Primellose®), MCC (Pharmacel® 102) and sodium starch glycolate (SSG) (Primojel®), HPMC K100MCR) (Methocel TM), Milli-Q water (resistivity 18.2 MΩ cm)	*In vitro* drug dissolution, content uniformity weight variation

24.	Acetaminophen (Khaled et al., 2015)	3DP technology	Capsule shell	PVA, 5–25% HPMC	Dissolution test
25.	Cinnarizine (Singh et al., 2021)	FDM	Tablet	PVA	Melting point, loss on drying weight variation, friability hardness, drug content
26.	Acetaminophen (Zhang et al., 2019)	Hot melt extrusion	Cellulose-based filaments	Hypromellose acetate succinate, HPMC, HPC, EC	Thermogravimetric analysis, differential scanning calorimetry (DSC) polarized light microscopy (PLM) Repka-Zhang test of the mechanical properties of filaments, Fourier-transform infrared spectroscopy (FTIR), XRPD, rheology analysis, tablet morphology, tablet strength, *in vitro* drug release
27.	Baclofen (Abdulkhaleq et al., 2023)	Hot melt extrusion and FDM	Gastro-floating drug-delivery dosage form tablet	Eudragit RS-100 and EC	Drug content, *in vitro* floating behavior, *in vitro* dissolution, DSC, FT-IR, *in vivo* radiographic study, weight variation,
28.	Verapamil hydrochloride (Qian et al., 2022)	FDM	Sustained-release gastric-floating	(Affinisol™ HPMC HME 100lv), Polyvinyl caprolactam-polyvinyl acetate-polyethylene glycol copolymer, PEG, Methanol	Weight, hardness, drug content
29.	Ketorolac (Khan et al., 2022)	Pneumatic-based microextrusion printing technology	Oral Thin Films	HPC, starch, carbopol, HPMC, Propylene glycol, BHA, BHP, vitamin E, acetate, sunset yellow, purified water	Viscosity, density, spreadability, moisture content tensile strength, disintegration, dissolution, uniformity of dosage

(*continued*)

TABLE 1.1 (Continued)
Work Done on 3D-printed Drug Delivery Systems

S.No	Drug	Technology	Formulation	Excipients	Parameters Studied
30.	Rivaroxaban (Shkara *et al.*, 2022)	Fused deposition modeling 3DP technique	Tablet	Kollidon® VA 64 (Vinylpyrrolidone-vinyl acetate copolymer), Soluplus® (polyvinyl caprolactampolyvinyl acetate-polyethylene glycol graft copolymer), Kollidon® 30 (Polyvinylpyrrolidone K30), and Kollidon® 12 PF (Polyvinylpyrrolidone K12), PEG 400, PEG 4000, and Mannitol, Poloxamer 407, Sodium starch glycolate and Croscarmellose sodium	Drug content, *in vitro* drug-release test, hardness friability
31.	Catechin (Tagami *et al.*, 2019)	Semi-solid extrusion-type 3D printer	Muco-Adhesive oral films	HPMC (METOLOSE 90SH-15000SR HPMC 2208 type), Mannitol, Tween 20, Tween 80, glycerol and ethanol	Dissolution test, viscosity, film weight and thickness
32.	Paclitaxel and rapamycin (Serris *et al.*, 2020)	Hot melt extrusion	PLGA Films	PLGA	*In vitro* drug-release kinetics
33.	Paracetamol (Rodríguez-Pombo *et al.*, 2023)	Tomographic volumetric 3D printing	Printlets	PEGDA, PEG, distilled water, lithium phenyl 246 trimethyl benzoyl phoshilate, isopropanol, acetonitrile 199.9% HPLC grade, methanol HPLC grade	Absorbance
34.	Metronidazole (Utomo *et al.*, 2022)	Semi-solid extrusion	Intravaginal devices	PCL copolymer of methyl vinyl ether and maleic anhydride	FTIR, SEM, thermal analysis, rheology, swelling kinetic measurements, bioadhesion tests on porcine skin.

35.	Carbamazepine (Hu *et al.*, 2023)	Semi-solid extrusion	Tablet	SSG, PVP K30	Hardness, disintegration time, friability
36.	Paracetamol (Domsta *et al.*, 2022)	Molding technique	Suppositories	PEG, hard fat	Breaking force, uniformity of mass, diameter, and drug content, drug-release studies
37.	Lidocaine (Chatzitaki T *et al.*, 2021)	Pressure assisted microsyringes technology	Suppositories (SNEDDS)	GeloilTM SC, Gelucire48/16, Kolliphor RH40	DSC, PXRD, FTIR, SEM, TEM disintegration time, self-emulsification time, droplet size & zeta potential drug loading, *in vitro* drug release
38.	Budesonide and Tofacitinib citrate (Awad *et al.*, 2023)	Semi-solid extrusion	Suppositories	Gelucire 44/14, coconut oil, N, N- Dimethylacetamide	Disintegration, dissolution

scientists are working on formulation development approaches using 3DP to meet patient needs. The domain of medical devices, prosthetics, implants, dentures, surgical accessories, regenerative medicine and tissue/organ fabrication have seen the utility value of 3DP technology for tailoring individual patient needs. Despite the significant advancements in medicine delivery facilitated by 3DP technology, there are numerous obstacles that necessitate careful consideration. Some factors comprise the type of AM technology suitable, the printing rate, the speed of the printing head, the time interval allocated to print each layer, selection of the polymer material for the printing process. In addition to the challenges inherent in the printing process, the cost of product development and the lack of built-in flexibility pose significant concerns in the context of 3D printing. From a manufacturing perspective and technique employed, a comprehensive understanding of various factors is necessary, for example, the powder rate of the binder liquid, the interaction between the binder and the powder, the processes of re-solidification and evaporation, as well as the dissolving of the powder. The troubleshooting varies with each material and method employed and the product in consideration for printing, especially pharmaceuticals where the stability of the drug candidate is important. As technology advances, the potential applications of 3DP in healthcare are likely to expand. The existing lacunae would be overcome leading to more innovative approaches for delivering healthcare services.

REFERENCES

Abdulkhaleq, N.M. and Ghareeb, M.M. 3D printing of baclofen gastro-floating drug delivery systems: a comparison study with in vitro and in vivo evaluation. *Research Journal of Pharmacy and Technology* 16(1) (2023) 363–72. doi: 10.52711/0974-360X.2023.00063.

Adamo, A., Beingessner, R.L., Behnam, M., Chen, J., Jamison, T.F. and Jensen, K.F. On-demand continuous-flow production of pharmaceuticals in a compact, reconfigurable system. *Science*, 352 (2016) 61–67.

Agarwal, S., Saha, S., Balla, V.K., Pal, A., Barui, A. and Bodhak S. Current developments in 3D bioprinting for tissue and organ regeneration – a review. *Frontiers in Mechanical Engineering*, 6 (2020) 589171.

Alhijjaj, M., Belton, P. and Qi, S. An investigation into the use of polymer blends to improve the printability of and regulate drug release from pharmaceutical solid dispersions prepared via fused deposition modeling (FDM) 3D printing. *European Journal of Pharmaceutics and Biopharmaceutics*, 108 (2016) 111–125.

Alhnan, M.A., Okwuosa, T.C., Sadia, M., Wan, K.W., Ahmed, W. and Arafat, B. Emergence of 3D printed dosage forms: opportunities and challenges. *Pharmaceutical Research*, 33 (2016) 1817–1832.

Ameeduzzafar, Alruwaili, N.K., Rizwanullah, M., Abbas Bukhari, S.N., Amir, M., Masood Ahmed, M. and Fazil, M. 3D printing technology in design of pharmaceutical products. *Current Pharmaceutical Design*, 24 (2018) 5009–5018.

Angeliki, S., Eleni,T., Rekkas D.M. and Marilena, V. 3D-printed modified-release tablets: a review of the recent advances. *Molecular Pharmacology* Intech Open, London, 2020. www.intechopen.com/chapters/70777

Awad, A., Fina, F., Trenfield, S.J., Patel, P., Goyanes, A. and Gaisford, S. 3D printed pellets (miniprintlets): a novel, multi-drug, controlled release platform technology. *Pharmaceutics*, 11 (2019) 148.

Awad, A., Hollis, E., Goyanes, A., Orlu, M., Gaisford, S. and Basit, A.W. 3D printed multi-drug-loaded suppositories for acute severe ulcerative colitis. *International Journal of Pharmaceutics: X*, 5(2023) 100165. https://doi.org/10.1016/j.ijpx.2023.100165

Awad, A., Madla, C.M., McCoubrey, L.E., Ferraro, F., Gavins, F.K., Buanz, A., Gaisford, S., Orlu, M., Siepmann, F., Siepmann, J. and Basit, A.W. Clinical translation of advanced colonic drug delivery technologies. *Advanced Drug Delivery Reviews*, 1 (2022) 114076.

Bácskay, I., Ujhelyi, Z., Fehér, P. and Arany, P. The evolution of the 3D-printed drug delivery systems: a Review. *Pharmaceutics*, 14(7) (2022) 1312. https://doi.org/10.3390/pharmaceutics14071312

Barazanchi, A., Li, K.C., Al-Amleh, B., Lyons, K. and Waddell, J.N. Additive technology: update on current materials and applications in dentistry. *Journal of Prosthodontics*, 26 (2017) 156–163.

Baylón, K., Rodríguez-Camarillo, P., Elías-Zúñiga, A., Díaz-Elizondo, J.A., Gilkerson, R. and Lozano, K. Past, present and future of surgical meshes: a review. *Membranes*, 7 (2017) 47.

Biglino, G., Hopfner, C., Lindhardt, J., et al. Perspectives on medical 3D printing at the point-of-care from the new European 3D Printing Special Interest Group, *3D Printing in Medicine*, 9(1) (2023) 14.

Calvo-Haro, J.A., Pascau, J., Asencio-Pascual, J.M., et al. Point-of-care manufacturing: a single university hospital's initial experience. *3D Printing in Medicine*, 7(1) (2021) 11. https://doi.org/10.1186/s41205-021-00101-z

Calvo-Haro, J.A., Pascau, J., Mediavilla-Santos, L., Sanz-Ruiz, P., Sánchez-Pérez, C., Vaquero-Martín, J. and Perez-Mañanes, R. Conceptual evolution of 3D printing in orthopedic surgery and traumatology: from "do it yourself" to "point of care manufacturing". *BMC Musculoskeletal Disorders*, 22(1) (2021 Dec) 360.

Caudill, C.L., Perry, J.L., Tian, S., Luft, J.C. and DeSimone, J.M. Spatially controlled coating of continuous liquid interface production microneedles for transdermal protein delivery. *Journal of Controlled Release*, 284 (2018) 122–132.

Chatzitaki, A.T., Tsongas, K., Tzimtzimis, E.K., Tzetzis, D., Bouropoulos, N., Barmpalexis, P., Eleftheriadis, G.K., Fatouros, D.G. 3D printing of patient-tailored SNEDDS-based suppositories of lidocaine. *Journal of Drug Delivery Science Technology*, 61(2021) 102292. https://doi.org/10.1016/j.jddst.2020.102292

Choi, Y.W., Ryoo, B.H. and Jeong, Y.M. Novel controlled release-niacin formulation. Google Patents (2009).

Cox, S.C., Jamshidi, P., Eisenstein, N.M., Webber, M.A., Hassanin, H. and Attallah, M.M. Adding functionality with additive manufacturing: fabrication of titanium-based antibiotic eluting implants. *Materials Science and Engineering C*, 64 (2016) 407–415.

Di Marzio, N., David, E., Tiziano, S. and Lorenzo M. Bio-fabrication: Convergence of 3D bioprinting and nano-biomaterials in tissue engineering and regenerative medicine. *Frontiers in Bioengineering and Biotechnology*, 8(2020), 326. doi: 10.3389/fbioe.2020.00326

Domsta, V., Krause, J., Weitschies, W. and Seidlitz, A. 3D Printing of paracetamol suppositories: an automated manufacturing technique for individualized therapy. *Pharmaceutics*, 14(2022) 2676. https://doi.org/10.3390/pharmaceutics14122676

Dumpa, N., Butreddy, A., Wang, H., Komanduri, N., Bandari, S. and Repka, M.A. 3D printing in personalized drug delivery: an overview of hot-melt extrusion-based fused deposition modelling. *International Journal of Pharmaceutics*, 600 (2021) 120501.

Elkanayati, R.M., Chambliss, W.G., Omari, S., Almutairi, M., Repka, M.A. and Ashour, E.A. Mucoadhesive buccal films for treatment of xerostomia prepared by coupling HME and

3D printing technologies. *Journal of Drug Delivery Science and Technology*, 75 (2022 Sep 1) 103660.

Elsayed, M., Ghazy, M., Youssef, Y. and Essa, K. Optimization of SLM process parameters for Ti6Al4V medical implants. *Rapid Prototyping Journal* 25 (2019) 433–447.

Eshkalak, S.K., Ghomi, E.R., Dai, Y., Choudhury, D. and Ramakrishna, S. The role of three-dimensional printing in healthcare and medicine. *Materials & Design*, 194(2020) 10894. https://doi.org/10.1016/j.matdes.2020.108940

Fu, J., Yu, X. and Y. Jin. 3D printing of vaginal rings with personalized shapes for controlled release of progesterone. *International Journal of Pharmaceutics*, 539 (2018) 75–82.

Ganguli, A., Pagan-Diaz, G. J., Grant, L., Cvetkovic, C., Bramlet, M., Vozenilek, J., Kesavadas, T. and Bashir, R. 3D printing for preoperative planning and surgical training: a review. *Biomedical Microdevices*, 20(3)(2018) 65. https://doi.org/10.1007/s10544-018-0301-9

Gioumouxouzis, C.I., Katsamenis, O.L., Bouropoulos, N. and Fatouros D.G. 3D printed oral solid dosage forms containing hydrochlorothiazide for controlled drug delivery. *Journal of Drug Delivery Science and Technology*, 40(2017) 164–171.

Greymi, T., Nicole, I., Essyrose, M., Aristides, D.T., Dimitrios, A.L. and Cynthia, Y.-W.-M. 3D printing in ophthalmology: from medical implants to personalised medicine. *International Journal of Pharmaceutics*, 625(2022), 122094.

Goyanes, A., Allahham, N., Trenfield, S.J., Stoyanovd, E., Gaisford, S. and Basit, A.W. Direct powder extrusion 3D printing: fabrication of drug products using a novel single-step process. *International Journal of Pharmaceutics*, 567 (2019) 118471.

Goyanes, A., Buanz, A.B. and Hatton, G.B. 3D printing of modified-release aminosalicylate (4-ASA and 5-ASA) tablets. *European Journal of Pharmaceutics and Biopharmaceutics*, 89 (2015) 157–162.

Goyanes, A., Chang, H. and Sedough, D. Fabrication of controlled-release budesonide tablets via desktop (FDM) 3D printing. *International Journal of Pharmaceutics*, 496 (2015) 414–420.

Goyanes, A., Det-Amornrat, U., Wang, J., Basit, A.W. and Gaisford, S. 3D scanning and 3D printing as innovative technologies for fabricating personalized topical drug delivery systems. *Journal of Controlled Release*, 234 (2016) 41–48

Goyanes, A., Kobayashi, M. and Martínez-Pacheco, R. Fused-filament 3D printing of drug products: microstructure analysis and drug release characteristics of PVA-based caplets. *International Journal of Pharmaceutics*, 514 (2016) 290–295.

Goyanes, A., Martinez, P. R., Buanz, A., Basit, A.W. and Gaisford, S. Effect of geometry on drug release from 3D printed tablets. *International Journal of Pharmaceutics*, 494 (2015) 657–663.

Gul, M., Arif, A. and Ghafoor, R. Role of three-dimensional printing in periodontal regeneration and repair: literature review. *Journal of Indian Society of Periodontology*, 33 (2019) 504–510.

Hassanin, H., Finet, L., Cox, S.C., Jamshidi, P., Grover, L.M. and Shepherd, D.E.T. Tailoring selective laser melting process for titanium drug-delivering implants with releasing micro-channels. *Additive Manufacturing*, 20 (2018) 144–155.

Hu, J., Fitaihi, R., Abukhamees, S. and Abdelhakim, H.E. Formulation and characterisation of carbamazepine orodispersible 3D-printed mini-tablets for paediatric use. *Pharmaceutics*, 15(1) (2023) 250.

Hua, S. Physiological and pharmaceutical considerations for rectal drug formulations. *Frontiers in Pharmacology*, 10 (2019) 1196.

Hua, S. Advances in oral drug delivery for regional targeting in the gastrointestinal tract-influence of physiological, pathophysiological and pharmaceutical factors. *Frontiers in Pharmacology*, 28 (2020) 524.

Iliescu, F.S., Paunica, S., Vrtacnik, D. and Bobei, A.R. A double softlithography method for processing of nono microneedles arrays. *UPB Scientific Bulletin B: Chemistry and Material Science*, 79 (2017) 121–132.

Ita, K. Transdermal delivery of drugs with microneedles-potential and challenges. *Pharmaceutics*, 7 (2015) 90–105.

Jamróz, W., Kurek, M. and Łyszczarz, E. 3D printed orodispersible films with Aripiprazole. *International Journal of Pharmaceutics*, 533 (2017) 413–420.

Jamróz, W., Szafraniec, J. and Kurek, M. 3D printing in pharmaceutical and medical applications – recent achievements and challenges. *Pharmaceutical Research*, 35 (2018) 176.

Jassim-Jaboori, A. and Oyewumi, M. 3D printing technology in pharmaceutical drug delivery: prospects and challenges. *Journal of Biomolecular Research & Herapeutics*, 4 (2015) 1–3.

Jin, Z., He, C., Fu, J., Han, Q. and He, Y. Balancing the customization and standardization: exploration and layout surrounding the regulation of the growing field of 3D-printed medical devices in China. *Bio-design and Manufacturing*, 5(2022) 580–606.

Katakam, P., Adiki, S.K. and Satapathy, S.R. Recent advancements of additive manufacturing for patient-specific drug delivery. In: *Additive Manufacturing Processes in Biomedical Engineering*, 1st Edition. Boca Raton: CRC Press; (2022) 1–26.

Keating, A.V., Soto, J., Tuleu, C., Forbes, C., Zhao, M. and Craig, D.Q.M. Solid state characterisation and taste masking efficiency evaluation of polymer based extrudates of isoniazid for paediatric administration. *International Journal of Pharmaceutics*, 536 (2018) 536–546.

Kempin, W., Domsta, V., Grathoff, G., Brecht, I. Semmling, B., Tillmann, S., Weitschies, W. and Seidlitz, A. Immediate release 3D-printed tablets produced via fused deposition modeling of a thermo-sensitive drug. *Pharmaceutical Research*, 35 (2018) 124.

Khaled, S.A., Burley, J.C. and Alexander, M.R. Desktop 3D printing of controlled release pharmaceutical bilayer tablets. *International Journal of Pharmaceutics*, 461 (2014)105–111

Khaled, S.A., Burley, J.C., Alexander, M.R., Yang, J. and Roberts, C.J. 3D printing of tablets containing multiple drugs with defined release profiles. *International Journal of Pharmaceutics*, 494(2) (2015) 643–650.

Khan, F.B., Kilor, V., Sapkal, N. and Dule, P. Formulation development of mouth dissolving printed film of ketorolac and in vitro evaluation. *International Journal of Applied Pharmaceutics*, 14(5) (2022) 128–136.

Kumar, P., Vatsya, P., Rajnish, R.K., Hooda, A., and Dhillon, M.S. Application of 3D printing in hip and knee arthroplasty: a narrative review. *Indian Journal of Orthopaedics*, 55 (2020) 14–26. https://doi.org/10.1007/s43465-020-00263-8

Lei, L., Yu, Y., Ke, T., Sun, W. and Chen, L. The application of three-dimensional printing model and platelet-rich fibrin technology in guided tissue regeneration surgery for severe bone defects. Journal of Oral Implantology, 45 (2019) 35–43.

Lewis, T. Could 3D printing solve the organ transplant shortage? *The Guardian*, 30 July (2017). www.theguardian.com/technology/2017/jul/30/will-3d-printing-solve-the-organ-transplant-shortage

Martinez, P.R., Goyanes, A. and Basit, A.W. Fabrication of drug-loaded hydrogels with stereolithographic 3D printing. *International Journal of Pharmaceutics*, 532 (2017) 313–317.

Mathew, E., Domínguez-Robles, J., Larrañeta, E. and Lamprou, D.A. Fused deposition modelling as a potential tool for antimicrobial dialysis catheters manufacturing: new trends vs. conventional approaches. *Coatings*, 9(2019) 515.

Mathew, E., Pitzanti, G., Larrañeta, E. and Lamprou, D.A. 3D printing of pharmaceuticals and drug delivery devices. *Pharmaceutics*, 12(3) (2020) 266. https://doi.org/10.3390/pharmaceutics12030266

McCoubrey, L.E., Favaron, A., Awad, A., Orlu, M., Gaisford, S. and Basit, A.W. Colonic drug delivery: formulating the next generation of colon-targeted therapeutics. *Journal of Controlled Release*, 1(2023) 1107–1126.

Melocchi, A., Parietti, F., Maroni, A., Foppoli, A., Gazzaniga, A. and Zema, L. Hot-melt extruded filaments based on pharmaceutical grade polymers for 3D printing by fused deposition modelling. *International Journal of Pharmaceutics*, 509 (2016) 255–263.

Mohanty, S., Larsen, L.B., Trifol, J., Szabo, P., Burri, H.V.R. and Canali, C. Fabrication of scalable and structured tissue engineering scaffolds using water dissolvable sacrificial 3D printed moulds. *Materials Science and Engineering, C*, 55 (2015) 569–578.

Musazzi, U.M., Selmin, F., Ortenzi, M.A., Mohammed, G.K., Franzé, S. and Minghetti, P. Personalized orodispersible films by hot melt ram extrusion 3D printing. *International Journal of Pharmaceutics*, 551 (2018) 52–59.

Muwaffak, Z., Goyanes, A., Clark, V., Basit, A.W., Hilton, S.T. and Gaisford, S. Patient-specific 3D scanned and 3D printed antimicrobial polycaprolactone wound dressings. *International Journal of Pharmaceutics*, 527 (2017) 161–170.

Norman, J., Madurawe, R.D., Moore, C.M.V., Khan, M.A. and Khairuzzaman, A. A new chapter in pharmaceutical manufacturing: 3Dprinted drug products. *Advanced Drug Delivery Reviews*, 108 (2017) 39–50.

Patel, A., Shah, T., Shah, G., Jha, V. and Ghosh, C. Preservation of bioavailability of ingredients and lack of drug-drug interactions in a novel five-ingredient polypill (Polycap ™). *American Journal of Cardiovascular Drugs*, 10 (2012) 95–103.

Patel, R., Sheth, T., Shah, S. and Shah, M. A new leap in periodontics: three-dimensional (3D) printing. *Journal of Advanced Oral Research*, 8 (2017) 1–7.

Pereira, B.C., Isreb, A., Forbes, R.T., Dores, F., Habashy, R. and J.B. Petit. Temporary Plasticiser: a novel solution to fabricate 3D printed patient-centred cardiovascular '*polypill*' architectures. European Journal Pharmaceutics and Biopharmaceutics, 135 (2019) 94–103.

Pieters, A., De Schrijver, H., Neefs, W. and Vertenten, W. 3D printing enables patient-specific medical devices for a better quality of care. 2022.

Pietrzak, K., Isreb, A. and Alhnan, M.A. A flexible-dose dispenser for immediate and extended release 3D printed tablets. *European Journal of Pharmaceutics and Biopharmaceutics*, 96 (2015) 380–387.

Point-of-Care 3D Solutions. 3dsystems.com. www.3dsystems.com/healthcare/point-of-care

Prasad, L.K. and Smyth, H. 3D printing technologies for drug delivery: a review. *Drug Development and Industrial Pharmacy*, 42 (2016) 1019–1031. doi: 10.3109/03639045.2015.1120743

Pravin, S. and Sudhir, A. Integration of 3D printing with dosage forms: a new perspective for modern healthcare. *Biomedicine & Pharmacotherapy*, 107 (2018) 146–154.

Qian, H., Chen, D., Xu, X., Li, R., Yan, G. and Fan, T. FDM 3D-printed sustained-release gastric-floating verapamil hydrochloride formulations with cylinder, capsule and hemisphere shapes, and low infill percentage. *Pharmaceutics*, 14(2) (2022) 281.

Rasperini, G., Pilipchuk, S.P., Flanagan, C.L., Park, C.H., Pagni, G. and Hollister S.J. 3D-printed bioresorbable scaffold for periodontal repair. Journal of Dental Research, 94 (2015) 153S–157S.

Rengier, F., Mehndiratta, A., von Tengg-Kobligk, H., Zechmann, C.M., Unterhinninghofen, R., Kauczor, H.U. and Giesel, F.L. 3D printing based on imaging data: review of medical applications. *International Journal of Computer Assisted Radiology and Surgery*, 5(4) (2010) 335–341. https://doi.org/10.1007/s11548-010-0476-x

Rodríguez-Pombo, L., Martínez-Castro, L., Xu, X., On, J.J., Rial, C., García, D.N., González-Santos, A., Flores-González, J., Alvarez-Lorenzo, C., Basit, A.W. and Goyanes, A. Simultaneous fabrication of multiple tablets within seconds using tomographic volumetric 3D printing. *International Journal of Pharmaceutics*, 5 (2023) 100166.

Salmoria, G., Klauss, P. and Zepon. K. Development of functionally graded reservoir of PCL/PG by selective laser sintering for drug delivery devices: selective laser sintering-fabricated drug delivery system that contains graded progesterone content. *Virtual and Physical Prototyping*, 7 (2012) 107–115.

Schweiger, J., Edelhoff, D. and Güth, J.F. 3D printing in digital prosthetic dentistry: an overview of recent developments in additive manufacturing. *Journal of Clinical Medicine*, 10 (2021): 2010. doi:10.3390/jcm10092010

Serrano, D.R., Kara, A., Yuste, I., Luciano, F.C., Ongoren, B., Anaya, B.J. and Molina, G. 3D printing technologies in personalized medicine, nanomedicines, and biopharmaceuticals. *Pharmaceutics*, 15 (2023) 313. http://dx.doi.org/10.3390/pharmaceutics15020313

Serris, I., Serris, P., Frey, K.M. and Cho, H. Development of 3D-printed layered PLGA films for drug delivery and evaluation of drug release behaviours. *AAPS PharmSciTech*, 21 (2020) 1–5.

Shkara, A.M. and Ghareeb, M.M. Formulation and in-vitro evaluation of rivaroxaban tablet by fused deposition modelling 3d printing technique. *International Journal of Drug Delivery Technology*, 12(1) (2022) 281–291.

Singh, S., Vinchurkar, K., Dixit, P. and Mishra, D.k. Formulation design and evaluation of 3D printed tablet of cinnarizine by fused deposition modeling technique. *IJCRT*, 9 (2021) 5881–5897.

Skowyra, J., Pietrzak, K. and Alhnan, M.A. Fabrication of extended-release patient-tailored prednisolone tablets via fused deposition modelling (FDM) 3D printing. *European Journal of Pharmaceutical Sciences*, 68 (2015) 11–17.

Solanki, N.G., Tahsin, M., Shah, A.V. and Serajuddin, A.T.M. Formulation of 3D printed tablet for rapid drug release by fused deposition modeling: screening polymers for drug release, drug polymer miscibility and printability. *Journal of Pharmaceutical Sciences*, 107 (2018) 390–401.

Strianese, O., Rizzo, F., Ciccarelli, M., Galasso, G., D'Agostino, Y., Salvati, A., Del Giudice, C., Tesorio, P. and Rusciano, M.R. Precision and personalized medicine: how genomic approach improves the management of cardiovascular and neurodegenerative disease. *Genes*, 11(7) (2020) 747. https://doi.org/10.3390/genes11070747

Tagami, T., Yoshimura, N., Goto, E., Noda, T. and Ozeki, T. Fabrication of muco-adhesive oral films by the 3D printing of hydroxypropyl methylcellulose-based catechin-loaded formulations. *Biological and Pharmaceutical Bulletin*, 42(11) (2019) 1898–1905.

Tappa, K. and Jammalamadaka, U. Novel biomaterials used in medical 3D printing techniques. *Journal of Functional Biomaterials*, 9 (2018) 17.

Turkyilmaz, I., and Wilkins, G. N. 3D printing in dentistry – exploring the new horizons. *Journal of Dental Ssciences*, 16(3) (2021) 1037–1038. https://doi.org/10.1016/j.jds.2021.04.004

Ursan, I.D., Chiu, L. and Pierce, A. Three-dimensional drug printing: a structured review. *Journal of the American Pharmacists Association*, 53(2013) 136–144.

Utomo, E., Domínguez-Robles, J., Anjani, Q.K., Picco, C.J., Korelidou A., Magee E., Donnelly, R.F. and Larrañeta, E. Development of 3D-printed vaginal devices containing metronidazole for alternative bacterial vaginosis treatment. *International Journal of Pharmaceutics: X*, 5(2022) 100142. doi: 10.1016/j.ijpx.2022.100142

Vaz, V.M. and Kumar, L. 3D printing as a promising tool in personalized medicine. *AAPS PharmSciTech*, 22(2021) 49. https://doi.org/10.1208/s12249-020-01905-8

Villota, I., Calvo, P.C., Campo, O.I., Villarreal-Gómez, L.J. and Fonthal, F. Manufacturing of a transdermal patch in 3d printing. *Micromachines (Basel)*, 13(2022) 2190. doi: 10.3390/mi13122190

Vithani, K., Goyanes, A., Jannin, V., Basit, A.W., Gaisford, S. and Boyd, B.J. An overview of 3D printing technologies for soft materials and potential opportunities for lipid-based drug delivery systems. Pharmaceutics Research, 36 (2018) 4.

Vukicevic, M., Mosadegh, B., Min, J.K., and Little, S.H. Cardiac 3D printing and its future Directions. *JACC: Cardiovascular Imaging*, 10(2) (2017) 171–184. https://doi.org/10.1016/j.jcmg.2016.12.001

Weisman, J.A., Ballard, D.H., Jammalamadaka, U., Tappa, K., Sumerel, J., D'Agostino, H.B., Mills, D.K. and Woodard, P.K. 3D printed antibiotic and chemotherapeutic eluting catheters for potential use in interventional radiology: *in vitro* proof of concept study. Academic Radiology, 26 (2019) 270–274.

Weisman, J.A., Nicholson, J.C., Tappa, K., Jammalamadaka, U., Wilson, C.G. and Mills, D.K. Antibiotic and chemotherapeutic enhanced three-dimensional printer filaments and constructs for biomedical applications. *International Journal of Nanomedicine*, 10 (2015) 357–370.

Zhang, J., Xu, P., Vo, A.Q., Bandari, S., Yang, F., Durig, T. and Repka, M.A. Development and evaluation of pharmaceutical 3D printability for hot melt extruded cellulose-based filaments. *Journal of drug delivery science and technology*, 52 (2019), 292–302.

2 Innovative and Modified Additive Manufacturing Processes

Extended Applications in the Pharmaceutical Industry

Popat Mohite, Sudarshan Kakad, and Anil Pawar

2.1 INTRODUCTION

Additive manufacturing (AM) or 3D printing has come a long way, and is now a game-changer in many different markets. Its industrial significance has grown, progressively displacing traditional production techniques like casting and milling. The advancement of AM technology creates new opportunities for distinctive material combinations, integrated functionality, and unmatched creative freedom. This change challenges the established linkages between cost, part count, complexity, tolerance, and shape that are governed by traditional manufacturing technologies, thereby significantly reshaping the dynamics of manufacturing. AM technologies bring about a paradigm change that calls for a different approach to product development and a methodical break from conventional thinking. The disruptive nature of AM calls for a fundamental rethinking of how goods are imagined and brought to life, not just a shift in tools. The capacity of 3D printing to create complex geometries layer-by-layer opens up new possibilities in terms of design and manufacturing. The benefits of this revolutionary technology include the potential for rapid prototyping, enhanced customization capabilities, and decreased material waste. Adopting AM necessitates a break from traditional manufacturing practices in favor of a more creative and flexible strategy. The move to AM signifies a break from the constraints of conventional production techniques and ushers in a new era of manufacturing opportunities (Höller et al., 2022).

The American Society for Testing and Materials (ASTM) F42 Technical Committee defines AM as fabricating objects from 3D model data by joining materials, usually layer-by-layer. This advanced approach is also known as direct additive processing, digital manufacturing, solid freeform fabrication, rapid prototyping, and quick manufacturing. It differs from subtractive manufacturing methods as it does not involve removing material (Guo & Leu, 2013). Any material, encompassing metals, polymers, ceramics, composites, etc., can undergo fabrication through AM. Its advantages include enhanced functionality, intricate designs, near-net shaping with minimal

DOI: 10.1201/9781003439509-3

post-processing, and reduced lead times. Various industries, such as jewellery, automotive, oil refining, maritime, construction, and aerospace, have integrated AM into their processes. However, challenges persist in the field, notably in developing alloys compatible with AM techniques and addressing premature material breakdown despite noticeable improvements in attributes. The nexus between structure and property, continual process innovation, and overall advancements remain focal points for further exploration in additive manufacturing (Prashanth & Wang, 2020).

Digital models can be used to produce three-dimensional solid objects using 3D printing, also known as additive manufacturing or fast prototyping. It was invented by Charles Hull in the early 1980s and gained widespread interest for its efficiency in transforming computer designs into tangible products. Utilizing computer-aided design (CAD) software or 3D scanners that record measurements and images for computer transmission, digital 3D models are created. Primarily employed in the manufacturing sector for producing prototypes, 3D printing offers unparalleled design freedom, allowing the construction of intricate structures to be impractical with traditional methods. Its application has extended to the pharmaceutical and medical industries, facilitating the development of customized medications, oral dosage forms, medical equipment, and tissue engineering. This technology involves layering thin material to construct the 3D object, with various 3D-printing technologies available in the market, each named after its specific process for creating the object (Tan et al., 2019). Academic and business circles are starting to take an interest in 3D printing as a cutting-edge manufacturing technique. Since the first stereolithography machine prototype was created 30 years ago, it has become clear that 3D printing has the potential to make substantial progress. While technology has much potential, it is unclear how it will affect current companies (Lu et al., 2015).

The design of formulation now in new directions with the use of 3D printing, including implants, controlled release formulations and personalized medications. From conceptualization to actual manufacturing, there are several phases in the creation of pharmaceutical products. Researchers and industry can now make products with increasingly complicated design and excellent quality control. Pharmaceutical AM classified the above main stages, modeling conceptualization and objective design, slicing the objects, preformulation, instrument set-up, building/printing, removal/cleaning, and post-processing (J. Zhang et al., 2018). It was unthinkable, even a few years ago, to imagine 3D printing being used in the formulation development pipeline for first in human preformulation. Furthermore, there is also research being done on use of 3D printing in front-line clinical trial settings to offer trial participants individualized care. The significant advancement of 3D printing in the pharmaceutical industry can be attributed to a substantial body of prior research, motivated by its wide range of possible applications (Sen et al., 2023). This book chapter provides an overview on methods of AM, their extended application, and challenges with AM in the pharmaceutical industry.

2.2 CLASSIFICATION OF ADDITIVE MANUFACTURING TECHNIQUES

AM techniques are diverse, with each method having distinct advantages and limitations. These techniques can be broadly categorized into several classes based on the underlying principles and processes. In this discussion, we will introduce the classification of AM techniques, providing an overview of the main categories and their key characteristics.

These techniques can be systematically classified based on their underlying principles and processes. A basic categorization is determined by the kind of substance utilized. We come across a number of categories in this classification, including polymer-based AM, which is frequently used in rapid prototyping and the fabrication of plastic parts. It works by layering objects together using thermoplastic filaments or liquid photopolymer resins. Metal-based AM, on the other hand, employs high-powered lasers or electron beams to selectively melt and fuse metal powders, making it particularly valuable for producing intricate and robust metal components. Emerging categories, like bioink-based AM for bioprinting tissues and organs and other specialized materials like concrete and food-based 3D printing, demonstrate the boundless potential of AM techniques. Understanding this classification based on materials is pivotal for selecting the most suitable AM method for a given application, whether in aerospace, healthcare, or even culinary arts. The classification of AM methods is shown in Figure 2.1.

2.3   3D PRINTING

3D printing, or AM, is a digital fabrication where a physical object is created using geometrical models and materials. This method is quickly employed for open-source design production and large-scale manufacturing in the pharmaceutical industry (Jadhav & Jadhav, 2022). Furthermore, scientists and scholars now have many possibilities thanks to 3D printing that enable them to construct intricate structures with the needed features. Unlike traditional production methods like machining, 3D printing allows for the creation of any size or shape (Sai Saran et al., 2022). 3D printing technology is not going to replace the well-established methods for producing solid dosage forms. However, it can be applied in the healthcare sector, where bulk output is not as crucial as quality, consistency, accuracy, and precision. Different types of 3D printing technologies exist, each with varying processing speeds, resolutions, and types of materials. These are a few 3D printing methods; however, most are inappropriate for pharmaceutical applications due to constraints in raw materials and production processes (Rahman et al., 2018).

1.   Binder jetting
2.   Material vaporization
3.   Vat – polymerization
4.   Direct energy deposition material extrusion

The two primary 3D printing methods are nozzle-based and light-based. In nozzle-based 3D printing, materials are extruded onto a platform. This method includes inkjet printing and extrusion. Light-based 3D printing methods include selective laser sintering, selective laser melting (SLM), digital light processing printing (DLP), and laser-assisted printing (SLS). Digital light processing and laser-assisted printing techniques employ photo-polymerization procedures, while in SLM and SLS,

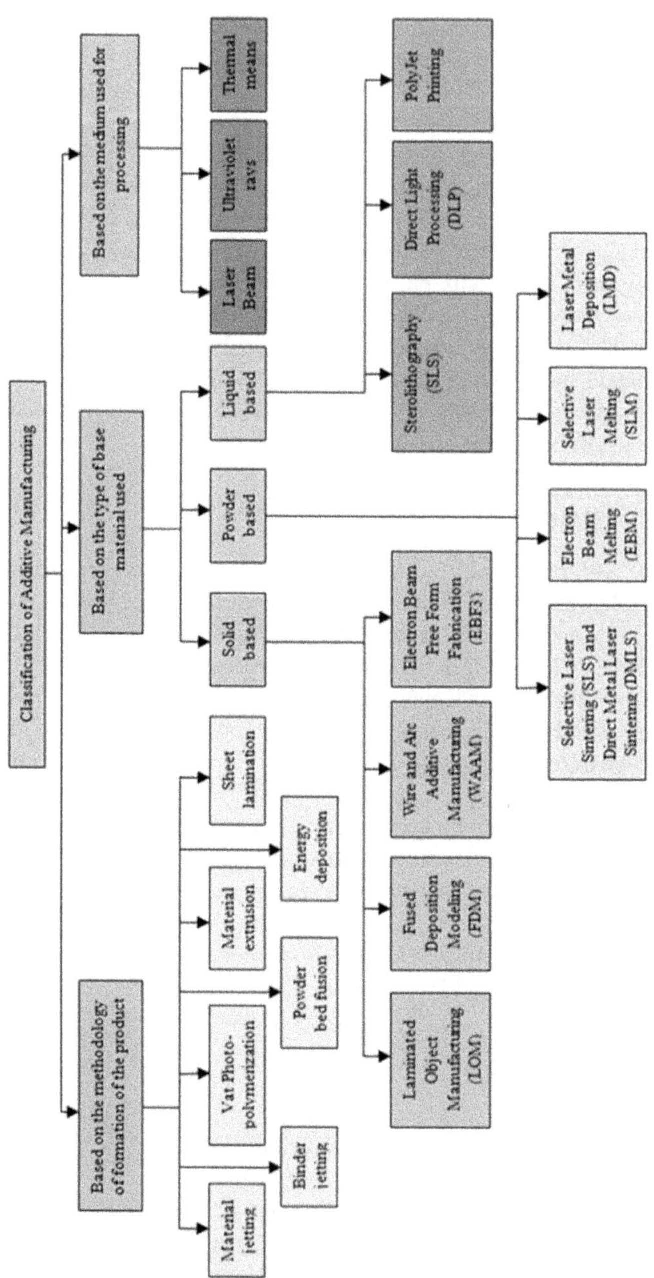

FIGURE 2.1 The categorization of additive manufacturing methods. (Adapted and reproduced from Alghamdi et al. (2021).)

material powders are melted using lasers at high temperatures and then molded (J. Zhang et al., 2020).

2.3.1 MATERIAL EXTRUSION (ME) METHOD

Material extrusion (ME) techniques build a component layer-by-layer by ejecting heated or pressured material through a nozzle along a predefined route. The thermoplastic or paste that has been extruded is then placed on the building platform, where it cools and solidifies. It is among the most widely used and reasonably priced methods for printing drug delivery systems. Material extrusion is distinguished by its high speed and reasonably low cost (Ngo et al., 2018). For extrusion and adhesion with previous layers, printed parts used in the famous ME method known as FDM must be thermoplastic (Figure 2.2). This technique was developed by Scott Crump in 1988 (Mwema & Akinlabi, 2020). This method mostly makes use of thermo-polymers. It prints a component layer-by-layer by melting an input filament and then using a traversing nozzle to deposit it on a printing platform. Printing a dosage form is one of the easiest and most economical methods. In addition, the printouts generated are mechanically robust and generally do not need any post-processing, which cuts down on the time needed to create a printed object (J. Zhang et al., 2017). Gels and pastes can also be extruded by applying pressure, as in the case of pneumatic or syringe extrusion (PE/SE) techniques. The ability to print a range of materials at lower temperatures without melting them is a benefit of pneumatic or syringe extrusion over FDM (Figure 2.3). Material extrusion is used in most drug administration modalities, such as rectal, vaginal, transdermal, oral, and transrectal (Lim et al., 2018). The FDM process is also

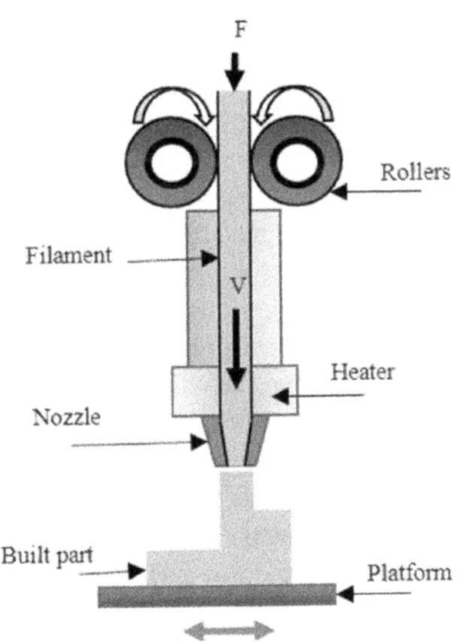

FIGURE 2.2 A graphic depicting the FDM extrusion process. (Adapted and reproduced from Herderick (2015).)

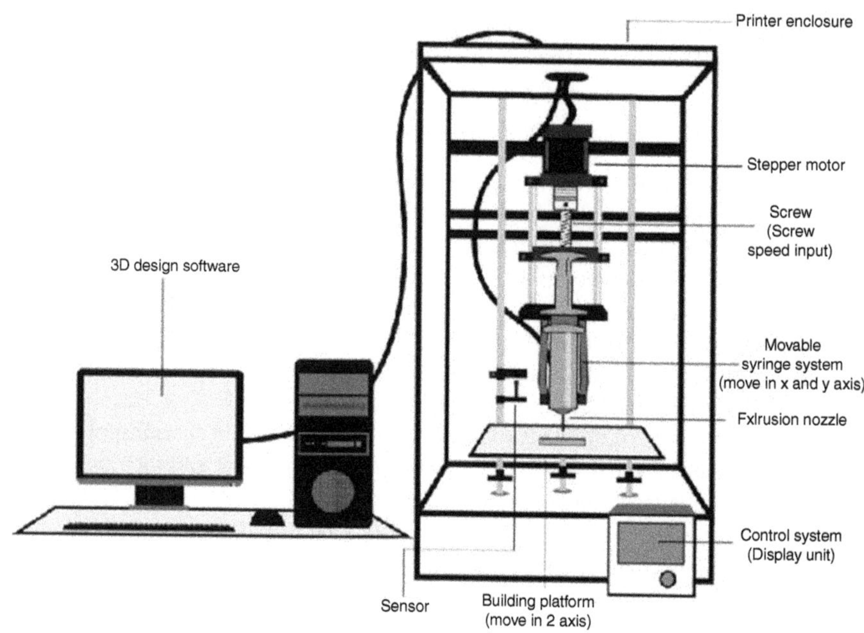

FIGURE 2.3   Diagram for syringe extrusion in a 3D printer. (Adapted and reproduced from Panraksa et al. (2020).)

widely used to create a variety of drug-loaded implants with various purposes. PLA has grown in popularity since it is easy to print on and has a long lifespan. To treat the ailments locally, a range of APIs have been packed into various implant shapes, including disc cages. The implants were able to carry out certain functions like bone attachment and the inhibition of bacterial biofilms because they had the best medication loading combination (Boetker et al., 2016; Weisman et al., 2019).

The FDM technique frequently involves heating materials to temperatures as high as 250 °C, deemed unsuitable for heat-sensitive drugs. The development of printed drug-loaded filaments is affected by other factors, such as defects in the cooling process. A 3D printing setup using semi-solid extrusion can be beneficial to tackle this issue. This technique involves feeding a mixture of powder or paste and printing it through a nozzle or syringe using either pressure or a screw at various temperature ranges. The SE method is superior to the FDM approach when working with low temperatures. Moreover, it enables a more significant drug load percentage without compromising the amount or quality of the medication (Khaled et al., 2014; Lu et al., 2010). It has been demonstrated that this process works well for creating polypills. This combination is a five-in-one dose polypill (Khaled et al., 2015). Most scientific study has been directed toward developing FDM-printed tablets with a controlled pharmacological profile, as is evident. For a medication to have a meaningful pharmacological effect on the human body, it must be released promptly. The patient's condition will determine which controlled medication release method needs to be employed. For example, continuous-release drugs are essential because their limited concentration range makes it difficult for the medicine to work as intended in the body. If the concentration is too high, the medication may not operate as intended, and if it is too low, then may show side effects. The 3D-printed tablets and caplets have complicated architectures, varying infill densities, and drug-loading ingredients to generate an instant or delayed release profile (Beck et al., 2017; Jamróz et al., 2017; Li et al., 2017).

2.3.2 Vat Polymerization

This method uses UV light to crosslink a selective photosensitive resin layer to a solid polymer. Subsequently, the photosensitive polymer is blended into the preceding layer; repeat this procedure till the portion is finished. After removing the cured portion from the tank, heating and cleaning improve the structure and strength. When compared to alternative technologies, this one is quite desirable and appealing due to its excellent quality and speed of printing. This approach is separated into two categories based on the different sources it cures: stereolithography (SLA) and digital light processing (DLP) (Mohammed et al., 2020). Rapid 3D printing technology called DLP has gained much traction in the TE sector thanks to its exceptional precision and versatility. The technology of 3D printing based on DLP originates from image projection technology. In this technique, chipsets relying on micro-electromechanical technology are employed for processing photosensitive materials and light sources (Figure 2.4). One crucial functional component is the digital micromirror, which comprises programmable, micro-sized mirrors. Light is projected onto photosensitive resin using a rotating digital micromirror device to adjust the light's path. The projection of the lens and plane, which DMD modifies, determines the resolution of 3D printing using DLP. This method provides high-resolution or micron-scale data (J. Zhang et al., 2020).

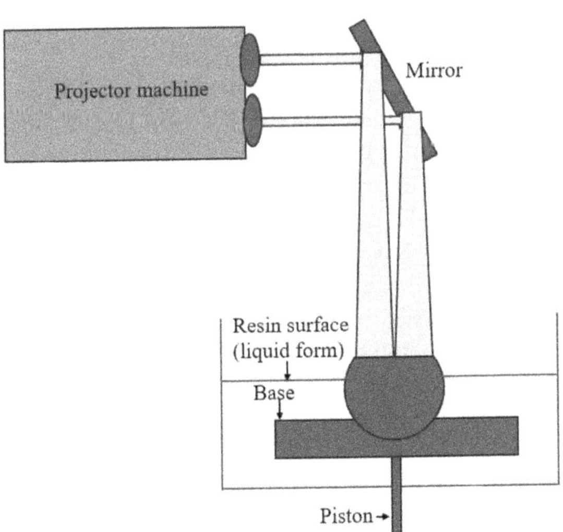

FIGURE 2.4   An outline of the digital light processing system.

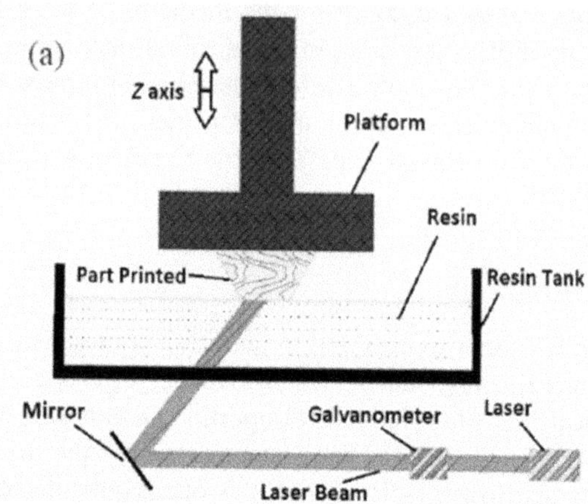

FIGURE 2.5 An outline depicting stereo-lithography. (Adapted and reproduced from Vaz & Kumar (2021).)

One necessary polymerization process is stereolithography. A solid polymer is created by scanning the liquid monomer's surface with an ultraviolet laser beam. The laser's route is controlled by a computer using a sliced CAD model. The liquid monomer tank is controlled by an elevator and moves up and down between each layer of the cured 2D in the plane construction. Consequently, the layer stack produces a three-dimensional polymer structure (Figure 2.5) (Y. Zhang et al., 2018).

The vat polymerization process can be used to modulate the drug-release kinetics in oral tablets and to fabricate more complex structures needed for transdermal administration systems (Mohammed et al., 2020).

2.3.3 BINDER JETTING

Emanuel Sachs developed binder jetting technology at the Massachusetts Institute of Technology, and it was patented in 1993. This 3D printing method is known as powder bed and inkjet head 3D printing. The development process involved using thermal bubble inkjet printheads to spray a gypsum-like powder and a glycerin/water binder. The powdered material is sprayed onto a layer and bound with a binder, often a polymeric liquid, to form the appropriate layer shape using the binder jetting process (Mostafaei et al., 2021). The creation of novel materials for biological and pharmaceutical applications, structurally reliable metallic structures, and the ability to create ceramics and other materials that might be difficult for alternative AM technologies are all made possible by the recent advancements in binder jetting techniques. This method offers a distinctive AM technology platform for the reasonably priced production of valuable goods with intricate geometry (Leary, 2020). An equipment design for binder retrieval is shown in Figure 2.6. The equipment comprises a storage container for powder alongside a construction surface. Initially, a flattening device applies a fine layer of powder to the surface. Then, the substance is locally activated and consolidated as the inkjet nozzle moves back and forth. The platform drops slightly

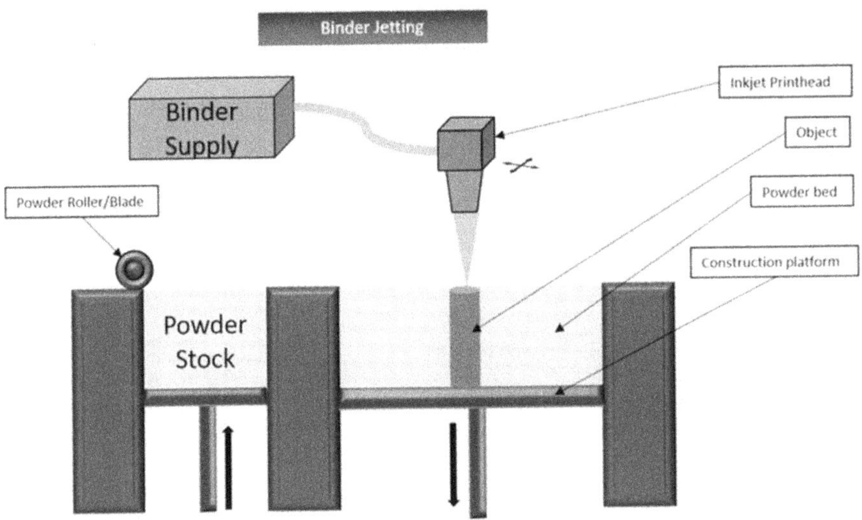

FIGURE 2.6 Diagram illustrating the binder jetting 3D printing process. (Adapted and reproduced from Leary (2020).)

after each powder layer is applied, and the binder injection process is repeated after a new layer is evenly distributed.

Sintering, consolidation, infiltration, and binder burning occur during heat treatment. A solid metallic object must cure for approximately 6–12 hours before undergoing a 24–36 hour heat treatment at a temperature higher than 1000 °C (Y. Zhang et al., 2018).

2.3.4 DEPOSITION OF DIRECT ENERGY

A particular kind of AM called DED entails applying an energy source, such as a laser beam, electron beam, plasma, or electrical arc, to a substrate while delivering feedstock material in the form of wire or powder. In doing so, a little melt pool is formed, enabling the layer-by-layer deposition of material (Svetlizky et al., 2021). Using this technique, high-performance super-alloys have been created. There are several names for direct energy deposition, including direct metal deposition (DMD), electron beam AM, laser solid forming (LSF), laser-engineered net shaping (LENSTM), and direct light fabrication (DLF). DED can be seamlessly integrated with traditional reduction methods to finalize the processing. This technology is frequently applied to titanium, stainless steel, aluminium, and similar metals for aerospace purposes. DED is typically distinguished by its rapidity, with speeds ranging from 0.5 kg/hr for lenses to 10 kg/hr for WAAM and up to 6 m × 1.4 m × 1.4 m for commercial printers, respectively, for substantial work envelopes (Ngo et al., 2018). DED is represented in Figure 2.7. However, additional techniques for supplying inert gases are required. This technology requires a vacuum and would not have significant oxidation difficulties and a laser system. Inert gas is frequently blasted from powder DED machines'

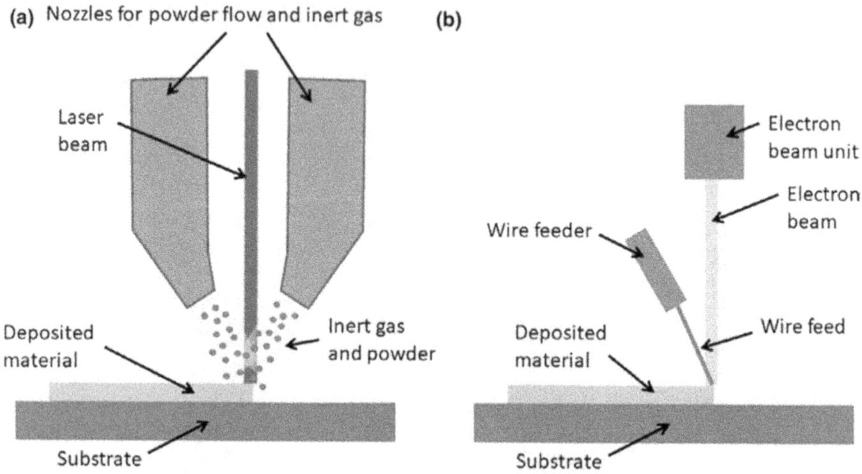

FIGURE 2.7 Schematic representation of the DED system using a laser. (Adapted and reproduced from Srivastava & Rathee (2021).)

nozzles with the powder, coating the molten surface and slowing the oxidation rate. Several nozzles enable the blending of various components to produce functionally graded materials (Sing et al., 2020).

Compared to other processes, this one has a lesser surface quality and accuracy of 0.25 mm and can make simpler pieces. For this reason, this technique is applied to both significant and straightforward components and important repair components. DED provides accurate composition control, controlled microstructure, and high mechanical qualities at a lower manufacturing cost (Ngo et al., 2018).

2.3.5 CHARACTERISTICS OF DIFFERENT AM PROCESSES

AM has completely changed the manufacturing process. It works by layer-by-layer building items in three dimensions, and it differs greatly from conventional sub-tractive manufacturing processes like milling and molding. AM is incredibly versatile due to its wide spectrum of processes, each with distinct qualities and capacities. This review explores the unique qualities of different AM methods. AM processes can be categorized according to the materials used, the methods used, and the intended uses. Grasping the key elements of each AM process, such as stereolithography (SLA), electron beam melting (EBM), selective laser sintering (SLS), and FDM, will help you get a deeper understanding of each one. We learn more about the astounding cross-industry possibilities of this technology. The qualities of various AM processes, such as accuracy, variety of materials, speed, and economy, open up new possibilities for creative applications in fields including aerospace, medicine, and fashion. This investigation lays the groundwork for a more thorough examination of the particulars of each AM approach and its applicability in other fields. The characteristics of different AM processes are shown in Table 2.1 (Salmi, 2021).

TABLE 2.1
Attributes of Several AM Techniques

AM Process	Short Description	Material Form	Plastics	Metals	Ceramics	Trade/Other Names
Powder bed fusion (PBF)	Parts of a powder bed are fused by thermal energy	Powder	+++	+++	+	Selective laser melting, direct metal laser sintering, and selective laser sintering (SLS, DMLS) (SLM)
Material extrusion (MEX)	Substance released by a nozzle	Filament, pellets, paste	+++	++	++	Fused filament fabrication (FFF), fused deposition modelling (FDM)
VAT photo-polymerization (VP)	Light cures liquid photopolymer in a vat	Liquid	+++	+	++	SLA, projection of digital light (DLP)
Material jetting (MJ)	Material droplets are placed in a specific order	Liquid	+++	+	+	PolyJet, NJP
Binder jetting (BJ)	A liquid bonding agent is selectively deposited	Powder	+++	++	+	ColorJet printing and 3D printing (3DP) (CJP)
Sheet lamination (SL)	Sheets of material are bonded	Sheets	++	++	-	Ultrasonic additive manufacturing and laminated object manufacture (LOM) (UAM)
Directed energy deposition (DED)	Concentrated heat energy is used during deposition to combine materials via melting	Powder, wire	-	+++	+	Ultrasonic additive manufacturing and laminated object manufacture (LOM) (UAM)

Note: +++, widely available/many studies exist; ++, available/several studies exist; +, R&D phase/studies exist; -, no studies exist.

2.4   HYBRID AM TECHNIQUE

The hybrid AM technique is used to increase productivity and quality. The possibilities provided by hybrid AM are changing the guidelines for material design and introducing a fresh perspective to the AM technique. Instead of focusing on processing optimization, the aim of most hybrid AM techniques is to increase part performance and quality. A cyclic process chain is characteristic of hybrid AM processes, which are differentiated from post-processing operations that fail to satisfy the fully linked criteria. The term hybrid AM and multilateral printing have been used interchangeably to refer to integrated machinery and combined processes (Sealy et al., 2018).

The following terms are frequently used in the literature to refer to various hybrid techniques (Schuh et al., 2009):

A. Hybrid materials, structures, or functions:
    1. Carbon fiber reinforced aluminum
    2. Hybrid circuits
    3. Composite layer printing
B. Hybrid machines
    1. Milling and turning centers
    2. 3D printers and milling machine
C. Hybrid processes
    1. Laser assisted machining
    2. Vibrated assisted machining
    3. Electrochemical grinding
    4. ECAP and extrusion

New hybrid AM technology is used for the preparation of polymer composite rain-forced with short fibers and nanotubes. The method utilizes thin films, or "buckypapers," that are directly applied to a layer of plastic and embedded into the 3D-printed structure. These films are made on the spot using a suspension (Gackowski et al., 2022). Hybrid AM is a technique that combines material jetting and material extrusion AM processes. In addition to printing non-Newtonian viscous silicone, this process speeds up fabrication by a factor of 10 to 20 when compared to standard extrusion techniques (Liravi & Toyserkani, 2018).

2.5   EXTENDED APPLICATIONS IN THE PHARMACEUTICAL INDUSTRY

Beyond conventional manufacturing procedures, AM, commonly referred to as 3D printing, is finding surprising popularity in the pharmaceutical sector. The following are a few extended applications of AM in the pharmaceutical industry:

- Personalized medicine: AM makes it possible to produce drugs that are specifically customized to meet the needs of each patient. This is beneficial for patients, such as children, the elderly, or those who have swallowing issues for whom regular dosage forms are inappropriate. The researchers examine the use of AM in pediatric medicine, where precise and individualized dosing is frequently crucial, in one of the case studies. Children may not always benefit from traditional medications because of differences in height, weight, and ability to swallow. The study shows that it is possible to manufacture individualized medicine dosage forms for pediatric patients using 3D printing technology. They also point out that 3D printing makes it possible to precisely manage dosage dimensions and can add flavor- masking chemicals to improve medicine adaptability and make it easier for children to use. The customized doses that met each patient's unique needs were generated with success. The study demonstrates how personalized medicine, made possible by AM, can transform the pharmaceutical business by enhancing medication adherence and therapeutic outcomes, particularly for vulnerable groups such as pediatric patients. This case study highlights the potential for AM to revolutionize healthcare, especially in the area of personalized medicine. It also provides an insight into the pharmaceutical industry's future, wherein each treatment can be specially customized to meet the demands of the individual patients.

- Complex dosage forms: AM enables the development of complex, multi-layered dosage forms that can deliver mixtures of active pharmaceutical ingredients in a single tablet or capsule or release medications at varying rates. This creates the path for medication delivery methods that work better. The objective of this case study is to produce a 3D-printed polypill or printlet that may be used to fulfil the intricate drug regimens that older people frequently need. Polypills simplify administration and increase adherence by combining several medications into a single dosage form. The article describes how to develop polypills using AM that release variable amounts of multiple APIs based on the therapeutic needs of individual medications. This is made possible by carefully regulating the 3D-printed tablets geometry and porosity. The case study shows how complicated dosage forms that are customized to each patient's need can be developed with 3D printing technology. This case study demonstrates the potential of AM to improve patient adherence and in the instance of elderly individuals, the management of numerous chronic illnesses by providing a solution for polymerization in a single, convenient dosage form. The emergence of 3D-printed polypills serves as an example of how AM can revolutionize the pharmaceutical sector by producing complex dosage forms that more effectively meet the various therapeutic needs of patients. This case study provides an intriguing look into the pharmaceutical industry's future, where drugs are custom-made to meet each patient's demands.

- Modified release system: the development of a modified release system is made possible by the exact control over the geometry and porosity of 3D-printed tablets. This can help to increase patient compliance for medications that need to be released gradually or continuously. This case study explores the development of 3D-printed tablets with customized release profiles for several medications. A key pharmacological technique for managing a drug's release rate and improving both patient adherence and efficacy is modified release. Here, controlled medication release is made possible by the distinctive geometries and porosities that are produced via AM. The research shows how tablets with precise engineering can release different medications in different ways;

certain agents release instantly, while others release over time. When handling complicated drug regimens or ailments that require time-specific dosage, this method is invaluable. The researchers demonstrated how modified release systems can be made using 3D printing technology, giving medical practitioners the ability to customize medication administration to meet the needs of each patient. These tablets are particularly helpful for treating long-term illnesses and improving outcomes from therapy. This case study highlights how AM has the ability to revolutionize the pharmaceutical sector by creating complicated dosage forms that have a substantial influence on patient care and treatment efficacy, particularly when several medications require customized release methods.

- Taste-masking: pharmaceuticals with better taste-masking qualities can be produced by AM, which will make prescriptions more appealing to patients, particularly those who are elderly or pediatric. The case study investigates how AM might disguise flavor, with a particular emphasis on orally disintegrating tablets (ODTs). ODTs are an ideal option for individuals who have trouble swallowing conventional pills because of their quick disintegration in the mouth. This case study shows how AM can revolutionize pharmaceutical formulation by providing novel techniques to improve patient pleasure and compliance by getting rid of some drugs' disagreeable tastes. In order to produce ODTs that conceal the bitter taste of active pharmaceutical ingredients, the study makes use of 3D printing technology. The researchers successfully eliminated the bitter taste from the 3D-printed tablets by carefully adding flavor-masking chemicals within the tablets.

- Clinical trials and research: in order to support the development of innovative medication formulations and therapies, AM is crucial in the development of modified dosage forms and drug-delivery devices for clinical trials and research. The use of 3D printing to produce exploratory dosage forms for clinical trials in the realm of pharmaceutical research is examined in this case study. Development of modified release dosage form is the main objective, in which two isomers of amino salicylates, 5-aminosalicylic acid and 4-aminosalicylic acid are model medications used to treat inflammatory bowel disease (IBD). In order to assess the pharmacokinetics and pharmacodynamics of novel drug formulations intended for the treatment of IBD, clinical trials including these medications are essential. The work demonstrates how precise fabrication of dosage forms with particular release profiles is made possible by 3D printing technology. To regulate the rate at which the medication is given, tablets with specific porosities and geometries should be produced. Pharmaceutical researchers can test medication delivery scenarios in clinical trial setting thanks to this degree of customization.

- Pharmaceutical prototyping: AM is used by pharmaceutical industries to quickly prototype new medication compositions. This lowers expenses and speeds up the development process. This case study investigates the quick creation of customized medicine dosage forms using 3D printing technology. This study's main focus is on developing customized drugs that are catered to each patient's need specifically. This is a topic that is becoming more and more important in contemporary healthcare to improve patient adherence and treatment outcomes. It also highlights how additive printing has the ability to revolutionize pharmaceutical prototypes. It lowers development costs, speeds up the process of creating novel medication formulations, and makes it possible to evaluate various drug-delivery scenarios. Because 3D printing is flexible, researchers can quickly produce prototype dosage forms and modify them to meet the needs of individual patients. Employing 3D printing technology, the researchers created and produced customized tablets with exact dosages and geometries suited to each patients unique needs. Through modifying characteristics such as tablet dimensions, shape and drug concentration, the research effectively showcased 3D printing's capacity to generate a wide range of modified dosage forms quickly.

- Dose optimization: drug dosages with accurate dimensions and concentration can be 3D printed, allowing patients to receive precisely optimized amounts based on their needs. The development of customized pediatric drugs is the main objective of this case study, with a focus on dose optimization. Due to differences in age, weight and developmental stages, pediatric patients frequently present special obstacles. For this reason, it is crucial to deliver exact medication dosages customized for each kids. The researchers produced customized pediatric prescriptions by using 3D printing technology. With this method, dosage measurements and drug concentration could be precisely controlled, guaranteeing that every child was given the right amount. To further improve dose optimization, researchers might fine-tune the medication release by modifying the geometry and porosity of the 3D-printed tablets.

These extended applications of AM in the pharmaceutical industry reshape drug development, manufacturing, and delivery. 3D printing is vital in improving patient outcomes and advancing pharmaceutical research and development by offering greater precision, personalization, and versatility.

2.6 ADVANTAGES OF AM

AM has several advantages such as below (Attaran, 2017). AM makes it possible for design flexibility, which is frequently impractical or prohibitively expensive to produce using conventional production methods. This creative freedom is beneficial for producing highly customized or specialized products (Mehrpouya et al., 2021). One significant technology for quick prototyping is AM. It makes it possible to produce prototypes and revisions quickly and affordably, cutting the time needed from design to testing and final product development (Campbell et al., 2012). Much material waste is frequently produced when extra material is removed during traditional subtractive manufacturing processes. On the other hand, because AM is an additive process, there is very little material waste (Devi et al., 2021). Parts with complex, bespoke, or detailed geometries may be more economically viable to produce via AM. Changing tools and going through several phases in traditional manufacturing methods may be necessary, which can be costly and time-consuming (Divakaran et al., 2022). AM works well for producing things that can be personalized and customized. This is especially useful in healthcare, where one may create prosthetics, implants, and other medical devices specifically suited to each patient's anatomy (Rommel & Fischer, 2013). Just-in-time or on-demand production is made possible by AM, which eliminates the need for large stocks. This may result in financial savings, cheaper storage expenses, and simpler supply chains (Rommel & Fischer, 2013). Manufacturing lead times are shortened when components and finished goods may be produced swiftly and locally. This is especially helpful for sectors where quick response times are essential (Kulkarni et al., 2021). Lattices and honeycomb patterns are examples of complex internal structures that can be created by AM and used to reduce weight without sacrificing structural integrity (Vranić et al., 2017). AM has the potential to be a more sustainable manufacturing technique since it reduces material waste and permits local production. Furthermore, using recyclable and biobased products adds even more to sustainability (Malshe et al., 2015).Various materials, including metals, ceramics, composites, and sophisticated polymers, can be used in AM. This adaptability makes it possible to produce pieces with specific material characteristics (Ma et al., 2021). AM makes it affordable to produce small quantities of parts. Prototypes, limited-edition goods, and niche markets will significantly benefit from this (Chaudhuri et al., 2021). Expensive mold dies and tooling are frequently needed in traditional manufacturing. These tooling expenditures are eliminated or decreased with AM (Attaran, 2017). By storing, retrieving, and duplicating digital data of components and goods as needed, physical warehouses are not required, and storage expenses are decreased (Devi et al., 2021; Lakshmanan et al., 2023). Even though AM has many benefits, it is vital to remember that it also has drawbacks and difficulties. These include material restrictions, post-processing needs, and specific speed and part size limitations. The particular needs and limitations of the intended application should guide the production method selection.

2.7 LIMITATIONS OF AM

AM has much potential, it has drawbacks and difficulties for the pharmaceutical sector (Araújo et al., 2021). A significant obstacle to AM in the pharmaceutical sector is the ever-changing and intricate regulatory environment. One of the biggest challenges is ensuring that 3D-printed medications adhere to strict regulatory standards, such as good manufacturing practices (GMP) (Chen et al., 2022). Regulatory agencies such as the FDA are still developing clear guidelines for the use of AM in the pharmaceutical industry (Tan & Choong, 2021). It may be challenging to ensure standardized production and consistent quality in AM. Because changes in 3D printing techniques, materials, and equipment may cause batch-to-batch variability in pharmaceutical goods, quality control is crucial (Mançanares et al., 2015). Finding suitable materials that are safe for human consumption and operate with the technology is one of the main issues in 3D printing. Ensuring the stability, purity, and biocompatibility of 3D-printed materials is crucial (Ngo et al., 2018). Assuring precise and consistent dosing for 3D-printed pharmaceuticals might be difficult. Precise calibration during the printing process is necessary due to the precise dose and medicine-release features (Trivedi et al., 2018). A conversion of small-scale 3D printing to large-scale manufacturing is also a challenge in the AM process. Another major challenge is to ensure the efficiency and scalability by considering the quality and legal compliance (Pignatelli & Percoco, 2022). Because digital design and 3D printing are so simple, issues with intellectual property, counterfeiting, and the unlicensed production of patented pharmaceuticals may come up (Kietzmann et al., 2015). To meet quality and safety standards, 3D-printed medications frequently must go through post-processing stages like coating, polishing, or machining. These extra measures may be expensive and time-consuming (Gutowski et al., 2017). Simple, small-molecule medications work better in 3D printing than complex biologics or combinations of multiple pharmaceuticals. Biologic formulation and 3D printing present a more difficult task (Borandeh et al., 2021). Not all medication types or dosage forms are appropriate candidates for AM. Compared to liquid or injectable formulations, solid oral dosage forms like tablets and capsules are more suitable for 3D printing (Trivedi et al., 2018). Although the concept of personalized medicine is intriguing, it presents difficulties for regulatory compliance, validation, and scaling up the manufacturing of customized pharmaceutical goods. Whereas AM presents intriguing opportunities for the pharmaceutical sector, the technology must overcome a number of regulatory, quality control, material selection, dosage precision, and scalability issues. To fully utilize 3D printing in medication production, pharmaceutical companies, government agencies, and technology suppliers must continue their research, development, and cooperation to overcome these obstacles (Wilts et al., 2019).

2.8 INDUSTRIAL SCALE, CURRENT PROGRESS AND CHALLENGES

2.8.1 Industrial Scale of AM

3D printing has grown significantly in several sectors, including aerospace, automotive, and healthcare. Its integration makes large-scale manufacture of complicated components possible, particularly in industries where complex structures and bespoke designs are beneficial. Moreover, AM has been essential in cutting lead times, enabling just-in-time production, and optimizing supply chains. The industrial uses of AM have developed due to the availability of various materials, such as metals, ceramics, polymers, and composites. The increasing demand for AM technologies and the significant decline in the cost of commercial 3D printers, materials, and accessories particularly in the healthcare industry are credited with the technologies' broad acceptance. From roughly $0.4 billion in 1996 to $1.4 billion in 2010, the global AM market experienced significant expansion. According to predictions, the market worth increased to $9 billion by 2019 and is expected to reach around $35 billion by 2024. AM sales show comparable growth trends, rising from over $71 million in 2001 to roughly $266 million in 2010, and are predicted to reach $8 billion by 2025. Since 2010, several factors have contributed to AM's quick rise. The widespread acceptance of AM technologies among academics, practitioners, and students has been made possible by affordable and easily accessible technology. Interest in AM has also increased due to the creation of efficient and user-friendly software and mobile applications for modeling and executing complex designs. By allowing users to create virtual 3D components, these tools encourage people to create physical goods. The extensive acceptance of AM has also been aided by its incorporation into curricula at universities and schools across the globe (Mohammed et al., 2020).

2.8.2 Current Progress in AM

AM has advanced significantly in recent years, particularly with regard to the 3D printing of metal. This has had a significant impact on the automotive and aerospace industries and made it possible to use materials like titanium and aluminum. On the other side, bioprinting has greatly advanced tissue engineering and regenerative medicine, and it has brought about a new age in healthcare by making it possible to 3D print functional organs and tissues. More and more design tools and software are making it easier to create intricate 3D-printed items. Furthermore, productivity is raised by hybrid manufacturing, which combines traditional procedures with AM. Particularly in the area of metal 3D printing, or AM, has advanced significantly in recent years. As a result, a wider variety of materials, such as titanium and aluminum, may now be used, revolutionizing sectors like automotive and aerospace. Through the use of 3D printing, bioprinting has made it possible to create functional organs and tissues, opening up new possibilities in the fields of tissue engineering and regenerative medicine. The process of creating complex 3D-printed parts is getting easier with every update to software and design tools. To further push the limits of what is feasible in manufacturing, hybrid manufacturing, which blends AM with conventional techniques is becoming more and more popular. It can be difficult to employ pharmaceutical-grade materials in SLS processes due to the risk of restricted laser energy absorption and thermal damage from high energy input. Increasing the energy transmission time by speeding up the laser or adding pharmaceutical excipients that are absorbent enough at the laser source's wavelength are two other ways to deal with this. Including a "design space" of process parameters becomes essential in order to account for heat deterioration, new materials used in 3D printing, and any changes to the processing environment (J. Zhang et al., 2018).

2.8.3 Challenges of AM

AM faces several significant obstacles despite its remarkable progress. One major challenge is ensuring law compliance, particularly in the aerospace and healthcare industries. It is essential to maintain strict quality control because processes can vary greatly. Continuous work is necessary to develop new materials requiring more advanced and specialized materials. Standardization becomes essential to ensure interoperability and quality standards between various AM systems. The post-processing stage may incur high costs and take an extended period. With 3D printing technology becoming more widely available, it is imperative to address issues like cost effectiveness, intellectual property, and the possibility of counterfeiting. In conclusion, even though AM has advanced significantly across industries and offers advantages like customized design, shorter lead times, and a variety of material options, obstacles in the areas of regulatory compliance, quality control, material development, and cost-effectiveness must be overcome if AM is to realize its transformative potential in the industrial landscape fully. To fully realize the potential of AM, several obstacles must be overcome (Satair, 2020, https://blog.satair.com/five-challenges-additive-manufacturing; Raja & John Rajan, 2023).

2.9 CONCLUDING REMARK

A disruptive environment with great promise for efficiency and innovation is revealed by investigating AM methods and their expanded applications in the pharmaceutical industry. Drug discovery and production have advanced to previously unheard-of levels thanks to 3D printing technologies, opening the door to customized treatment plans, intricate dosage forms, and improved drug delivery systems. The ability to produce drugs in a different way and overcome conventional limitations is made possible by the variety of AM, which includes processes like powder bed fusion and hot-melt extrusion. This study's result highlights the enormous potential of AM to transform the pharmaceutical industry and the creation of new drugs. AM is positioned as a cornerstone for the future of pharmaceuticals, opening the door for more effective, patient-centric, and sustainable methods to drug design and manufacture thanks to the synergistic interaction of technology, science, and industry expertise.

ACKNOWLEDGMENTS

The authors are thankful to St. John Institute of Pharmacy and Research, Palghar, Maharashtra for the technical support for writing the chapter.

REFERENCES

Alghamdi, S., John, S., Roy Choudhury, N., & Dutta, N. (2021). Additive manufacturing of polymer materials: Progress, promise and challenges. *Polymers*, 13(5), 753. https://doi.org/10.3390/polym13050753

Araújo, N., Pacheco, V., & Costa, L. (2021). Smart additive manufacturing: The path to the digital value chain. *Technologies*, 9(4), 88.

Attaran, M. (2017). The rise of 3-D printing: The advantages of additive manufacturing over traditional manufacturing. *Business Horizons*, 60(5), 677–688.

Beck, R. C. R., Chaves, P. S., Goyanes, A., Vukosavljevic, B., Buanz, A., Windbergs, M., Basit, A. W., & Gaisford, S. (2017). 3D printed tablets loaded with polymeric nanocapsules: An innovative approach to produce customized drug delivery systems. *International Journal of Pharmaceutics*, 528(1), 268–279. https://doi.org/10.1016/j.ijpharm.2017.05.074

Boetker, J., Water, J. J., Aho, J., Arnfast, L., Bohr, A., & Rantanen, J. (2016). Modifying release characteristics from 3D printed drug-eluting products. *European Journal of Pharmaceutical Sciences*, 90, 47–52. https://doi.org/10.1016/j.ejps.2016.03.013

Borandeh, S., van Bochove, B., Teotia, A., & Seppälä, J. (2021). Polymeric drug delivery systems by additive manufacturing. *Advanced Drug Delivery Reviews*, 173, 349–373.

Campbell, I., Bourell, D., & Gibson, I. (2012). Additive manufacturing: Rapid prototyping comes of age. *Rapid Prototyping Journal*, 18(4), 255–258.

Chaudhuri, A., Gerlich, H. A., Jayaram, J., Ghadge, A., Shack, J., Brix, B. H., Hoffbeck, L. H., & Ulriksen, N. (2021). Selecting spare parts suitable for additive manufacturing: a design science approach. *Production Planning & Control*, 32(8), 670–687.

Chen, Z., Han, C., Gao, M., Kandukuri, S. Y., & Zhou, K. (2022). A review on qualification and certification for metal additive manufacturing. *Virtual and Physical Prototyping, 17*(2), 382–405.

Devi, A., Mathiyazhagan, K., & Kumar, H. (2021). Additive manufacturing in supply chain management: A systematic review. *Advances in Manufacturing and Industrial Engineering: Select Proceedings of ICAPIE 2019*, Delhi, India, December 20–21, 2019, 455–464.

Divakaran, N., Das, J. P., Pv, A. K., Mohanty, S., Ramadoss, A., & Nayak, S. K. (2022). Comprehensive review on various additive manufacturing techniques and its implementation in electronic devices. *Journal of Manufacturing Systems, 62*, 477–502.

Gackowski, B. M., Phua, H., Sharma, M., & Idapalapati, S. (2022). Hybrid additive manufacturing of polymer composites reinforced with buckypapers and short carbon fibres. *Composites Part A: Applied Science and Manufacturing, 154*, 106794. https://doi.org/10.1016/j.compositesa.2021.106794

Guo, N., & Leu, M. C. (2013). Additive manufacturing: technology, applications and research needs. *Frontiers of Mechanical Engineering, 8*(3), 215–243. https://doi.org/10.1007/s11465-013-0248-8

Gutowski, T., Jiang, S., Cooper, D., Corman, G., Hausmann, M., Manson, J. A., Schudeleit, T., Wegener, K., Sabelle, M., & Ramos-Grez, J. (2017). Note on the rate and energy efficiency limits for additive manufacturing. *Journal of Industrial Ecology, 21*(S1), S69–S79.

Herderick, E. D. (2015). Progress in additive manufacturing. *JOM, 67*(3), 580–581.

Höller, C., Karanovic, S., Wiltsche, M., & Klug, A. (2022). Value creation through insourcing – Additive manufacturing as efficient in-house production technology. *Procedia CIRP, 107*, 1391–1396. https://doi.org/10.1016/j.procir.2022.05.163

Satair (2020). Five challenges of additive manufacturing in the aviation industry Technology, Industry trends, Mar 18. https://blog.satair.com/five-challenges-additive-manufacturing.

Jadhav, A., & Jadhav, V. S. (2022). A review on 3D printing: An additive manufacturing technology. *Materials Today: Proceedings, 62*, 2094–2099. https://doi.org/10.1016/j.matpr.2022.02.558

Jamróz, W., Kurek, M., Łyszczarz, E., Szafraniec, J., Knapik-Kowalczuk, J., Syrek, K., Paluch, M., & Jachowicz, R. (2017). 3D printed orodispersible films with Aripiprazole. *International Journal of Pharmaceutics, 533*(2), 413–420. https://doi.org/10.1016/j.ijpharm.2017.05.052

Khaled, S. A., Burley, J. C., Alexander, M. R., & Roberts, C. J. (2014). Desktop 3D printing of controlled release pharmaceutical bilayer tablets. *International Journal of Pharmaceutics, 461*(1), 105–111. https://doi.org/10.1016/j.ijpharm.2013.11.021

Khaled, S. A., Burley, J. C., Alexander, M. R., Yang, J., & Roberts, C. J. (2015). 3D printing of five-in-one dose combination polypill with defined immediate and sustained release profiles. *Journal of Controlled Release, 217*, 308–314. https://doi.org/10.1016/j.jconrel.2015.09.028

Kietzmann, J., Pitt, L., & Berthon, P. (2015). Disruptions, decisions, and destinations: Enter the age of 3-D printing and additive manufacturing. *Business Horizons, 58*(2), 209–215.

Kulkarni, P., Kumar, A., Chate, G., & Dandannavar, P. (2021). Elements of additive manufacturing technology adoption in small-and medium-sized companies. *Innovation & Management Review, 18*(4), 400–416.

Lakshmanan, R., Nyamekye, P., Virolainen, V.-M., & Piili, H. (2023). The convergence of lean management and additive manufacturing: Case of manufacturing industries. *Cleaner Engineering and Technology, 13*(2), 100620.

Leary, M. (2020). Chapter 13 – Binder jetting. In M. Leary (Ed.), *Design for Additive Manufacturing* (pp. 335–339). Elsevier. https://doi.org/10.1016/B978-0-12-816 721-2.00013-0

Li, Q., Wen, H., Jia, D., Guan, X., Pan, H., Yang, Y., Yu, S., Zhu, Z., Xiang, R., & Pan, W. (2017). Preparation and investigation of controlled-release glipizide novel oral device with three-dimensional printing. *International Journal of Pharmaceutics*, *525*(1), 5–11. https://doi.org/10.1016/j.ijpharm.2017.03.066

Lim, S. H., Kathuria, H., Tan, J. J. Y., & Kang, L. (2018). 3D printed drug delivery and testing systems – a passing fad or the future? *Advanced Drug Delivery Reviews*, *132*, 139–168. https://doi.org/10.1016/j.addr.2018.05.006

Liravi, F., & Toyserkani, E. (2018). A hybrid additive manufacturing method for the fabrication of silicone bio-structures: 3D printing optimization and surface characterization. *Materials & Design*, *138*, 46–61. https://doi.org/10.1016/j.matdes.2017.10.051

Lu, B., Li, D., & Tian, X. (2015). Development trends in additive manufacturing and 3D printing. *Engineering*, *1*(1), 085–089. https://doi.org/10.15302/J-ENG-2015012

Lu, X., Lee, Y., Yang, S., Hao, Y., Evans, J. R. G., & Parini, C. G. (2010). Solvent-based paste extrusion solid freeforming. *Journal of the European Ceramic Society*, *30*(1), 1–10. https://doi.org/10.1016/j.jeurceramsoc.2009.07.019

Ma, J., Li, Z., Zhao, Z.-L., & Xie, Y. M. (2021). Creating novel furniture through topology optimization and advanced manufacturing. *Rapid Prototyping Journal*, *27*(9), 1749–1758.

Malshe, H., Nagarajan, H., Pan, Y., & Haapala, K. (2015). *Profile of sustainability in additive manufacturing and environmental assessment of a novel stereolithography process*. ASME 2015 International Manufacturing Science and Engineering Conference, June 8–12, 2015, Charlotte, North Carolina, USA, Conference Sponsors: Manufacturing Engineering Division. Volume 2: Materials; Biomanufacturing; Properties, Applications and Systems; Sustainable Manufacturing. ISBN: 978-0-7918-5683-3

Mançanares, C. G., de Senzi Zancul, E., & Miguel, P. A. C. (2015). Sustainable manufacturing strategies: a literature review on additive manufacturing approach. *Product: Management and Development*, *13*(1), 47–56.

Mehrpouya, M., Vosooghnia, A., Dehghanghadikolaei, A., & Fotovvati, B. (2021). The benefits of additive manufacturing for sustainable design and production. In *Sustainable Manufacturing* (pp. 29–59). Elsevier.

Mohammed, A., Elshaer, A., Sareh, P., Elsayed, M., & Hassanin, H. (2020). Additive manufacturing technologies for drug delivery applications. *International Journal of Pharmaceutics*, *580*, 119245. https://doi.org/10.1016/j.ijpharm.2020.119245

Mostafaei, A., Elliott, A. M., Barnes, J. E., Li, F., Tan, W., Cramer, C. L., Nandwana, P., & Chmielus, M. (2021). Binder jet 3D printing – Process parameters, materials, properties, modeling, and challenges. *Progress in Materials Science*, *119*, 100707. https://doi.org/ 10.1016/j.pmatsci.2020.100707

Mwema, F. M., & Akinlabi, E. T. (2020). Basics of fused deposition modelling (FDM). In F. M. Mwema & E. T. Akinlabi (Eds.), *Fused Deposition Modeling: Strategies for Quality Enhancement* (pp. 1–15). Springer International. https://doi.org/10.1007/978-3-030-48259-6_1

Ngo, T. D., Kashani, A., Imbalzano, G., Nguyen, K. T. Q., & Hui, D. (2018). Additive manufacturing (3D printing): A review of materials, methods, applications and challenges. *Composites Part B: Engineering*, *143*, 172–196.

Panraksa, P., Udomsom, S., Rachtanapun, P., Chittasupho, C., Ruksiriwanich, W., & Jantrawut, P. (2020). Hydroxypropyl methylcellulose E15: A hydrophilic polymer for fabrication of orodispersible film using syringe extrusion 3D printer. *Polymers*, *12*: 2666. https://doi. org/10.3390/polym12112666

Pignatelli, F., & Percoco, G. (2022). An application-and market-oriented review on large format additive manufacturing, focusing on polymer pellet-based 3D printing. *Progress in Additive Manufacturing, 7*(6), 1363–1377.

Prashanth, K. G., & Wang, Z. (2020). Additive manufacturing: Alloy design and process innovations. *Materials, 13*(3), 542.

Rahman, Z., Barakh Ali, S. F., Ozkan, T., Charoo, N. A., Reddy, I. K., & Khan, M. A. (2018). Additive manufacturing with 3D printing: Progress from bench to bedside. *AAPS Journal, 20*(6), 101. https://doi.org/10.1208/s12248-018-0225-6

Raja, S., & John Rajan, A. (2023). Challenges and opportunities in additive manufacturing polymer technology: A review based on optimization perspective. *Advances in Polymer Technology, 2023,* 8639185. https://doi.org/10.1155/2023/8639185

Rommel, S., & Fischer, A. (2013). Additive manufacturing – A growing possibility to lighten the burden of spare parts supply. In G. L. Kovács & Kochan, D. (Eds), Digital Product and Process Development Systems. NEW PROLAMAT 2013. IFIP Advances in Information and Communication Technology, vol 411. Springer, Berlin, Heidelberg. https://doi.org/10.1007/978-3-642-41329-2_13

Sai Saran, O., Prudhvidhar Reddy, A., Chaturya, L., & Pavan Kumar, M. (2022). 3D printing of composite materials: A short review. *Materials Today: Proceedings, 64,* 615–619. https://doi.org/10.1016/j.matpr.2022.05.144

Salmi, M. (2021). Additive manufacturing processes in medical applications. *Materials (Basel, Switzerland), 14*(1). https://doi.org/10.3390/ma14010191

Schuh, G., Kreysa, J., & Orilski, S. (2009). Roadmap "Hybride Produktion": Wie 1+1=3-Effekte in der Produktion maximiert werden können. *Fraunhofer IPT, 104*(5). https://doi.org/10.3139/104.110072

Sealy, M. P., Madireddy, G., Williams, R. E., Rao, P., & Toursangsaraki, M. (2018). Hybrid processes in additive manufacturing. *Journal of Manufacturing Science and Engineering, 140*(6). https://doi.org/10.1115/1.4038644

Sen, K., West, T. G., & Chaudhuri, B. (2023). History and present scenario of additive manufacturing in pharmaceuticals. In S. Banerjee (Ed.), *Additive Manufacturing in Pharmaceuticals* (pp. 1–44). Springer Nature Singapore. https://doi.org/10.1007/978-981-99-2404-2_1

Sing, S. L., Tey, C. F., Tan, J. H. K., Huang, S., & Yeong, W. Y. (2020). 2–3D printing of metals in rapid prototyping of biomaterials: Techniques in additive manufacturing. In R. Narayan (Ed.), *Rapid Prototyping of Biomaterials* (Second Edition) (pp. 17–40). Woodhead Publishing. https://doi.org/10.1016/B978-0-08-102663-2.00002-2

Srivastava, M., & Rathee, S. (2021). Additive manufacturing: recent trends, applications and future outlooks. *Progress in Additive Manufacturing, 7,* 261–287. https://doi.org/10.1007/s40964-021-00229-8

Svetlizky, D., Das, M., Zheng, B., Vyatskikh, A. L., Bose, S., Bandyopadhyay, A., Schoenung, J. M., Lavernia, E. J., & Eliaz, N. (2021). Directed energy deposition (DED) additive manufacturing: Physical characteristics, defects, challenges and applications. *Materials Today, 49,* 271–295. https://doi.org/10.1016/j.mattod.2021.03.020

Tan, D., Nokhodchi, A., & Maniruzzaman, M. (2019). 3D and 4D printing technologies: Innovative process engineering and smart additive manufacturing. In Mohammed Maniruzzaman (ed), *3D and 4D Printing in Biomedical Applications* (pp. 25–52). Wiley. https://doi.org/10.1002/9783527813704.ch2

Tan, H. W., & Choong, Y. Y. C. (2021). Additive manufacturing in COVID-19: recognising the challenges and driving for assurance. *Virtual and Physical Prototyping, 16*(4), 498–503.

Trivedi, M., Jee, J., Silva, S., Blomgren, C., Pontinha, V. M., Dixon, D. L., Van Tassel, B., Bortner, M. J., Williams, C., & Gilmer, E. (2018). Additive manufacturing of pharmaceuticals for precision medicine applications: A review of the promises and perils in implementation. *Additive Manufacturing*, *23*, 319–328.

Vaz, V. M., & Kumar, L. (2021). 3D printing as a promising tool in personalized medicine. *AAPS PharmSciTech*, *22*(1), 49. https://doi.org/10.1208/s12249-020-01905-8

Vranić, A., Bogojevic, N., Ćirić Kostić, S., Croccolo, D., & Olmi, G. (2017). Advantages and drawbacks of additive manufacturing. *IMK-14 - Istraživanje i razvoj*, *23*(2), 57–62. DOI: 10.5937/IMK1702057V

Weisman, J. A., Ballard, D. H., Jammalamadaka, U., Tappa, K., Sumerel, J., D'Agostino, H. B., Mills, D. K., & Woodard, P. K. (2019). 3D printed antibiotic and chemotherapeutic eluting catheters for potential use in interventional radiology: In vitro proof of concept study. *Academic Radiology*, *26*(2), 270–274. https://doi.org/10.1016/j.acra.2018.03.022

Wilts, E. M., Ma, D., Bai, Y., Williams, C. B., & Long, T. E. (2019). Comparison of linear and 4-arm star poly (vinyl pyrrolidone) for aqueous binder jetting additive manufacturing of personalized dosage tablets. *ACS Applied Materials & Interfaces*, *11*(27), 23938–23947.

Zhang, J., Feng, X., Patil, H., Tiwari, R. V., & Repka, M. A. (2017). Coupling 3D printing with hot-melt extrusion to produce controlled-release tablets. *International Journal of Pharmaceutics*, *519*(1), 186–197. https://doi.org/10.1016/j.ijpharm.2016.12.049

Zhang, J., Hu, Q., Wang, S., Tao, J., & Gou, M. (2020). Digital light processing based three-dimensional printing for medical applications. *International Journal of Bioprinting*, *6*(1), 242. https://doi.org/10.18063/ijb.v6i1.242

Zhang, J., Vo, A. Q., Feng, X., Bandari, S., & Repka, M. A. (2018). Pharmaceutical additive manufacturing: A novel tool for complex and personalized drug delivery systems. *AAPS PharmSciTech*, *19*(8), 3388–3402. https://doi.org/10.1208/s12249-018-1097-x

Zhang, Y., Jarosinski, W., Jung, Y.-G., & Zhang, J. (2018). 2 – Additive manufacturing processes and equipment. In J. Zhang & Y.-G. Jung (Eds.), *Additive Manufacturing* (pp. 39–51). Butterworth-Heinemann. https://doi.org/10.1016/B978-0-12-812155-9.00002-5

Section II

Quality Characteristics' Challenge in 3D Printing of Pharmaceutical Products

3 Navigating the Terrain of 3DP for Pharmaceutical Products
Quality Conundrums and Solutions

Kanaka Durga Devi Nelluri, Sk. Abdul Rahaman, Vijaya Lakshmi Marella, Kakani Anil Kumar, and Kondabrolu Naga Bhargavi

3.1 INTRODUCTION

With the arrival of three-dimensional printing (3DP) technology, the pharmaceutical production industry has undergone tremendous change. This novel approach has transformed conventional medication manufacturing by enabling the development of detailed and personalized dosage forms, as well as highly accurate and flexible medical equipment (Awad *et al.*, 2018). As the potential for 3DP to revolutionize the pharmaceutical sector grows, new opportunities and obstacles must be thoroughly investigated (Alhnan *et al.*, 2016). The discussion, titled "Navigating the Terrain of 3DP for Pharmaceutical Products: Quality Conundrums and Solutions," focuses on the delicate connection between the cutting-edge world of 3DP and the strict needs of pharmaceutical quality assurance. As this field evolves, it is critical to gain a better knowledge of the issues it brings and the solutions it necessitates (Alhnan *et al.*, 2016). The goal of this investigation is not only to shed light on existing obstacles, but also to find novel solutions to overcome them, ensuring the quality and effectiveness of pharmaceutical goods created with 3DP. In this context, the introduction serves as a jumping-off point for a thorough examination of the landscape. It sets the scene for an investigation of the complications that lie ahead by discussing the relevance of 3DP's impact on pharmaceuticals. The introduction emphasizes 3DP's critical role in revolutionizing the pharmaceutical sector, as well as how it has overcome traditional manufacturing limits. Yet it recognizes the complications that come with this technological transformation, particularly in terms of preserving the high quality, safety, and effectiveness that pharmaceutical products demand.

This discussion will go into the numerous elements of this topic in the next parts, including the challenges that occur in assuring the quality of 3D-printed medications.

This inquiry intends to not only identify the impediments but also propose proactive solutions that can lead the pharmaceutical sector in exploiting the full potential of 3DP through a complete investigation of these quality conundrums (Basit *et al.*, 2022; Sen *et al.*, 2021). Each component, from material selection and process validation to testing procedures and regulatory compliance, is a vital jigsaw piece that must be solved in order to effectively utilize the transformative power of 3DP in pharmaceuticals (Ho *et al.*, 2020; Mostafaei *et al.*, 2021; Sankar *et al.*, 2017).

3.2 THE PROMISE AND PERILS OF 3DP IN PHARMACEUTICALS

By applying layers one at a time, 3DP, sometimes referred to as additive manufacturing, enables the accurate creation of complex shapes (Gupta *et al.*, 2021; Goyanes *et al.*, 2017). This technology has the ability to completely alter drug delivery and formulation in the pharmaceutical sector. A few of the promises that 3DP holds include personalized medicines, complex drug-release patterns, and customizable dose forms (Pérez-Sanpablo *et al.*, 2021; Oblom *et al.*, 2019).The convergence of 3DP and pharmaceuticals is a captivating prospect, heralding a new era of tailored therapeutic interventions. Personalized medicine, a cornerstone of modern healthcare, becomes even more achievable with 3DP (Chatzitaki *et al.*, 2021). Through the precise deposition of pharmaceutical ingredients, patient-specific dosage forms can be fabricated, aligning drug delivery with an individual's unique needs. This not only enhances treatment efficacy but also minimizes potential side effects, effectively revolutionizing the paradigm of medication.

Furthermore, the potential for 3DP to engineer complex drug-release patterns offers unprecedented control over pharmacokinetics. Tailoring the release profile of a drug can be crucial in optimizing therapeutic outcomes, especially for conditions requiring sustained or targeted delivery (Gioumouxouzis *et al.*, 2020; Genina *et al.*, 2017). The technology enables the creation of intricate structures within dosage forms, allowing drugs to be released in specific sequences or at varying rates. This opens doors to innovative treatments, such as combination therapies within a single dosage form or the synchronization of multiple drug administrations. Customizable dose forms represent another frontier unlocked by 3DP. Traditional dosage forms often necessitate compromises between mass production efficiency and patient-specific requirements. But due to 3DP's inherent adaptability, medications can be precisely tailored to individual patient needs (Goyanes *et al.*, 2017). This is particularly promising in paediatrics, geriatrics, and cases where conventional dosage forms present challenges. However, it is not simple to incorporate 3DP into the pharmaceutical industry. Assurance of the uniformity and quality of 3D-printed pharmaceutical items is one of the main challenges. 3DP must follow the regulatory standards and quality assurance procedures that have been developed for traditional manufacturing techniques. The quality, stability, and performance of the finished product are also substantially impacted by factors including material choice, printing conditions, and postprocessing procedures. As we navigate these promises, it is essential to acknowledge the perils that accompany such transformative technology. Regulatory frameworks must adapt to address the unique aspects of 3DP, ensuring patient safety without stifling innovation (Khaled *et al.*, 2017). Material selection becomes an intricate dance

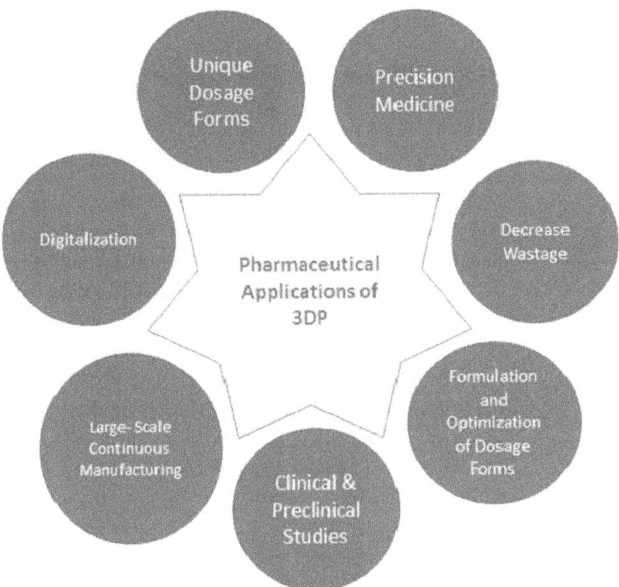

FIGURE 3.1 Pharmaceutical applications of 3DP.

between compatibility, stability, and regulatory compliance. Printing conditions and parameters introduce a layer of complexity to manufacturing processes, necessitating meticulous optimization and validation efforts (Krause *et al.*, 2021).

In summary, the intersection of 3DP and pharmaceuticals unveils remarkable promises that have the potential to redefine healthcare. From personalized medicine to intricate drug-release strategies, the possibilities are captivating. Pharmaceutical applications of 3DP were shown in Figure 3.1. Yet, these promises are entwined with challenges that demand thoughtful solutions (Liang *et al.*, 2018; Li *et al.*, 2018). By embarking on this journey with cautious optimism, the pharmaceutical industry can unlock a future where medications are as unique as the individuals they treat.

3.3 METHODS OF 3DP OF PHARMACEUTICAL PRODUCTS

Table 3.1 shows the different types of 3DP processes with their working procedure and their applications in pharmaceuticals.

3.4 QUALITY CONUNDRUMS IN 3D-PRINTED PHARMACEUTICALS

The choice of materials for 3DP emerges as a critical quality conundrum. Unlike conventional pharmaceutical materials, the spectrum of materials used in 3DP ranges from polymers to metals, introducing complexity to compatibility and stability assessments (Norman *et al.*, 2017; Mostafaei *et al.*, 2021). The solution lies in innovative material development, crafting materials specifically tailored to the

TABLE 3.1
Different Methods of 3DP of Pharmaceutical Products

S.No	Working Methods	Mode of Action	Pharmaceutical Applications
1.	Binder jet printing	The x-y axis-moving nozzle that contains a binder liquid sprays the liquid onto a flat powder surface. The layer solidifies as a result of the liquid's ability to bind the powder particles together. Then the vertical z-axis is used to lower the manufacturing build plate. To create a 3D-printed drug, the procedure is successively repeated while a thin powder layer is applied on top.	1. Ability to create formulations with zero order release and delayed release. 2. Utilized to create the first 3D-printed pharmaceutical that the USFDA has approved. 3. Ability to create formulations with both quick and sustained release. 4. Complex geometries can be created thanks to great resolution.
2.	Fused deposition modelling	A heated nozzle extrudes a drug-filled filament. The molten extrudate is ejected from the printer head along the x-y axis and solidifies on a build plate at room temperature. To create a 3D-printed drug, the build plate is gradually lowered along the vertical z-axis.	1. Capable of creating formulations with both immediate and sustained release. 2. May enhance formulations for prolonged release and solubility. 3. May make poorly soluble medicines more soluble. 4. Having several printing nozzles. 5. Low-cost system. 6. Being lightweight, portable, and convenient.
3.	Semi-solid extrusion	Using a syringe-based tool head, a drug-loaded semi-solid material (such as gel or paste) is extruded. To release the extrudate, which solidifies at room temperature onto a build plate, the printer head is moved along the x, y, and z axes.	1. Can be used to create palatable and chewable compositions. 2. Able to create a variety of formulation types, such as oral films, polypills, and dose forms with controlled and immediate releases.
4.	Direct powder extrusion	A drug-loaded formulation blend is introduced into a powder hopper using an extrusion-based method. The print head's heated single screw extruder creates a molten extrudate by feeding material from the hopper, which solidifies onto a build plate at room temperature. A 3D-printed drug can be created layer-by-layer sequentially lowering the build plate along the vertical z-axis.	1. Ability to create formulations with both quick and sustained release. 2. Can make poorly soluble pharmaceuticals more soluble and scale-up-ready.

TABLE 3.1 (Continued)
Different Methods of 3DP of Pharmaceutical Products

S.No	Working Methods	Mode of Action	Pharmaceutical Applications
5.	Stereo-lithography	By utilizing a laser to trace a precise pattern on the powder bed, selective partial or full melting of the powder particles is achieved during the selective laser sintering process. After the sintered layer has been sintered, a roller distributes a fresh layer of powder on top of it. A 3D-printed drug is created by repeating the process layer-by-layer.	Able to create a variety of formulations, from controlled release to immediate release dosage forms, as well as medical devices; high-resolution process enables creation of complex geometries; suitable for polypill production.
6.	Selective laser sintering	To cause polymerization and solidification, the procedure includes exposing a photopoly merisable resin to high-intensity light. Each time the resin hardens to a specified depth, the platform is then lowered vertically along the z-axis, and the created layer is recoated to construct a 3D-printed medication.	Widely investigated for the manufacture of medical devices and sustained release medicinal products; high resolution and accuracy allow the manufacture of complex geometries; can increase the solubility of poorly soluble pharmaceuticals; appropriate for the manufacture of multilayered polypills.

demands of 3DP for pharmaceuticals. These materials must uphold drug stability, release kinetics, and patient safety without compromise. Process control and optimization represent a pathway to ensuring accuracy in 3DP. Balancing the intricacies of printing specifications, such as material deposition and temperature control, is crucial to maintain consistent drug distribution and release profiles. Through real-time monitoring and meticulous parameter adjustment, the industry can achieve both regulatory compliance and the precision that 3DP promises (Gioumouxouzis *et al.*, 2018). Furthermore, the cooperation between industry and regulatory bodies stands as a linchpin solution. Industry stakeholders must implement stringent quality-control measures while regulators adapt frameworks to accommodate the unique challenges posed by 3DP. This collaboration paves the way for innovative guidelines that balance safety and innovation, creating an environment where advancements can thrive without compromising product integrity. Some of the quality conundrums faced during printing of 3D pharmaceuticals are elaborated in Table 3.2.

TABLE 3.2
Different Quality Challenges Faced During 3DP of Pharmaceutical Products

Sr. No.	Quality Challenge	Description	Pharmaceutical Applications
1.	Choice of materials and compatibility	Selecting suitable 3DP materials and ensuring compatibility with pharmaceuticals.	Enables customization; offers diverse materials.
2.	Printing specification and accuracy	Balancing precision and accuracy in 3DP specifications to achieve consistent drug distribution and release.	Ensures dosing consistency; allows for tailored printing.
3.	Processing and quality assurance	Post-processing impact on quality, uniform drug distribution, and stability; importance of quality-control methods.	Achieves uniformity; stabilizes structures.
4.	Regulation complying with standards	Balancing regulatory compliance with 3DP's innovation, considering unique attributes and safety of the products.	Fosters innovation; aligns with regulatory frameworks.
5.	Pharmaceutical manufacturing and regulatory rules	Meeting strict regulatory standards while adopting advanced technologies like 3DP in pharmaceutical manufacturing.	Adheres to regulatory standards; integrates advanced tech.

3.4.1 CHOICE OF MATERIALS AND COMPATIBILITY

The integration of 3DP into pharmaceutical production holds immense potential, but it brings forth a perplexing challenge: the selection of suitable materials and their compatibility. Unlike traditional pharmaceutical manufacturing, 3DP employs a diverse range of polymers, metals, and ceramics, each with unique properties. This diversity offers unprecedented customization but introduces a conundrum regarding material safety, stability, and interaction with pharmacological agents. The choice of material is critical, as it directly influences drug stability, release kinetics, and overall product performance (Lin *et al.*, 2021; Xu *et al.*, 2021). Rigorous testing is imperative to ensure that the chosen materials not only facilitate precise printing but also maintain their integrity throughout a product's shelf life. Compatibility with active pharmaceutical ingredients is paramount, demanding comprehensive studies to guarantee that interactions do not compromise therapeutic efficacy or patient safety (Reddy Dumpa *et al.*, 2020). Overcoming these quality conundrums necessitates multidisciplinary collaboration between material scientists, pharmaceutical experts, and regulatory bodies. Through meticulous material selection, robust testing, and validation processes, the pharmaceutical industry can mitigate risks and unlock the full potential of 3DP while upholding the highest standards of product quality and patient care.

3.4.2 Printing Specification and Accuracy

In the realm of 3D-printed pharmaceuticals, the pursuit of precision and accuracy presents a perplexing challenge that demands thorough consideration. The intricate interplay of printing specifications and the imperative for utmost accuracy defines a critical quality conundrum. As each layer is meticulously deposited to form a dosage form, the adherence to exact specifications becomes paramount to ensure consistent drug distribution and release. Printing specifications encompass a complex array of variables, ranging from material properties and layer thickness to print speed and temperature control. These parameters intricately influence the structural integrity and performance of the final pharmaceutical product. Any deviation from the specified parameters can lead to undesirable variations in drug-release kinetics, jeopardizing the intended therapeutic outcomes (Robles-Martinez *et al.*, 2019). Moreover, the quest for accuracy delves deeper into the realm of dimensional precision. In pharmaceuticals, even minute deviations from the intended geometry can have profound consequences on dosing accuracy, dissolution profiles, and ultimately, patient well-being. Striking a balance between rapid production and impeccable accuracy becomes a tightrope walk in 3D-printed pharmaceutical manufacturing.

Navigating these quality conundrums necessitates a meticulous approach. Robust validation processes, encompassing comprehensive testing and monitoring, are indispensable. Close collaboration between material scientists, engineers, and pharmaceutical experts is pivotal to determine optimal printing specifications that align with pharmaceutical requirements. In the intricate dance between printing specifications and accuracy, the pharmaceutical industry is tasked with not only achieving regulatory compliance but also realizing the full potential of 3DP's customization capabilities. This conundrum, while formidable, invites innovation in manufacturing techniques, quality control, and the convergence of diverse expertise to sculpt a future where 3D-printed pharmaceuticals are defined by their precision as much as their potential.

3.4.3 Processing Thereafter and Quality Assurance

Post-processing procedures like curing, drying, or coating can have a big impact on the quality of the finished item. In order to spot errors, inconsistencies, and deviations from the specified specifications, it is crucial to implement efficient quality-control methods both during and after printing (Seoane-Viaño *et al.*, 2021). In the realm of 3D-printed pharmaceuticals, a nexus of challenges awaits beyond the printing process itself. The crucial phase of post-processing emerges as a significant quality conundrum. Achieving uniform drug distribution and the desired drug-release profiles demands meticulous attention. Moreover, ensuring the stability and integrity of printed structures throughout their lifecycle adds complexity. These intricacies amplify the importance of robust quality assurance protocols tailored to 3DP. Navigating these conundrums is pivotal, bridging the gap between innovative manufacturing and the steadfast standards of pharmaceutical excellence, thereby unlocking the full potential of 3DP in advancing healthcare.

3.4.4 REGULATION COMPLYING WITH STANDARDS

In the field of 3D-printed medications, the pursuit of innovation walks hand in hand with the imperative of quality assurance. As this novel manufacturing method continues to reshape drug production, the intricate interplay between regulatory compliance and maintaining high standards becomes paramount. Ensuring the safety, efficacy, and consistency of 3D-printed pharmaceuticals presents a multifaceted challenge. Regulatory bodies must evolve to address the unique attributes of 3DP while upholding established pharmaceutical standards. Striking the right balance between fostering innovation and safeguarding patient welfare remains a conundrum. The diverse materials, intricate geometries, and intricate manufacturing processes of 3DP demand an adapted framework that can guarantee product integrity. Comprehensive validation procedures, rigorous material characterization, and meticulous process control are essential to navigate these quality challenges successfully. By aligning regulations with the transformative potential of 3DP, the pharmaceutical industry can embrace advancements while upholding its commitment to patient-centric excellence. Pharmaceutical manufacturing procedures must adhere to strict regulations set by regulatory organisations like the FDA and EMA. It can be difficult to follow these rules while utilizing cutting-edge technology like 3DP. It takes considerable consideration to ensure consistency in quality, safety, and efficacy while adhering to regulatory requirements.

3.5 SOLUTIONS TO ENSURE QUALITY IN 3D-PRINTED PHARMACEUTICALS

3.5.1 CONTEMPORARY MATERIAL DEVELOPMENT

In the dynamic landscape of 3D-printed pharmaceuticals, the quest for unwavering quality finds a promising ally in contemporary material development. The intricacies of this innovative manufacturing process demand materials that seamlessly blend compatibility, stability, and regulatory compliance. Cutting-edge materials, purposefully engineered for pharmaceutical applications, hold the potential to address the unique challenges posed by 3DP (Smith *et al.*, 2020). Table 3.3 shows that solutions for different quality challenges faced during 3DP of pharmaceutical products.

The development of materials tailored to the demands of 3DP is a pivotal solution to ensure quality. These materials must not only exhibit suitable mechanical properties but also facilitate precise drug release and maintain stability over time. Incorporating pharmaceutical ingredients without compromising their efficacy further amplifies the complexity. By crafting materials with meticulous precision, researchers can circumvent potential pitfalls and setbacks (Sadia *et al.*, 2018). New materials that work with 3DP technology and can ensure drug stability are continuously being researched. This entails creating polymers, binders, and excipients especially suited for use in 3DP applications for the pharmaceutical industry (Zheng *et al.*, 2021). Moreover, these innovative materials can lay the groundwork for optimized printing parameters and enhanced post-processing techniques. As the field advances, the collaboration between material scientists, pharmacologists, and regulatory bodies becomes

TABLE 3.3
Solutions for Different Quality Challenges Faced During 3DP of Pharmaceutical Products

Sr. No.	Solution	Description	Pharmaceutical Applications
1.	Contemporary material development	Innovative materials tailored for 3D-printed drugs.	Precise drug release, stability, tailored formulations.
		Address challenges of 3DP with quality materials.	Customized drug delivery, enhanced efficacy.
2.	Process control and optimization	Adjusting printing parameters for consistent quality.	Uniform drug release, high-quality products.
		Guarantee drug release and quality through control.	Enhanced efficiency, minimized risk of defects.
3.	Monitoring and quality control	Real-time monitoring during 3DP process.	Early error detection, intervention capability.
		Rigorous quality-control protocols for final products.	Structural integrity, reliable drug-release profiles.
4.	Cooperation of industry and regulators	Collaborative effort between industry and regulators.	Robust quality control, adaptable regulatory frameworks.
		Ensure innovative potential while maintaining safety.	Flexible guidelines, alignment with technological shifts.

paramount. Ultimately, contemporary material development emerges as a key enabler to harmonize the ground-breaking potential of 3D-printed pharmaceuticals with the rigorous standards that the industry demands.

3.5.2 Process Control and Optimisation

It is crucial to adjust printing parameters through process optimization and control. To guarantee consistent drug-release profiles and high-quality products, printing conditions can be identified with the aid of machine learning and modeling tools. When it comes to 3D-printed medications, the intricate challenge of ensuring uncompromised quality finds its solutions through rigorous process control and optimization strategies. The unique manufacturing intricacies of 3DP demand a dynamic approach that guarantees uniformity and efficacy (Trenfield *et al.*, 2018). Process control emerges as a linchpin in this endeavor, mandating real-time monitoring of every production step. By closely tracking variables like material deposition, temperature, and layer adhesion, deviations can be swiftly identified and rectified, averting potential quality compromises. Process optimization further fine-tunes the manufacturing workflow, enhancing consistency and efficiency. Through meticulous parameter adjustment and material selection, the risk of defects is minimized, bolstering product integrity. Incorporating quality-by-design principles, where robustness is built into the production process, proves essential. This approach anticipates potential challenges and mitigates them pre-emptively, resulting in dependable and reproducible outcomes (Wang *et al.*, 2021). By synergizing process control with optimization, the pharmaceutical industry can harness the full potential of 3DP, offering patients innovative, and high-quality treatments while maintaining unwavering safety and efficacy standards.

3.5.3 Monitoring in Progress and Quality Control

Real-time monitoring during the printing process can aid in the early detection of errors and deviations. Improved process control can be achieved by using techniques like spectroscopy, imaging, and thermal analysis to get insights into the behavior of materials. In the evolving field of 3D-printed drugs, ensuring unwavering quality demands proactive strategies that go beyond conventional norms. A pivotal approach to meet this challenge involves real-time monitoring in progress and rigorous quality control protocols. Implementing continuous monitoring during the 3DP process is a cornerstone solution. By integrating sensors and advanced imaging technologies, manufacturers can scrutinize critical parameters like layer deposition, temperature, and material consistency. This real-time insight allows for immediate intervention if discrepancies arise, ensuring that the final product adheres to the desired specifications (Trenfield *et al.*, 2021).

Simultaneously, robust quality-control protocols are indispensable. Adapting existing pharmaceutical standards to the unique intricacies of 3DP is essential. Rigorous testing, including structural integrity assessments, drug-release profiles, and mechanical strength evaluations, must be established. Additionally, thorough material characterization and compatibility studies are pivotal in ensuring that chosen materials align with pharmacological requirements. In this evolving landscape, solutions that emphasize continuous monitoring and stringent quality control act as safeguarding measures, bolstering confidence in the reliability and efficacy of 3D-printed pharmaceuticals. By embracing these strategies, the industry paves the way for transformative advancements while upholding its commitment to patient well-being.

3.5.4 The Cooperation of the Industry and the Regulators

In the dynamic landscape of 3D-printed pharmaceuticals, ensuring unwavering quality necessitates a collaborative effort between industry stakeholders and regulatory authorities. To effectively harness the innovative potential of this technology while maintaining patient safety, a symbiotic partnership is crucial. Industry players can contribute by implementing robust quality-control measures throughout the manufacturing process. This includes stringent material testing, precise printing protocols, and comprehensive post-processing validation. Concurrently, regulators must adapt existing frameworks to accommodate the nuances of 3DP. By actively engaging with manufacturers and staying abreast of technological advancements, regulators can craft flexible guidelines that address emerging challenges. Cooperation between industry and regulators becomes the linchpin in this endeavor, fostering an environment where innovation thrives without compromising quality. This synergy promises a future where 3D-printed pharmaceuticals offer unparalleled benefits while adhering to the highest standards of safety and efficacy (Wilsdon *et al.*, 2018). To create regulations that take into account the particular difficulties posed by 3DP, regulatory organizations and pharmaceutical businesses must work closely together. The creation of industry standards and improved regulatory processes may result from this partnership.

3.6 CONCLUSION

The advantages of 3DP in the pharmaceutical industry led to a future scope of customization where a personalized treatment is possible by producing individualized doses depending on a patient's exact needs. This could result in more precise dosing, enhanced patient adherence, and better treatment outcomes. 3DP can enable medications to be produced on-demand, eliminating the need for large-scale manufacturing, inventory management, and supply chain difficulties. This could result in cost reductions and improved access to pharmaceuticals in rural areas. 3DP has the potential to combine numerous medications or even therapeutic cells into a single-dose form. This has the potential to revolutionize combination therapy development and delivery by providing for exact control over medication ratios and release characteristics. Yet, to ensure the safety, efficacy, and quality of 3D-printed pharmaceutical items, extensive regulation will be required to address issues, such as material quality, precision, and repeatability. Meeting regulatory criteria requires ensuring reproducibility and consistency in the production process.

Overall, the future of 3DP in the pharmaceutical field shows great potential in terms of enhancing medicine effectiveness, patient care, and expanding pharmaceutical product research and production procedures. However, resolving present obstacles and setting regulatory norms will be critical for its successful implementation.

ACKNOWLEDGEMENTS

The authors are very much thankful to Management and Principal of KVSR Siddhartha College of Pharmaceutical Sciences, Vijayawada for their support and constant encouragement.

REFERENCES

Alhnan MA, Okwuosa TC, Sadia M, Wan KW, Ahmed W, Arafat B, Forbes RT. Emergence of 3D printed dosage forms: Opportunities and challenges. *Pharmaceutical Research.* 2016;**33**(8):1817–32.

Alhnan MA, Okwuosa TC, Sadia M, *et al.* Emergence of 3D pinted dosage forms: Opportunities and challenges. *Pharmaceutical Research.* 2016;**33**:1817–32.

Alomari M, Mohamed FH, Basit AW, *et al.* Personalised dosing: Printing a dose of one's own medicine. *International Journal of Pharmaceutics.* 2015;**494**:568–77.

Awad A, Trenfield SJ, Gaisford S, *et al.* 3D printed medicines: A new branch of digital healthcare. *International Journal of Pharmaceutics.* 2018;**548**:586–96.

Awad A, Trenfield SJ, Goyanes A, *et al.* Reshaping drug development using 3D printing. *Drug Discovery Today.* 2018;**23**:1547–55.

Awad A, Trenfield SJ, Pollard TD, *et al.* Connected healthcare: Improving patient care using digital health technologies. *Advanced Drug Delivery Reviews.* 2021;**178**:113958.

Basit A, Trenfield S. 3D printing of pharmaceuticals and the role of pharmacy. *International Journal of Drug Development and Research.* 2022;**308**:7959.

Berman, B. 3-D printing: The new industrial revolution. *Business Horizons.* 2012;**55**(2):155–62.

Bhowmick S, Dey S, Biswas D, Maiti S, Bhattacharjee D, Das P, Paul S. 3DP in pharmaceutical drug delivery: Challenges and opportunities. *Journal of Controlled Release.* 2021;**340**:556–72.

Chatzitaki A-T, Tsongas K, Tzimtzimis EK, *et al.* 3D printing of patient-tailored SNEDDS-based suppositories of lidocaine. *Journal of Drug Delivery Science and Technology.* 2021;**61**:102292.

Elbadawi M, Gustaffson T, Gaisford S, *et al.* 3D printing tablets: Predicting printability and drug dissolution from rheological data. *International Journal of Pharmaceutics.* 2020;**590**:119868.

Elbadawi M, Muñiz Castro B, Gavins FKH, *et al.* M3DISEEN: A novel machine learning approach for predicting the 3D printability of medicines. *International Journal of Pharmaceutics.* 2020;**590**:119837.

FabRx and Gustave Roussy enter into an agreement to develop a novel, personalised, multi-drug dosage form for the treatment of patients with early-stage breast cancer. FabRx. 2021. www.fabrx.co.uk/2021/06/25/fabrx-and-gustave-roussy-enter-into-an-agreement-to-develop-a-novel-personalised-multi-drug-dosage-form-for-the-treatment-of-patients-with-early-stage-breast-cancer

Florence AT, Lee VHL. Personalised medicines: More tailored drugs, more tailored delivery. *International Journal of Pharmaceutics.* 2011;**415**:29–33.

Genina N, Boetker JP, Colombo S, *et al.* Anti-tuberculosis drug combination for controlled oral delivery using 3D printed compartmental dosage forms: From drug product design to in vivo testing. *Journal of Controlled Release.* 2017;**268**:40–Gioumouxouzis CI, Baklavaridis A, Katsamenis OL, *et al.* A 3D printed bilayer oral solid dosage form combining metformin for prolonged and glimepiride for immediate drug delivery. *European Journal of Pharmaceutical Sciences.* 2018;**120**:40–52.

Gioumouxouzis CI, Tzimtzimis E, Katsamenis OL, *et al.* Fabrication of an osmotic 3D printed solid dosage form for controlled release of active pharmaceutical ingredients. *European Journal of Pharmaceutical Sciences.* 2020;**143**:105176.

Goyanes A, Fina F, Martorana A, *et al.* Development of modified release 3D printed tablets (printlets) with pharmaceutical excipients using additive manufacturing. *International Journal of Pharmaceutics.* 2017;**527**:21–30.

Goyanes A, Scarpa M, Kamlow M, *et al.* Patient acceptability of 3D printed medicines. *International Journal of Pharmaceutics.* 2017;**530**:71–8.

Goyanes A, Wang J, Buanz A, *et al.* 3DP of medicines: Engineering novel oral devices with unique Design and drug release characteristics. *Molecular Pharmaceutics.* 2015;**12**(11):4077–84.

Gupta A, Kumar S. 3DP technology: A comprehensive review of its applications in drug delivery and pharmaceuticals. *AAPS PharmSciTech.* 2021;**22**(5):175.

Ho CM, Ng, SH. 3D printed drug delivery devices: Perspectives and challenges. *Pharmaceutics.* 2020;**12**(1):14.

Jacob J, Coyle N, West TG, Monkhouse DC, Surprenant HL, Jain NB. Rapid disperse dosage form containing levetiracetam. U.S. Patent US20140271862A1, 17 May 2016.

Khaled SA, Alexander MR. Computer-aided design and 3DP of polymers for tissue engineering. In *Tissue Engineering* (pp. 1–27). CRC Press; 2017.

Khaled SA, Burley JC, Alexander MR, *et al.* 3D printing of five-in-one dose combination polypill with defined immediate and sustained release profiles. *Journal of Controlled Release.* 2015;**217**:308–14.

Khaled SA, Burley JC, Alexander MR, *et al.* 3D printing of tablets containing multiple drugs with defined release profiles. *International Journal of Pharmaceutics.* 2015;**494**:643–50.

Krause J, Müller L, Sarwinska D, *et al.* 3D printing of mini tablets for pediatric use. *Pharmaceuticals.* 2021;**14**:143.

Liang K, Carmone S, Brambilla D, *et al.* 3D printing of a wearable personalized oral delivery device: A first-in-human study. *Science Advanced.* 2018;**4**: eaat2544. DOI:10.1126/sciadv.aat2544

Li Q, Guan X, Cui M, *et al.* Preparation and investigation of novel gastro-floating tablets with 3D extrusion-based printing. *International Journal of Pharmaceutics.* 2018;**535**:325–32.

Lin X, Fu H, Hou Z, *et al.* Three-dimensional printing of gastro-floating tablets using polyethylene glycol diacrylate-based photocurable printing material. *International Journal of Pharmaceutics.* 2021;**603**:120674.

Marques AC, Santos HA. 3DP in pharmaceutics: A new tool for medication personalization and therapeutic innovation. *Advanced Healthcare Materials.* 2015;**4**(5):745–48.

Mostafaei A, Elliott AM, Barnes JE, Li F, Tan W, Cramer CL, Nandwana P, Chmielus M. Binder jet 3D printing—Process parameters, materials, properties, modeling, and challenges. *Progress in Materials Science.* 2021;**119**:100707.

Norman J, Madurawe RD, Moore CMV, *et al.* A new chapter in pharmaceutical manufacturing: 3D-printed drug products. *Advanced Drug Delivery Reviews.* 2017;**108**:39–50.

Öblom H, Zhang J, Pimparade M, *et al.* 3D-printed isoniazid tablets for the treatment and prevention of tuberculosis—Personalized dosing and drug release. *AAPS PharmSciTech.* 2019;**20**(2):52. doi: 10.1208/s12249-018-1233-7. PMID: 30617660; PMCID: PMC6373414

Pérez-Sanpablo A, Romero-Ávila E, González-Mendoza A. Three-dimensional printing in healthcare. *Revista Mexicana de Ingeniería Biomédica.* 2021;**42**(2):32–48. https://doi.org/10.17488/RMIB.42.2.3

Reddy Dumpa N, Bandari S, A. Repka M. Novel gastroretentive floating pulsatile drug delivery system produced via hot-melt extrusion and fused deposition modeling 3D printing. *Pharmaceutics.* 2020;**12**:52.

Robles-Martinez P, Xu X, Trenfield SJ, *et al.* 3D printing of a multi-layered polypill containing six drugs using a novel stereolithographic method. *Pharmaceutics.* 2019;**11**:274.

Sadia M, Isreb A, Abbadi I, *et al.* From 'fixed dose combinations' to 'a dynamic dose combiner': 3D printed bi-layer antihypertensive tablets. *European Journal of Pharmaceutical Sciences.* 2018;**123**:484–94.

Sankar PL, Parker LS. The precision medicine initiative's all of us research program: An agenda for research on its ethical, legal, and social issues. *Genetics in Medicine.* 2017;**19**:743–50.

Sen K, Mehta T, Sansare S, Sharifi L, Ma AW, Chaudhuri B. Pharmaceutical applications of powder-based binder jet 3D printing process–A review. *Advanced Drug Delivery Reviews.* 2021;**177**:113943.

Seoane-Viaño I, Ong JJ, Luzardo-Álvarez A, *et al.* 3D printed tacrolimus suppositories for the treatment of ulcerative colitis. *Asian Journal of Pharmaceutical Sciences.* 2021;**16**:110–9.

Smith A, Hasan S, Pradel P, *et al.* 3D printed oral drug delivery systems: A perspective on the expanding role of additive manufacturing in the pharmaceutical industry. *International Journal of Pharmaceutics.* 2020;**586**:119584.

Trenfield SJ, Goyanes A, Gaisford S, *et al.* Editorial: Innovations in 2D and 3D printed pharmaceuticals. *International Journal of Pharmaceutics.* 2021;**605**:120839.

Trenfield SJ, Awad A, Goyanes A, *et al.* 3D printing pharmaceuticals: Drug development to frontline care. *Trends in Pharmacological Sciences.* 2018;**39**:440–51.

Ventola CL. Progress in 3DP technology and its medical applications. *PT.* 2014;39(10):704–11.

Wang J, Zhang Y, Aghda NH, *et al.* Emerging 3D printing technologies for drug delivery devices: Current status and future perspective. *Advanced Drug Delivery Reviews.* 2021;**174**:294–31.

Wilsdon T, Edwards G, Lawlor R. The benefits of personalised medicine to patients, society and healthcare systems. EBE Biopharma. 2018.

Xu X, Goyanes A, Trenfield SJ, *et al.* Stereolithography (SLA) 3D printing of a bladder device for intravesical drug delivery. *Materials Science and Engineering: C.* 2021;**120**:111773.

Yu D-G, Shen XX, Branford-White C, Zhu LM, White K, Yang XL. Novel oral fast-disintegrating drug delivery devices with predefined inner structure fabricated by three-dimensional printing. *Journal of Pharmacy and Pharmacology.* 2009;**61**:323–29.

Yu DG, Yang XL, Huang WD, Liu J, Wang YG, Xu H. Tablets with material gradients fabricated by three-dimensional printing. *Pharmaceutical Sciences.* 2007;**96**:2446–56.

Zheng Y, Deng F, Wang B, *et al.* Melt extrusion deposition (MED™) 3D printing technology – A paradigm shift in design and development of modified release drug products. *International Journal of Pharmaceutics.* 2021;**602**:120639.

Section III

Extrusion-Based 3D Printing in Pharmaceutics

4 Extrusion-Based 3D Printing in Pharmaceuticals

Aastha Singh, Mohit Agrawal,
Vijay Kumar Sharma, Hema Chaudhary,
Aakriti Patel, Shivendra Kumar, Sunam Saha,
and Md. Sadique Hussain

4.1 INTRODUCTION

3 Dimensional Printing (3DP) is a novel approach for creating rapid 3D items from digital models by melting or depositing materials in successive stages, allowing for the layer-by-layer creation of structures with different geometrics. Additionally this process is known as rapid prototyping, solid free-form fabrication, and additive manufacturing (Goole *et al.*, 2016). The implementation of a 3DP approach in the pharmaceutical industry has the potential to alter fundamental assumptions about how drugs are developed, produced, and consumed by the general public (Lim *et al.*, 2018). A 3D object is created using the additive manufacturing process known as 3DP, in which successive layers of material are applied and cemented (Ventola *et al.*, 2014). Since the Food and Drug Administration (FDA) authorized the very first 3D-printed medication, Spritam®, in 2015 (Fitzgerald *et al.*, 2015), interest in 3DP has significantly expanded in the pharmaceutical industry. Levetiracetam, an anti-epileptic medication known as Spritam®, was created by Aprecia Pharmaceuticals (Skowyra *et al.*, 2015). This method creates a highly porous tablet that, in an emergency, can be quickly dissolved by the patient's saliva (ZipDose Technology, 2018).

In a number of sectors, such as plastic surgery, 3DP has shown to be a game-changing technology due to the bio-printing of organs and tissues, and the use of organ models for surgical training, as well as the production of prosthetics that are more personalized and affordable (Choonara *et al.*, 2016). The results of the investigations suggest that 3DP helps to achieve composition flexibility with complex release profiles, which explains the technology's capacity to build complex and workable drug-device geometries (Prasad *et al.*, 2016 and Katstra *et al.*, 2000). 3DP drug devices have early encouraging outcomes (Rowe *et al.*, 2000). Researchers have been inspired to investigate the capacity of numerous types of 3DP approaches to fabricate various dosage forms and bring advanced, complex drug devices, such as polypill (Khaled *et al.*, 2015) and dynamic dose combination (Sadia *et al.*, 2018), as a result of the creation of a BDDS with controlled release. Scientists have investigated

DOI: 10.1201/9781003439509-7

a number of 3DP approaches, including SLS, binder deposition, stereolithography, inkjet printing, and extrusion-based printing, to create novel drug devices that accomplish tasks that are challenging to accomplish utilizing the conventional techniques recently used in the pharmaceutical industries (Gross *et al.*, 2014 and Algahtani *et al.*, 2018). In numerous scientific fields, different approaches have made significant advancements. Each technique has its own specialties and limitations that have an influence on the printing process and the finished product when used in the pharmaceutical industry. The 3DP process known as stereolithography is capable of creating intricate and difficult structures. However, the expansion of this approach is constrained by the absence of biocompatible photo-sensitive polymers (Katstra *et al.*, 2000).

4.1.1 Advantages

SSE-based 3DP is the most advantageous approach for bio-printing since it can print a wide variety of materials because the printing method does not need a higher temperature (Khalil *et al.*, 2005). This method has a number of benefits for creating pharmacological dosage forms, which makes it a useful method. For a researcher who is not frequently exposed to 3DP technology, it is simple to deploy. The excipients that were typically utilized to create dosage forms using the traditional approach can be extruded.

4.1.2 Limitation

SE-based 3P is less advantageous than other 3DP technologies in various ways. Typically, the limiting printing resolution is <100 m. This resolution cap is substantially lower than the 3D printing technologies that are already in use. Excipients deteriorate in the presence of solvents, making this technique less suited for APIs. Additionally, the drying process needs to be handled carefully because solvent evaporation could cause the printed dosage form to shrink. In few circumstances, drying by using oven or vacuum as well as a specific amount of humidity needed to prevent the printed dosage from deforming (Khaled *et al.*, 2015 and Algahtani *et al.*, 2018).

4.2 EXTRUSION-BASED 3D APPROACHES

There are two different types of approaches which are used in pharmaceuticals. Semi-solid extrusion (SSE) and fused deposition modeling (FDM) are the two extrusion-based 3DP approaches. Both have different properties, process of printing, advantages, limitations as well as applications in pharmaceuticals.

Utilizing computer-aided design (CAD) software, the 3DP process begins with developing the necessary 3D object. The software and the hardware make up the two integrated components of the SSE printer. The software program regulates the robotic motions of the hardware. The pressure that is delivered and numerous factors have an impact on the printing process. The stage and syringe are the two primary components of the hardware. The components are loaded into the syringe for the

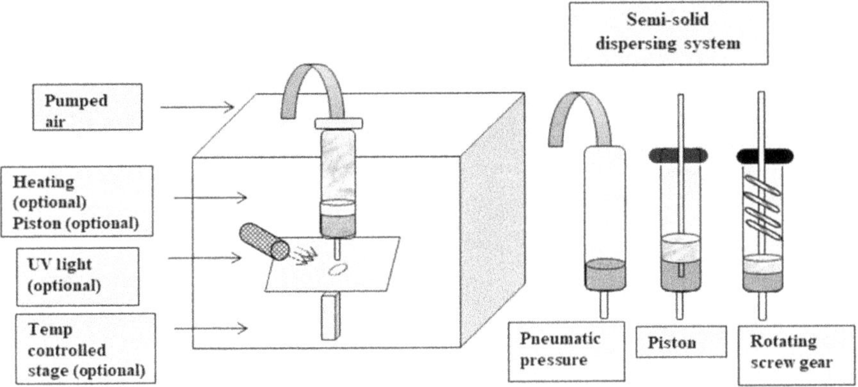

FIGURE 4.1 Diagrammatic representation of SSE.

extrusion operation. Pneumatic pressure, a piston, mechanism is used for extruding the semi-solid materials via a micrometer nozzle during material dispensing from the syringe. To extrude, the pneumatic pressure system pumps air through a syringe of semi-solid substances via the attached nozzle. This approach is favored because it is straightforward and has excellent control (Khalil *et al.*, 2005). The materials are pushed out through the attached nozzle by the screw-driven system using spinning screw gears (Figure 4.1). The stage moves in the C or ABC directions or is fixed (Figure 4.1).

4.2.1 PROCESS OF SSE PRINTING

The SSE printing process initially resembles FDM in that the substance is heated, extruded, and subsequently hardens to take the desired form. The intended structure is also constructed using a CAD programme, as with any kind of 3D printing, and imported into the printer software to facilitate item manufacturing. Although the shared process between the two is easily seen. The variances are mostly caused by the feedstock utilized, particularly because it is semi-solid.

4.2.2 EXTRUSION

The extrusion procedure is what distinguishes a SSE printer. The material is created utilizing a type of syringe and starts off as a gel or paste, unlike other kinds of 3DP. Due to the fact that the substance is held in a syringe, heating can take place either internally, just before printing, or outside, possibly while another syringe is being used. However, while heating, caution must be used because it can make the material too liquid to support any structure when deposited. Therefore, optimization is necessary to determine the appropriate temperature needed to print with various materials. Pneumatic, mechanical, or solenoid-based systems can all be used to power the material's extrusion (Ozbolat, 2016).

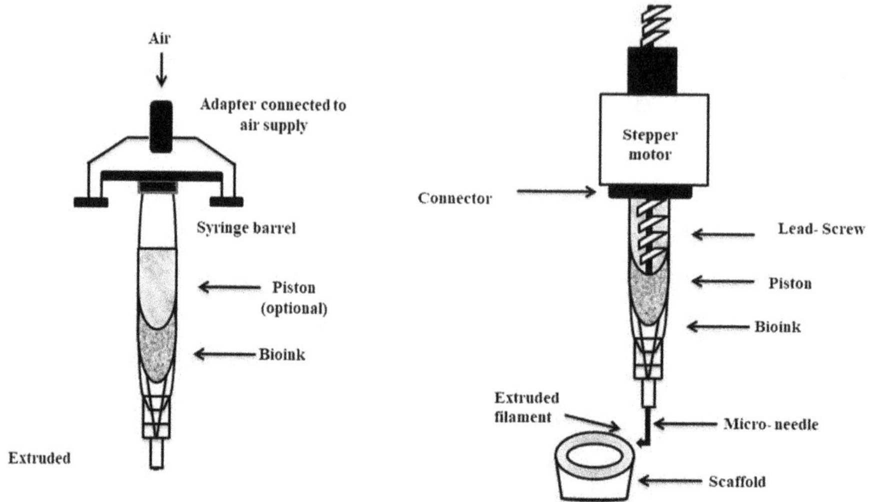

FIGURE 4.2   (A) Pneumatic micro-extrusions. (B) Mechanical micro-extrusions.

- Using the power of air to depress the syringe, which subsequently extrudes the goods, this pneumatic system uses air pressure to operate (Figure 4.2A). To prevent the material from being discharged when no force is applied, this mechanism frequently uses a valve on the nozzle. As a result of employing compressed gas, these methods have been linked to a delay between beginning, dispensing, and extrusion. Also, when employing small amounts, it may be challenging to ensure the precision of the material administered.

- As the name implies, mechanical-based devices (Figure 4.2B) exert mechanical force on the syringe directly. In general, these systems offer a far more straightforward mechanism when compared to the pneumatic process and can manage gel extrusion using either a piston- or screw-based structure. These devices' portability has been significantly enhanced because they do not require large compressed gas equipment. Since the screw-based printing method can be hampered by pressure variations, piston-based printing is thought to offer high control over the extrusion flow.

- Electrical pulses are sent to the valve by solenoid micro-extrusion printers (Figure 4.3). A floating ferromagnetic plunger and a ferromagnetic ring are attracted to one another magnetically, but the pulse breaks that attraction. The printers may distribute material in sub-L volumes thanks to this technology. The mechanism, which is mostly employed in bio-printing, can occasionally be difficult to reproduce.

4.2.3 Printing

The SS substance is extruded via a nozzle at the syringe's base to begin the printing process. Here, the substance's viscosity can have a significant influence on how things function; if the substance is too liquid, the structure will not maintain its shape,

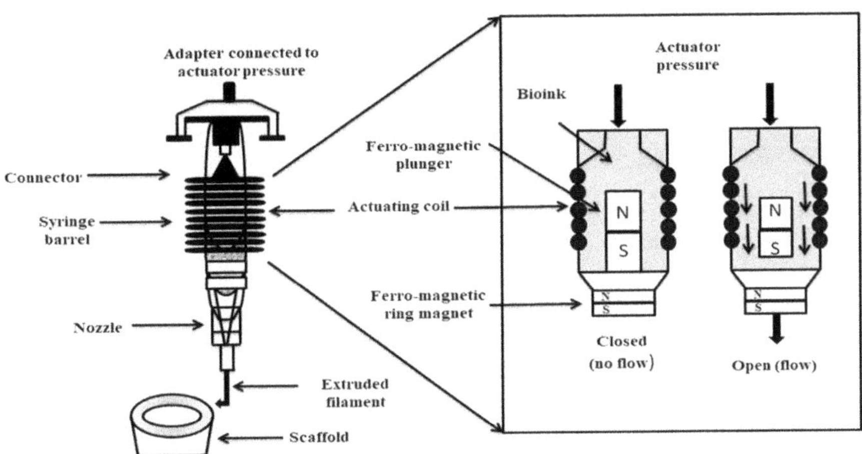

FIGURE 4.3 Solenoid micro-extrusions.

which clog the nozzle and somehow harm the extrusion mechanism if it is excessively viscous (Ozbolat, 2016). This can be fixed by modifying the formulation of the substance to change its physical characteristics and improve its fluidity. Alternatively, the feedstock's viscosity can be decreased by heating up the syringe or employing a bigger nozzle head that can prevent clogging. The area between the bedplate to the viscosity of the substance must also be calibrated, but in certain cases, this is done automatically. After the head has been calibrated, the printer will print any form to guarantee a constant flow of material, which is frequently first halted by air bubbles gathering in the syringe's nozzle. A computer-controlled motor system is used to position the nozzle, enabling the printer head to move along the a, b and c point. When printing, the bed can potentially result in several problems. The first extruded layer must both adhere to the bed and be simple to remove when the procedure is finished for the subsequent layers of material to be placed. This can be accomplished by heating the print bed to reduce tension in the base layers and minimize material warping, which could result in the premature release of the manufactured object. But once more, it is important to carefully regulate this temperature to make sure the material can solidify properly and keep its shape (Firth *et al.*, 2018).

4.2.4 SSE Benefits

When using SSE technology, the ease of medication loading is instantly noticeable. As long as the compound is combined evenly and its potency is not lost during printing, this method makes it much easier to determine the drug's composition. Also, it should be noted that the gel's composition might have a significant impact on its viscosity. Important factors like the pH are changed when different components' concentrations are changed. The major promise of SSE is seen in its quick printing as well as its low heating temperature. Due to their degree of thermolability, many pharmaceutically active substances deteriorate at the working temperatures of few 3D printers. Apart

from that, the feedstock for SSE needs substantially low heat to obtain a printable viscosity. Thus, additional thermolabile chemicals may be used by decreasing the heat
supplied to the material.

4.2.5 SSE Drawback

The poor resolution at which SSE can print is a glaring restriction on its useful-
ness. The nozzle heads of SSE printers are frequently substantially broader than the
extrusion orifices of conventional printers because they have to be able to accommodate a highly viscous substance. This low resolution may make it more difficult to
produce tablets accurately, which could result in an incorrect dosage or dissolving
profile. The low resolution enables the technology to print at the fast pace mentioned
earlier. Because the feedstock is semi-solid, post-printing drying is frequently necessary to make sure the 3D-printed tablets have dried thoroughly enough to maintain
structural viability and preserve form when stored. When creating some less viscous
pharmaceutical formulations, a drying stage might be necessary because there is a
chance that the structure will collapse before it has cooled enough. The Roberts group
discovered that hoover drying at 40°C for 24 hours was necessary to verify that complete hardening had taken place (Khaled *et al.*, 2015 and Khaled *et al.*, 2015). The
fact that this was not needed when formulating the controlled-release bilayer tablets
is intriguing, suggesting that maybe highly viscous formulations do not need such a
step (Khaled *et al.*, 2014).

4.3   3DP OF PHARMACEUTICALS DOSAGE FORMS BASED ON SSE BASED 3DP: RECENT RESEARCH AND APPLICATIONS

The most often utilized method for tissue engineering has been SSE, which has also
been employed for organ repair, preoperative surgical treatment planning, disease
models, and vascular micro-fabrication (Zhang *et al.*, 2016, Jang *et al.*, 2016, Ploch
et al., 2016 and Malheiro *et al.*, 2016). This is because a variety of materials may
be extruded without the requirement for heating. The 3DP approach, which is SSE-
based, is also utilized to create a variety of pharmacological dosage forms. Examples
of innovative dose forms made possible by SSE-based 3DP technology are shown in
Table 4.1.

4.3.1 Immediate Release Tablets

In order to obtain satisfactory industrial operation and patient usage with the traditional tablet pressing utilized in the pharmaceutical industry, a significant percentage
of excipients must be added to the API (Jivraj *et al.*, 2000). With large API doses,
the tablet's overall size increases and becomes difficult for patients to swallow.
Additionally, the efficiency of the treatment is decreased and the likelihood of side
effects is increased (Tucker *et al.*, 2017). There is a great desire for more customized
medication tablets because they use less excipient. Using SSE printing, Khaled *et al.*
created an immediate release paracetamol tablet with substantial drug loading (Kaialy

TABLE 4.1
Illustrations of Innovative Dosage Forms Created by Utilizing 3DP Technologies Based on SSE

Sr. No.	Formulation /Dosage Form	API	Excipients Used in the Preparation	Outcomes	Ref.
1	Local delivery patches for the treatment of ductal carcinoma	5–fluorouracil	PCL, poly (lactic-co-glycolic acid)	Adaptable patch (4 week release window)	Yi *et al.*, 2016
2	Multi-active tablets	Captopril, nifedipine, glipizide	Cellulose acetate, cellulose microcrystalline, HPMC, polyvinylpyrrolidone, sodium srach glycolate, lactose, Mannitol and PEG 6000	Captopril is released in zero-order through the osmotic pump, whereas nifedipine and glipizide have sustained release characteristic.	Khaled *et al.*, 2015
3	Gastro floating tablets	Dipyridamole	MCC, HPMC, PVPI, Lactose	The tablets design demonstrates a floating capacity of more than 12 hrs. The infill percentages and the release profile were connected.	Li *et al.*, 2018
4	Polypill	Asprine, hydrochlorothiazide, pravasttaion, atenclol, ramipril	HPMC, Polyvinyl pyrrolidine, sodium starch glycolate, cellulose acetate, mannitol, lactise and PEG 6000	Aspirin and hydrochlorothiazide have a quick release profile, whereas pravastatin, atebolol and Ramipril have a sustained release profile.	Khaled *et al.*, 2018
5	Immediate release tablets	PCM	Croscarmellose sodium, polyvinylpyrrolidone	Eighty percent medication loading was attained a five-minute time frame for a quick medication release.	Jivraj *et al.*, 2000.

et al., 2014). By utilizing SSE printing, a high-loaded pcm tablet (80%) was created. The tablet's physical characteristics are in accordance with USP specifications. Additionally, testing revealed that neither the printing nor the excipients of choice had an impact on the paracetamol. Less than 60 seconds are needed for the pill to dissolve, and during the first 10 minutes, 90% of the medication is delivered into the dissolution media. This work exhibits SSE's capabilities to create a tablet with a large drug-loading capacity, a dose that is programmable, and that complies with USP criteria (Khaled *et al.*, 2015).

4.3.2 Cancer Patches for Local Drug Delivery

Anticancer medications were made to target cancerous cells, but it can be challenging to do so systemically without also killing healthy cells, which can have major side effects. To improve the medicine's ability to target tumors, a variety of drug-delivery methods were investigated, including nanotechnology. A local medication delivery patch for pancreatic cancer growth inhibition was produced by Yi *et al.* (2016). The patch is made to administer 5-fluorouracil to the pancreatic cancer tissue over a lengthy period (4 weeks). According to the study, the geometry of the printed patch directly affects how quickly a medicine is released. The growth of the cancer tissue is suppressed after the patch is applied to a mouse subcutaneous pancreatic cancer xenograft. According to this study, making chemotherapeutic drug patches for local treatment of cancer using SSE-based 3DP technology is a practical option. (Yi *et al.*, 2016 and Health *et al.*, 2008), intratumor infusion (Lammers et al., 2006), and brain cancer implanted wafers (Panigrahi *et al.*, 2011).

4.4 FDM

FDM is a method of additive manufacturing. To create a 3D item, molten materials are extruded one layer at a time onto a platform. The most used 3DP technology worldwide is called FDM. Originally only used for engineering and prototyping, this approach is now being applied to the pharmaceutical industry due to improvements in the manufacture of filaments and the broad range of substances that may be printed on FDM printers have two incorporated components (software and hardware), just like SSE printers do. The 3D drawing was produced by utilizing CAD software. The software on the computer, connected to the printer is then used to slice the design to a printable layer. The printing process is controlled by the software component. The platform, the robotic arm which moves the printer head and filament feeder make up the hardware in most cases. An appropriate filament is utilized to fabricate the dosage forms. This filament is obtained from the market or is made using the hot melt extrusion method. The API is loaded with the filaments for the available filaments. The API and polymer beads must first be mixed. Driving gears force thermoplastic filament through the printer head to maintain a steady substance supply. The printer head is comprised of a heating matter and a metal nozzle. The heated component is in-charge of delivering the necessary heat to melt the filament that will be extruded by the nozzle. Extruded substances bond to the preceding solid layer as they cool. An

A- and B-moving robotic arm is used to control the printer head. This area is capable of accurate C movement. The area descended to enable the deposition of the subsequent layer when each layer's printing was finished, and so on until the necessary 3D object was finished (Algahtani *et al.*, 2018)

4.5 3DP OF PHARMACEUTICALS DOSAGE FORMS BASED ON FDM-BASED 3DP: RECENT RESEARCH AND APPLICATIONS

Since 1988, 3DP on an FDM platform has been widely employed in a variety of manufacturing companies, including robots, electronics, instructional models, fast prototyping, bespoke manufacturing, and medical. The popularity of FDM-based 3DP technology is attributed to its use, range of substances for varied purposes, and reasonably priced printers (Novakova-Marcincinova, 2012). The field of drug distribution is not an exception; the fabrication of drug devices utilizing FDM printing is thought to be the most researched. Here, we discussed a few instances of different drug-dosage forms developed by the FDM-based 3DP. This topic concludes systems, i.e., wearable, customized drug devices, bilayer, intragastric, drug-loaded implants, and instant release, modulated release, and release systems. Examples of innovative dose forms made possible by FDM-based 3DP technology are shown in Table 4.2.

4.5.1 MODIFIED RELEASED TABLETS

To achieve greater drug efficacy and improve patient convenience, the time or place where a drug is released may need to be changed in specific therapeutic situations. The FDM-based printers can produce patient-tailored preparation because they can produce tablets in a variety of geometries and because the polymers needed to modify medication release are readily available (Algahtani *et al.*, 2018). In some therapeutic circumstances, it may be necessary to alter the time or location where a medicine is released in order to increase pharmacological efficacy and enhance patient convenience. A layer of enteric polymer is subsequently applied to the finished caplet. The production caplets' dissolution was contrasted with that of the commercially available budesonides, Cortiment® and Entocort®.The pH of the digestive tract was intended to be mimicked by the dissolving medium (Goyanes *et al.*, 2015).

4.5.2 INTERMEDIATE-RELEASE TABLETS

Sadia *et al.* (2018) created channelled tablets as a novel method of accelerating the disintegration process without the use of disintegrates. Using printing techniques based on FDM. Making channels inside the manufactured tablet is intended to facilitate faster drug release. The hydrochlorothiazide tablet was created with various alignments and channel sizes. The channels' width and depth had an impact on the release pattern. Hydrochlorothiazide was discharged from the numerous channels with shorter depths than from the longer channels. This method demonstrates how to create channelled tablets using FDM printing for quick medication release without the use of disintegrates.

TABLE 4.2
Illustrations of Innovative Dosage forms Created using 3DP

Sr. No.	Formulation/ Dosage Form	API	Excipients Used in the Preparation	Outcomes	Ref.
1	Orodispersible film	Aripiprazole	PVA	The poorly water soluble drugs rate of dissolution is accelerated by the amorphization of aripiprazole during the creation of the printed film, which creates a porous structure.	Roberts *et al.*, 2014
2	Discs, beads, catheter constructs	Gentamicin methotrexate	PLA	The cytostatic and effective antibacterial and cancer growth-inhibiting properties were present in the all 3D-printed construction.	Weisman *et al.*, 2015
3	Hallow capsules (size 9)	Radiolabelled with fluorodeoxiyglucose	Hydroxypropyl cellulose, ethylcellulose, PVA-PEG graftcopolymer and hypromellose acetate succinate	No capsules emptied from the stomach, according to rat *in vivo* tests.	Goyanes *et al.*, 2018
4	T-shaped intrauterine device	Indomethacin	Poly (caprolactone)-	Drug diffusion from the apparatus regulated the drug release.	Hollander *et al.*, 2016
5	Vaginal rings contraceptive	Progesterone	Poly ethylene glycol, Polycaprolactone, poly lactic acid	Use diffusion-controlled release to demonstrate persistent progesterone release for more than seven days.	Fu *et al.*, 2018

4.6   3DP OF DRUGS USING EXTRUSION: THE ROLE OF POLYMER

Additional functional excipients or groups of are also utilised in either FDM or SSE 3DP. (Zidan *et al.*, 2019 and Kempin *et al.*, 2018) However, a significant amount of each constituent is present in the polymer. As a result, the polymer is crucial in creating a drug-polymer matrix that is appropriate for dosing and has a high degree of material process ability.

4.6.1   ETHYL-CELLULOSE

In recent years, ethyl cellulose is frequently used as an effective polymer in the preparation of pharmaceutical medications and also 3DP medications have begun to use EC. It is a water-insoluble thermoplastic polymer. To make use of these qualities, the pharmaceutical industry uses EC in FDM 3DP. Due to its ability to provide a longer release, it is commonly used as a polymer in pharmaceutical formulations (Cellulosics *et al.*, 2005). EC needs to undergo some type of sample preparation before being used in FDM printing, such as acetone dissolving or the inclusion of a plasticizer (Kempin *et al.*, 2017).

4.6.2   HYDROXYPROPYL CELLULOSE (HPC)

The polymer HPC is malleable and water soluble. The building block of HPC is a monomer consisting of a glucose molecule with several hydroxypropyl substituents. Rapid temperature changes and overheating have a significant impact on HPC's viscosity and stability. Due to moisture levels that range from about 10 to 1%, HPC has a low glass transition temperature in the region of 25 to 0 °C (Picker *et al.*, 2007). It can be utilized in melting and extrusion processes because of its exceptional thermo stability.

4.6.3   POLYCAPROLACTONE (PCL)

PCL is semi-crystalline, biocompatible polyester with a Tg of around 54 °C and a melting point of 55–60 °C (Goyanes *et al.*, 2016). In organic solvents, it is extremely soluble. Because of its incredibly low *in vivo* degradation, it is used for long term implant delivery systems (Ulery *et al.*, 2011).

4.6.4   POLYVINYL ALCOHOL (PVA)

A synthetic polymer that is biocompatible, expandable, and water-soluble is called polyvinyl alcohol (PVA) (Goyanes *et al.*, 2016 and Morita *et al.*, 2000). It also has a Tg of 85 °C, melting points between 180 and 228 °C (Goole *et al.*, 2016 and Konta *et al.*, 2017). It acts as a thermoplastic polymer as well. FDM makes extensive use of it (Gupta *et al.*, 2011). PVA dissolves more easily in hydrochloric acid, making it appropriate for immediate-release tablets.

4.6.5 CARBOPOL

Crosslinked polyacrylic acid polymers with high molecular weight are known as carbopol® homopolymers (Azad *et al.*, 2020). Alkyl sucrose or allyl pentaerythritol are used for cross-linking. PAM 3DP is compatible with Carbopol® 971P and 974P. Carbopol® 971P is a slightly crosslinked polymer with a viscosity range of 4000–11,000 cP (0.5 wt% suspension), and it flows like honey in a semi-solid formulation (Azad *et al.*, 2020). It is appropriate for suspension, oral liquids, and controlled-release tablets. Known for producing exceptionally viscous gels, Carbopol® 974P is a strongly crosslinked polymer (Ulery *et al.*, 2011).

4.7 CONCLUSION

3DP has significantly increased in tissue engineering over the past decade due to the invention of new materials. Extrusion-based 3DP, or fused deposition modeling, was first invented by S. Scott Crump in 1988 to create a toy for his daughter. The major extrusion-based 3DP approaches are SSE and FDM. SSE is a versatile approach for bio-printing, allowing for the creation of pharmacological dosage forms without higher temperatures SSE-based 3DP has been used in tissue engineering, organ repair, preoperative surgical treatment planning, disease models, and vascular micro fabrication. It has also been used to create pharmacological dosage forms, such as immediate-release tablets and cancer patches for local drug delivery. FDM, a 3D additive manufacturing method, is now being applied to the pharmaceutical industry due to improvements in filament manufacturing and the broad range of substances that can be printed on FDM printers. The most recent findings about the association of pharmaceutical 3DP technology demonstrate that it is still in its early stages and that its full potential has not yet been realized. It is projected that the pharmaceutical industry will use 3DP as a scalable, digital technology to create completed drug products with unique dosages and patient-specific drug-release characteristics. It is anticipated that shortly, small-scale customized medication manufacturing will replace mass production using conventional manufacturing techniques thanks to 3D technology.

REFERENCES

Algahtani MS, Mohammed AA, Ahmad J. Extrusion-based 3D printing for pharmaceuticals: Contemporary research and applications. *Current Pharmaceutical Design*. 2018 Nov 1;24(42):4991–5008.

Azad MA, Olawuni D, Kimbell G, Badruddoza AZ, Hossain MS, Sultana T. Polymers for extrusion-based 3D printing of pharmaceuticals: A holistic materials–process perspective. *Pharmaceutics*. 2020 Feb 3;12(2):124.

Cellulosics D. Ethocel Ethylcellulose Polymers Technical Handbook. Dow Chemical Company. 2005 Sep.

Choonara YE, du Toit LC, Kumar P, Kondiah PP, Pillay V. 3D-printing and the effect on medical costs: A new era?. *Expert Review of Pharmacoeconomics & Outcomes Research*. 2016 Jan 2;16(1):23–32.

Deshpande RD, Gowda DV, Mahammed N, Maramwar DN. Bi-layer tablets-An emerging trend: A review. *International Journal of Pharmaceutical Sciences and Research*. 2011 Oct 1;2(10):2534.

Firth J, Basit AW, Gaisford S. The role of semi-solid extrusion printing in clinical practice. *3D Printing of Pharmaceuticals*. 2018;31:133–151.

Fitzgerald S. FDA approves first 3D-printed epilepsy drug experts assess the benefits and caveats. *Neurology Today*. 2015 Sep 17;15(18):26–7.

Fu J, Yu X, Jin Y. 3D printing of vaginal rings with personalized shapes for controlled release of progesterone. *International Journal of Pharmaceutics*. 2018 Mar 25;539(1–2):75–82.

Goole J, Amighi K. 3D printing in pharmaceutics: A new tool for designing customized drug delivery systems. *International Journal of Pharmaceutics*. 2016 Feb 29;499(1–2):376–94.

Goyanes A, Chang H, Sedough D, Hatton GB, Wang J, Buanz A, Gaisford S, Basit AW. Fabrication of controlled-release budesonide tablets via desktop (FDM) 3D printing. *International Journal of Pharmaceutics*. 2015 Dec 30;496(2):414–20.

Goyanes A, Det-Amornrat U, Wang J, Basit AW, Gaisford S. 3D scanning and 3D printing as innovative technologies for fabricating personalized topical drug delivery systems. *Journal of Controlled Release*. 2016 Jul 28;234:41–8.

Goyanes A, Fernández-Ferreiro A, Majeed A, Gomez-Lado N, Awad A, Luaces-Rodríguez A, Gaisford S, Aguiar P, Basit AW. PET/CT imaging of 3D printed devices in the gastrointestinal tract of rodents. *International Journal of Pharmaceutics*. 2018 Jan 30;536(1):158–64.

Goyanes A, Kobayashi M, Martínez-Pacheco R, Gaisford S, Basit AW. Fused-filament 3D printing of drug products: Microstructure analysis and drug release characteristics of PVA-based caplets. *International Journal of Pharmaceutics*. 2016 Nov 30;514(1):290–5.

Gross BC, Erkal JL, Lockwood SY, Chen C, Spence DM. Evaluation of 3D printing and its potential impact on biotechnology and the chemical sciences. *Analytical Chemistry*. 2014;86:3240–3253.

Gupta S, Webster TJ, Sinha A. Evolution of PVA gels prepared without crosslinking agents as a cell adhesive surface. *Journal of Materials Science: Materials in Medicine*. 2011 Jul;22:1763–72.

Heath JR, Davis ME. Nanotechnology and cancer. *Annual Review of Medicine*. 2008; 59:251–65.

Holländer J, Genina N, Jukarainen H, Khajeheian M, Rosling A, Mäkilä E, Sandler N. Three-dimensional printed PCL-based implantable prototypes of medical devices for controlled drug delivery. *Journal of Pharmaceutical Sciences*. 2016 Sep 1;105(9):2665–76.

Jang J, Yi HG, Cho DW. 3D printed tissue models: Present and future. *ACS Biomaterials Science & Engineering*. 2016 Oct 10;2(10):1722–31.

Jivraj M, Martini LG, Thomson CM. An overview of the different excipients useful for the direct compression of tablets. *Pharmaceutical Science & Technology Today*. 2000 Feb 1;3(2):58–63.

Kaialy W, Larhrib H, Chikwanha B, Shojaee S, Nokhodchi A. An approach to engineer paracetamol crystals by antisolvent crystallization technique in presence of various additives for direct compression. *International Journal of Pharmaceutics*. 2014 Apr 10;464(1–2):53–64.

Katstra WE, Palazzolo RD, Rowe CW, Giritlioglu B, Teung P, Cima MJ. Oral dosage forms fabricated by Three Dimensional Printing™. *Journal of Controlled Release*. 2000 May 3;66(1):1–9.

Kempin W, Domsta V, Grathoff G, Brecht I, Semmling B, Tillmann S, Weitschies W, Seidlitz A. Immediate release 3D-printed tablets produced via fused deposition modeling of a thermo-sensitive drug. *Pharmaceutical Research*. 2018 Jun;35:1–2.

Kempin W, Franz C, Koster LC, Schneider F, Bogdahn M, Weitschies W, Seidlitz A. Assessment of different polymers and drug loads for fused deposition modeling of drug loaded implants. *European Journal of Pharmaceutics and Biopharmaceutics*. 2017 Jun 1;115:84–93.

Khaled SA, Alexander MR, Wildman RD, Wallace MJ, Sharpe S, Yoo J, Roberts CJ. 3D extrusion printing of high drug loading immediate release paracetamol tablets. *International Journal of Pharmaceutics*. 2018 Mar 1;538(1–2):223–30.

Khaled SA, Burley JC, Alexander MR, Yang J, Roberts CJ. 3D printing of tablets containing multiple drugs with defined release profiles. *International Journal of Pharmaceutics*. 2015 Oct 30;494(2):643–50.

Khaled SA, Burley JC, Alexander MR, Yang J, Roberts CJ. 3D printing of five-in-one dose combination polypill with defined immediate and sustained release profiles. *Journal of Controlled Release*. 2015 Nov 10;217:308–14.

Khaled SA, Burley JC, Alexander MR, Roberts CJ. Desktop 3D printing of controlled release pharmaceutical bilayer tablets. *International Journal of Pharmaceutics*. 2014 Jan 30;461(1–2):105–11.

Khalil S, Nam J, Sun W. Multi-nozzle deposition for construction of 3D biopolymer tissue scaffolds. *Rapid Prototyping Journal*. 2005 Feb 1;11(1):9–17.

Konta AA, García-Piña M, Serrano DR. Personalised 3D printed medicines: Which techniques and polymers are more successful?. *Bioengineering*. 2017 Sep 22;4(4):79.

Lammers T, Peschke P, Kühnlein R, Subr V, Ulbrich K, Huber P, Hennink W, Storm G. Effect of intratumoral injection on the biodistribution, the therapeutic potential of HPMA copolymer-based drug delivery systems. *Neoplasia*. 2006 Oct 1;8(10):788–95.

Li Q, Guan X, Cui M, Zhu Z, Chen K, Wen H, Jia D, Hou J, Xu W, Yang X, Pan W. Preparation and investigation of novel gastro-floating tablets with 3D extrusion-based printing. *International Journal of Pharmaceutics*. 2018 Jan 15;535(1–2):325–32.

Lim SH, Kathuria H, Tan JJ, Kang L. 3D printed drug delivery and testing systems—a passing fad or the future?. *Advanced Drug Delivery Reviews*. 2018 Jul 1;132:139–68.

Malheiro A, Wieringa P, Mota C, Baker M, Moroni L. Patterning vasculature: The role of biofabrication to achieve an integrated multicellular ecosystem. *ACS Biomaterials Science & Engineering*. 2016 Oct 10;2(10):1694–709.

Matijašić G, Gretić M, Vinčić J, Poropat A, Cuculić L, Rahelić T. Design and 3D printing of multi-compartmental PVA capsules for drug delivery. *Journal of Drug Delivery Science and Technology*. 2019 Aug 1;52:677–86.

Morita R, Honda R, Takahashi Y. Development of oral controlled release preparations, a PVA swelling controlled release system (SCRS): I. Design of SCRS and its release controlling factor. *Journal of Controlled Release*. 2000 Feb 3;63(3):297–304.

Novakova-Marcincinova L. Application of fused deposition modeling technology in 3D printing rapid prototyping area. *Manufacturing and Industry Engineering*. 2012;11(4):35–7.

Ozbolat IT, Hospodiuk M. Current advances and future perspectives in extrusion-based bioprinting. *Biomaterials*. 2016 Jan 1;76:321–43.

Panigrahi M, Das PK, Parikh PM. Brain tumor and Gliadel wafer treatment. *Indian Journal of Cancer*. 2011 Jan 1;48(1):11–7.

Pawar VK, Kansal S, Garg G, Awasthi R, Singodia D, Kulkarni GT. Gastroretentive dosage forms: A review with special emphasis on floating drug delivery systems. *Drug Delivery*. 2011 Feb 1;18(2):97–110.

Picker-Freyer KM, Dürig T. Physical mechanical and tablet formation properties of hydroxypropylcellulose: In pure form and in mixtures. *AAPS PharmSciTech*. 2007;8:82.

Ploch CC, Mansi CS, Jayamohan J, Kuhl E. Using 3D printing to create personalized brain models for neurosurgical training and preoperative planning. *World Neurosurgery*. 2016 Jun 1;90:668–74.

Prasad LK, Smyth H. 3D printing technologies for drug delivery: A review. *Drug Development and Industrial Pharmacy*. 2016 Jul 2;42(7):1019–31.

Roberts ER, Green D, Kadam UT. Chronic condition comorbidity and multidrug therapy in general practice populations: A cross-sectional linkage study. *BMJ Open*. 2014 Jul 1;4(7):e005429.

Rowe CW, Katstra WE, Palazzolo RD, Giritlioglu B, Teung P, Cima MJ. Multimechanism oral dosage forms fabricated by three dimensional printing™. *Journal of Controlled Release*. 2000 May 3;66(1):11–7.

Sadia M, Arafat B, Ahmed W, Forbes RT, Alhnan MA. Channelled tablets: An innovative approach to accelerating drug release from 3D printed tablets. *Journal of Controlled Release*. 2018 Jan 10;269:355–63.

Sadia M, Isreb A, Abbadi I, Isreb M, Aziz D, Selo A, Timmins P, Alhnan MA. From 'fixed dose combinations' to 'a dynamic dose combiner': 3D printed bi-layer antihypertensive tablets. *European Journal of Pharmaceutical Sciences*. 2018 Oct 15;123:484–94.

Skowyra J, Pietrzak K, Alhnan MA. Fabrication of extended-release patient-tailored prednisolone tablets via fused deposition modelling (FDM) 3D printing. *European Journal of Pharmaceutical Sciences*. 2015 Feb 20;68:11–7.

Thakral S, Thakral NK, Majumdar DK. Eudragit®: A technology evaluation. Expert Opinion on Drug Delivery. 2013 Jan 1;10(1):131–49.

Tucker GT. Personalized drug dosage–closing the loop. *Pharmaceutical Research*. 2017 Aug;34(8):1539–43..

Ulery BD, Nair LS, Laurencin CT. Biomedical applications of biodegradable polymers. *Journal of Polymer Science Part B: Polymer Physics*. 2011 Jun 15;49(12):832–64.

Ventola CL. Medical applications for 3D printing: Current and projected uses. *Pharmacy and Therapeutics*. 2014 Oct;39(10):704.

Weisman JA, Nicholson JC, Tappa K, Jammalamadaka U, Wilson CG, Mills DK. Antibiotic and chemotherapeutic enhanced three-dimensional printer filaments and constructs for biomedical applications. *International Journal of Nanomedicine*. 2015;10:357.

Yi HG, Choi YJ, Kang KS, Hong JM, Pati RG, Park MN, Shim IK, Lee CM, Kim SC, Cho DW. A 3D-printed local drug delivery patch for pancreatic cancer growth suppression. *Journal of Controlled Release*. 2016 Sep 28;238:231–41.

Zhang YS, Duchamp M, Oklu R, Ellisen LW, Langer R, Khademhosseini A. Bioprinting the cancer microenvironment. *ACS Biomaterials Science & Engineering*. 2016 Oct 10;2(10):1710–21.

Zidan A, Alayoubi A, Coburn J, Asfari S, Ghammraoui B, Cruz CN, Ashraf M. Extrudability analysis of drug loaded pastes for 3D printing of modified release tablets. *International Journal of Pharmaceutics*. 2019 Jan 10;554:292–301.

ZipDose Technology, Spritam, Aprecia. 2018. Available from: www.aprecia.com/technology/zipdose.

5 Extrusion-Based 3D Printing Technology

A Revolution in Pharmaceutical Drug Manufacturing

Kiranmai Mandava, Sneha Thakur, Keerthi Kadimcharla, and Prakash Katakam

5.1 INTRODUCTION

Additive manufacturing (AM) technology, popularly 3D printing, is described as "the process of deforming materials into 3D model data generally through layered fashion which is layer upon layer" (Norman *et al.*, 2017). The AM technology is categorized into three types relying on the physical identity of raw material at the beginning of AM, such as solid (filament, wire, or others), paste (a suspension of granular material), granules and powder. Extrusion-based AM technology (EB3D printing) is a user-friendly set up suitable in microscale even with low-cost investment and energy (Firth *et al.*, 2018, Trenfield *et al.*, 2018). As a result, this technology has wide acceptance in diversified sectors right from amateurs to large-scale producers of industry. The popular EB3D techniques include layered construction of 3D prototypes and parts with most intricate and embedded designs (Gonzalez-Gutierrez *et al.*, 2018). EB3D technique entails nozzle extrusion of material that are using a piston or plunger equipped with a screw system for venting hot material where feed stock is thus reducing viscosity sufficiently feeding out (Rutz *et al.*, 2015, Jung *et al.*, 2016). Recent advancements in EB3D printing during the last decade include sophistication of friendly printing materials, and sophisticated AM capacity for large printing and heading towards high temperatures for capacitative building and expansion of huge print-head temperatures and for acquiring faster building with wide expansion of various feedstock material for improvement of printed integrity of layered parts (Lee *et al.*, 2017). EB3D printing has potential acceptance in aerospace, building, medical, food technology, and power sectors as well (Liu *et al.*, 2017). Biomaterials are proving advancement in a quick fashion compared to other material classes due to strong demand from the healthcare industry (Sears *et al.*, 2017). For example, the 100 $ billion market will be foreseen by skin bioprinting between 2018and 2040 (Li *et al.*, 2021). This techniques encompasses the production of goods from a variety materials, such as polymers, food materials, solid construction

DOI: 10.1201/9781003439509-8

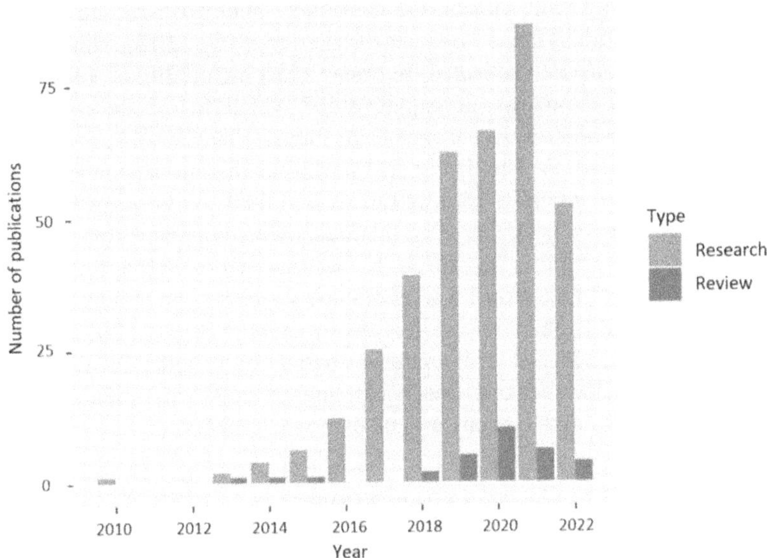

FIGURE 5.1 Contribution of high-impact publications each year in EB3D technology. (Altıparmak *et al.,* 2022.)

materials, photo-polymers, ceramics, biocompatible, and biomaterials (Altıparmak *et al.,* 2022). Figure 5.1 elaborates the results of research work done on/by the Scopus Database scholarly search and presents the reviews and research papers in each of the utility modes, materials, and developments of EB3D printing. Many efforts can be put forward on the comprehensive research (Figure 5.1) of the methodology to prove the capacity of using EB3D printing for novel drug therapeutics and other AM constructing processes (Hospodiuk *et al.,* 2018). Figure 5.1 shows the research work analysis relevant to the Scopus bibliographic study of impactful publications, which is cited as it enhances EB3D advantages and its application in therapeutics.

5.2 FUNDAMENTALS OF EXTRUSION-BASED 3D PRINTING (EB3D)

Advancements in AM technology or EB3D (approved as ISO/ASTM 52900:2015) have identified EB3D printing as a solid state AM processhas been widely adopted for easy use, precision, design of complex geometries with CAD, multiple solidification of polymeric materials (Norman *et al.,* 2017). This high-performance technique was operational in 1990 though patented in 1980 (Firth *et al.,* 2018). EB3D printing involves both fusion deposition melting (FDM) and pressure-assisted microsyringe (PAM) in the fabrication of hollow products that are suitable to pharmaceutical manufacturing (Trenfield *et al.,* 2018). The growing research interest in EB3D printing has contributed 45% of impactful publications from2015to date. The polymers involved in the fabrication are versatile in designing solid-state pharmaceuticals pertaining to API with functional excipient and polymers. Accurate polymeric consistency is obtained by mixing with solvent and extruding using syringe with mechanical, pneumatic, or solenoid systems (Gonzalez-Gutierrez *et al.*, 2018), which involve a curing step (chemical/photo activated) to ensure biocompatibility of a large number of materials. The entire process is computer aided, which reduces the cost, time, and labor and exploits modalities to enhance clear imaging in MRI, CT, and ultrasound printing (Rutz *et al.*, 2015). The rheological properties that influence the EB3D phenomenon indeed have an effect on drug release and final solid dosage forms. These include, density, specific heat, viscosity, thermal conductivity, and alpha main relaxation of polymers (Tagami *et al.*, 2019a, b, Goyanes *et al.*, 2015a, b). Rheological tests include flow test, thixotropic test, amplitude sweep test and yield stress, which affects the processibility and fabrication of the structure (Lee *et al.*, 2012). Figure 5.2 shows the various mechanisms of extrusion-based 3D printing involving various types of polymeric and other materials depending on the process parameters, which are functional in deciding the geometry and extrusion process.

5.2.1 Fusion Deposition Modeling (FDM)

It is a simple and versatile 3D printing technique utilized in pharmaceuticals and bioengineered foods. FDM operates on the principle of depositing layered solid material over a plate by extruding the melted thermoplastic polymer through a high-temperature nozzle (Infanger *et al.*, 2019). Figure 5.2 demonstrates an FDM printer working a principle printer. The API in the pharmaceuticals is admixed with the thermoplastic polymer using a suitable solvent and melted together at certain temperature before extrusion onto the filament board. This low-cost manufacturing process offers complex geometries in designing pharmaceuticals with high mechanical strength that offers less resistance to drug release (Table 5.1). The limitation with high-temperature decomposition can be overcome with use of biodegradable polymers with low viscosity (Lee *et al.*, 2017). Two types of working principles that are used in FDM printing based on the drive are Bowden type and direct ink type, which are detailed below:

- Bowden type: the printer head is small and present at the extrusion point, which is decoupled from the moving hot point that mobilizes the filament using the Bowden tube. Due to the less distance between the extrusion and hot end point, there is disturbance in the filament distribution, which is a limitation for flexible filament materials.
- Direct ink printing: the extruder is directly placed over the printer head that decreases the distance between and lays down a short filament path, enabling usage of flexible filament materials.

5.2.2 Pressure-Assisted Microsyringe (PAM)

PAM is also a nozzle-based system (Table 5.2) for deposition of layers with viscous and semi-liquid materials that are extruded from microsyringes (Liu W *et al.*, 2017, Li *et al.*, 2021). The syringe is similar to the printer head, which moves to and fro and the half of the liquid fluidic is extruded using air under pressure. The microstructure

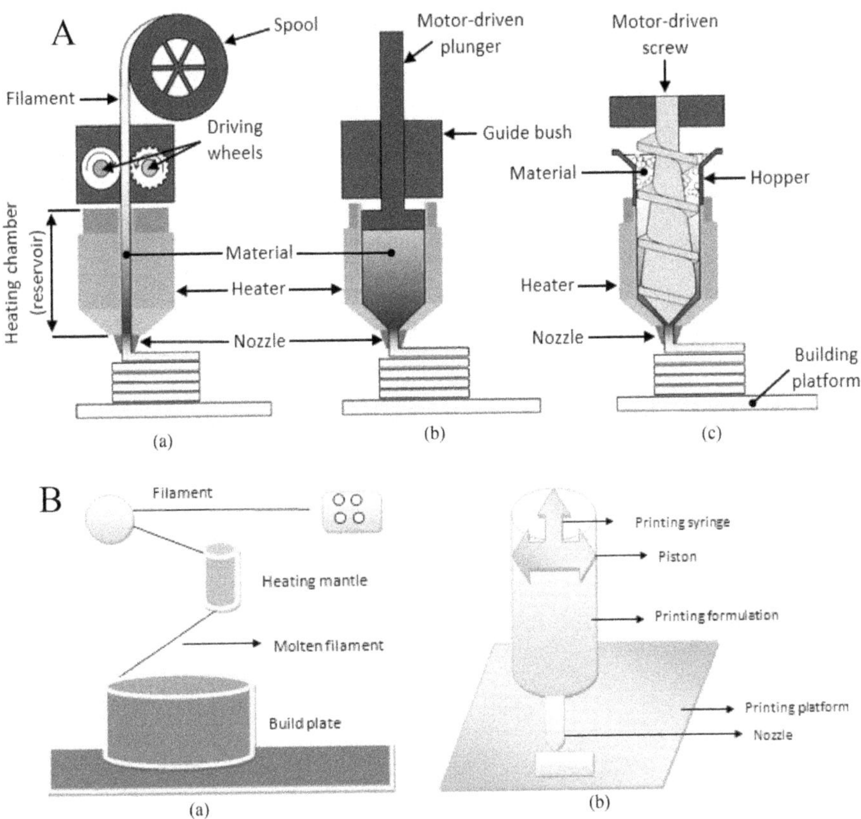

FIGURE 5.2 (A) Types of extrusion-based systems with syringe systems like (a) filament type, (b) syringe type or plunged, (c) screw based. (B) Working principle of EB3D printers (a) FDM printer, (b) pressure-assisted micro-syringe system. (Gonzalez-Gutierrez *et al.*, 2018.)

layer has a thickness of less than 5–10μ allowing the fabrication of complex drug-delivery systems with an advantage over conventional methods due to its continuous operation mode at room temperature (Sears *et al.*, 2017). The hindrance is choice of suitable solvents during manufacturing. The latest modification as PAM is rapid process using a motor stepper to extrude polymer instead of compressed air. The factors that influence the process are reported in Table 5.3. Tables 5.1, 5.2 and 5.3 have been demonstrative to make observations on the strategic working of printer, process parameters sensible to suit the materials and device novel geometries. The parameters have been listed after analyzing the information from relevant publication works and inputs have been tabulated for better understanding.

5.3 EXCIPIENT AND DRUG FORMULATIONS

The 3D extrusion based printing has expanded wide applications in drug delivery. Following are the examples with applications (Table 5.4). EB3D printing has a

TABLE 5.1

Various Processes Involved in AM Manufacturing by EB3D Printing Mechanisms

Sr. No.	Extrusion AM Process	Principle	Limitation	Advantage
1	FDM	The process is conducted in a closed insulated thermal chamber maintained at constant processing temperature in order to produce high mechanical strength, layer adhesion.	Number of layers are limited	Most common method
2	Fusion filament fabrication (FFF) modified extruders of the FFF syringe FFF Ram FFF	Preheated process compartment is entangled with deposition material to propose uniform deposition	Build size	Widely used, low cost
3	Screw-based FDM	The extrusion of hardened material is layered by means of rotating screw	Enhanced material flow	Widely used for hard materials

TABLE 5.2

Types of EB3D Printers Based on the FDM Principle

Sr. No	Type	Resolution (μ)	Extrusion Aid	Advantages
1	Pneumatic	250–330	Compressed air supplier which is connected to a syringe barrel mediated by an on/off valve	High precision, specialized for low viscous bioinks, hydrogels and rapid extrusion
2	Mechanical	100–1200	Mechanical force applied on syringe (piston/screw based)	Simpler process, offers spatial flow with screw and controlled flow by piston mechanisms, rapid process, cheap and easy to maintain
3	Solenoid	200–450	Electrical pulse system connected to a syringe to open and close the valve	Use is limited due to less reproducibility and uneven deposition of material

Sources: Altıparmak *et al.* (2022); Hospodiuk *et al.* (2018).

TABLE 5.3
The Factors That Influence the Extrusion-Printed Scaffolds

Classification	Factors	References
Process based	Radius of nozzle orifice	Tagami *et al.,* 2019
	Heat condition	Goyanes *et al.,* 2015a, b
	Rate of cooling	Lee *et al.,* 2012
	Pressure of extrusion	Infanger *et al.,* 2019
	Traveling rate	Boehm *et al.,* 2014
	Cad module	
	Feeding rate	
	Feed stock fill %	
	Layered spacing	
Material based	Material type	Infanger *et al.,* 2019
	Physical properties	Boehm *et al.,* 2014
	Plasticizer properties	
	Polymer/API ratio,	
	Radial link.	
	Solvent used	

wide acceptance of excipients and application. In the realm of bioelectronics, SSE 3D printing is gaining popularity, especially for the creation of biosensors that can measure physiological data or as a way to start the release of drugs from medical devices. SSE is particularly pertinent for bioprinting applications because of the design constraints of the feedstock material. The syringes (disposable) and cartridges (pre filled) are used in EB3D technology, which help it to achieve the crucial quality standards required by regulatory agencies. SSE extrusion printer with the aid of CAD software converts into STL file and then printed. There can be multiple changes that can be incorporated before the final stage of printing by simply changing the CAD file. Exclusive technology for developing novel NCE and enhancing market designs is Hot-melt extrusion (HME) especially for BCS class II drugs. The fact that many patents and publications till recent times have listed HME technology as a revolutionary pharmaceutical formulation method which shows that it also provides a chance to acquire intellectual property (Huang *et al.,* 2010). FDM is one of the advanced and widely exploited AM techniques. Using the FDM technique, polymers, polymer matrix composites (PMC), bio-composites or polymer ceramic composites (PCC), nanocomposites, and fiber-reinforced composites (FRC) all can be prototyped. The most widely used polymers are reported in Table 5.4. Further the FDM technique allows for the incorporation of a wide variety of reinforcement elements like graphene, carbon nanotubes iron fillers and copper (Wickramasinghe *et al.,* 2020). Table 5.4 demonstrates the novel drug formulations and its application formulated based on the type extrusion modeling working principle subjected. Furthermore, the advantages of the various types of extrusion methods has improved the bioavailability, therapeutic efficacy, and the release pattern of the dosage forms based on the type of excipient profile.

TABLE 5.4
Application of EB3D Printing in Drug Delivery Systems

Sr. No.	Type of Extrusion Technique	Excipient	Drug Formulation	Application	Reference
1	3D extrusion	HPMC K4M, HPMC E15, MCC PH101	Gastro-retentive tablets (8h floating)	Improved bioavailability and therapeutic efficacy	Haleem *et al.,* 2021
2	Semi-solid material extrusion	Hypromellose (HPMC), sugar alcohols (mannitol, xylitol)	Lyophilized ophthalmologic patches	Personalized multiple drugs were incorporated	Li *et al.,* 2018
3	HME and FDM	PVA	Topical or transdermal drug delivery.	Increased swallowing in pediatric, geriatric and dysphagia	Tagami *et al.,* 2022
4	FDM	PVA	ASA or 5-ASA	Modified release	Goyanes *et al.,* 2015a, b
5	FDM	PVA	Budesonide Caplets	Controlled release	Goyanes *et al.,* 2015a, b

5.4 PHARMACEUTICAL APPLICATIONS OF EXTRUSION-BASED 3D PRINTING

5.4.1 Personalized Medicine and Dosage Forms

The FDM technology was used to make improved release (IR) tablets, most likely due to its ease of fabrication (Infanger *et al.,* 2019, Katakam *et al.,* 2015). The FDM technology was used to successfully construct a low-dose dosage form made of thermoplastic polyurethane and loaded with 60% medication. An EB3D printer was used to create the IR tablet, which contained an extremely high dose of 80% paracetamol. Using an EB3D printer was also used to generate three near controlled zero release p-ephedrine HCl formulation. The API release rates were altered with different proportions of HPMC and Kollidon while keeping production parameters constant. The ability of EB3D to produce gastro retentive tablet formulations has also demonstrated a high correlation (Park *et al.,* 2021). Poly pills were created for the treatment of patients with diabetes who have hypertension, a polypill comprising nifedipine, captopril, and glipizide was created using EB3D printing (Derossi *et al.*, 2017). This polymer tablet contained sustained-release compartments for nifedipine, glipizide, and captopril as well as an osmotic compartment in which captopril was active. The connecting layer of the polymer pill instantly disintegrates after being swallowed, resulting in the separation of the captopril polymer pill's and release zone. The release zones have glipizide and nifedipine drugs diffusing from the layered gels that remained constant, while the designed captopril with zero-order kinetics based on osmotic pressure via porous shell with controlled release. A strong association between their *in vitro* dissolving profiles and pharmacokinetics at clinical level was also shown by the potential of EB3D printing to create gastro-floating tablet formulations. Thus tailored drug formulations with different release profiles were obtained. Further, the five API poly pill was also synthesized using a 3D extrusion printer.

5.4.2 NOVEL DRUG DELIVERY SYSTEMS

EB3D printing has wide applications as it conducts the spatial deposition of various biopolymers (Karavasili *et al.*, 2020). The sequential release of drugs with high therapeutic index were designed by PLGA core structures with alginate sheath for model drugs such as flourescien and rhodamine (hydrophilic and hydrophobic) (Silva *et al.*, 2022). Implants of human skin models have been synthesized that addresses the tissue rejection problem as donors will not be hindering necessarily, customized skin or tissue models of humans would cut skin transplantation waiting periods (Wickramasinghe *et al.*, 2020). Complex tissue that scaffolds for bone TB therapy were produced using 3D printers for bone defect healing by mixing calcium phosphate cement in combination with hydrogel strands containing vascular endothelial growth factor (VEGF)-loaded (Jang *et al.*, 2021).

5.4.3 POINT-OF-CARE MANUFACTURING AND DECENTRALIZED DRUG PRODUCTION

The EB3D technology for polymeric microneedles with complicated geometries, created by combining EB3D-based hydrogel using casting or deformative procedures (Seiti *et al.*, 2023). The EB3D technique substantially increased the resolution limit of EB3D printing by producing micro-needles with sharp tips of 9.6 m or radius of curvature, utilized for vaccine distribution (Abo El-Enin *et al.*, 2022). CLIP (continuous liquid interface production) has also been created to form 3D constructs like triangles, pillars, and numerous complex constructs utilizing photo reactive resin and UV light. Recent improvements in EB3D technology laid the speedy production of bio-mimetic constructions. It would take the place of preclinical animal models at various phases of the development of novel drugs. Additionally, it has been proposed that 3DP technology might be used to develop DNA biosensors that are more selective against a DNA target that is not complimentary (Reddy & Sharma, 2020).

5.5   MATERIAL SELECTION AND FORMULATION CONSIDERATIONS

5.5.1   Criteria for Selecting Printable Materials

Printable material is the one that has a character, which allows the matter to be handled by stability of design and ability owing to its weight. In EB3D printing, printable material needs to comply with specific printable characteristics like pressure-driven extrusion flow, bead formation, and its functionality of the component (Seiti *et al.*, 2023). Along with these specified characteristics, printable materials shall fit into any given printable model.The viscoelastic model is one such model where printable materials are classified based on processing parameters like deposition temperature, shear rate, flow rate, head speed, nozzle diameter, etc. Four types of printable materials described here are elastic solids, viscoelastic solids, viscoelastic liquids, and viscous liquids. Key parameters used to assess printability are rheology (Reddy & Sharma, 2020), material composition and concentration, computer simulation/modeling, nozzle variables, grid geometry, resolution, pore and filament dimensions, shape fidelity and its correlation with printing angle and concentration of oxygen in 3D printing environment.

5.5.2   Optimization of Drug Formulation for EB3D Printing

Various optimization techniques have been reported for drug formulations using EB3DP. Table 5.5 reports the various optimization techniques in EB3D printing for various manufactureddrug formulations.

5.5.3   Drug-Excipient Compatibility

Drug-excipient compatibility is the prerequisite for any novel drug-dosage system (NDDS). Fabrication of these NDDS using EB3D printing shall be studied under three categories, one is SSE, the second is FDM, and the third technique is melt extrusion

---

TABLE 5.5

Optimization Techniques in EB3D Printing for Drug Formulations

Sr. No.	Optimization Technique	Advantages/Details	Reference
1	Quality by design (QbD)	Egglets which are immediate release and abuse deterrent	Nukala *et al.*, 2019
2	Statistical design	Impact of formulation excipient on drug release	Tian *et al.*, 2021
3	Multi-stage optimization	Fabrication of bone tissue scaffolds	Yang *et al.*, 2017
4	Machine learning (ML) assisted optimization	Graphical user interface/ industrial enabled	Rahmani *et al.*, 2022
5	Pressure-assisted microsyringe-polarity optimization	Shell design for drug (paste) delivery/personalized medicine	Mohammed *et al.*, 2021

TABLE 5.6
API–Excipient Compatibility in Novel Drug Dosage Forms using EB3D

Sr. No.	API	Excipients	NDDS	Reference
1	5-Fluorouracil	Polycaprolactone, PLGA	Biodegradable local patch for controlled release	Shim *et al.,* 2017
2	Ciprofloxacin HCl	HPC, POLYOXTM, WSR N10 (resin)	Occular inserts (coupling hot melt extrusion)	Alzahrani *et al.,* 2023
3	Paracetamol	Eudragit, Soluplus, PVPVA, PVA	Solid dosage forms-binary mixtures, solid dosage forms-binary mixtures	Silva*et al.,* 2022, Mahato & Narang, 2019
4	Metaprolol tartrate	Eudragit, Soluplus, PVPVA, PVA	1.	2.

deposition (MED). Analytical tools like differential exploratory calorimetry (Wang *et al.*, 2021), and derivative thermo gravimetric analysis are reliable ones to assess compatibility between API and excipient in formulation stage I (preformulation) studies. Compatibility (Table 5.6) can be rationally explored using 3D printing optimization techniques. Pharmaceutical polymers (HPC, Eudragit RS, Kollidon VA64 (PVP/VA), Soluplus (SLP), RL (EuRL) and disintegrants, cross carmellose sodium, crospovidone, sodium starch glycolate, low substituted hydroxyl propyl cellulose and microcrystalline cellulose compatibility validated step wise by HME and FDM (Mwema *et al.*, 2020). Table 5.6 functionalizes the API–excipient compatibility of a few commercial marketed formulations using EB3D printing and respective novel drug delivery systems, which have been derived based on the combinations.

5.5.4 RHEOLOGICAL PROPERTIES OF FORMULATIONS

Nowadays, a pressure-assisted microsyringe is employed in pharmaceutical applications. EB3D printing is generally relying on a pneumatic, solenoid, and mechanical piston. Optimized mixture of functional ingredients, polymers, solvent, and other excipients having necessary rheological properties that can make a semi-solid and it is suitable for 3D printing. Polymer rheology factors show influence on structure (rectilinear, hexagonal, or honeycomb) formation and the process of printing. Another important technique of 3D printing is FDM 3D printingto achieve an optimum ability to process, and printed filaments need to have suitable rheological and mechanical properties (Alzahrani A *et al.*, 2023, Long *et al.*, 2019). Being an important rheological property viscosity, yield stress in compression and shear, as well as viscoelastic characteristics shall play a significant role in getting reproducibility of 3D structural designs. Viscosity is largely dependent on temperature. Typically, high temperatures are employed in FDM 3D modeling of pharmaceuticals (Shahrjerdi *et al.*, 2023, Chakka *et al.*, 2023). Low to optimal temperatures with an increase in viscosity were tried by a few researchers. There is still some ambiguity that exists in exploring the proper correlations with respect to printing capacity. High temperature causes thermal degradation whereas lower than optimal temperature causes nozzle block and low bond strength between layers (Mwema *et al.*, 2020).

5.5.5 STABILITY AND DEGRADATION CONSIDERATIONS

Drug formulations are intended to be designedand can get the maximum physico-chemical nature in terms of stability of the API contained therein, in correlation with bioavailability and manufacturing constraints. The research functionalizes around the molecular structure and process formulation parameters; but also to develop functional mechanistic aspects like its causes, which helps designing mitigation constraints for development and commercialization of product (Long *et al.*, 2019). In 3D printing using API, drug product stability is an area of focus on the availability (Mahato & Narang 2017) and dosage form manufacturability. In this context, drug product instability is an area of focused research not only due to the diversity in molecular structure and formulation variables; but also in the development of fundamental mechanistic aspects like its causes, which help in designing mitigation strategies for successful drug product development and commercialization (Long *et al.*, 2019). Stability of vascularization network within the bioinks (Cui *et al.*, 2021) is another concern to obtain the long-term effect from biomaterials. The phase transition that happens in the filament material as a result of heating it (above the melting point), melting it in the nozzle, and then resolidifying it after feed stock extrusion. Elevated temperatures can lead to polymer degradation, which can result in thermally unstable flaws and structural alterations from random cleavages or depolymerization. Chain breakage, increased viscosity, and decreased molecular weight are the thermo-mechanical degradation effects that may occur under the influence of high temperatures. Polymer deterioration (due to photochemical, thermal, and hydrolytic causes) may take place even while employing printouts (Pugliese *et al.*, 2021). The material's characteristics and structure are impacted by this. It is crucial to assess the thermal stability of polymers. A heated sample's constant rate of mass change can be evaluated with the aid of thermo gravimetric analysis (TGA) (Ding *et al.*, 2019). TGA helps to ascertain the initial degradation temperature and the thermal stability of the tested polymer's volatile component fractions. Commercial filaments for 3D printers generally made of nylon, polylactic acid (PLA), polyethylene terephthalate (PET), and acrylonitrile butadiene styrene (ABS), must undergo thermal degradation studies (Cao *et al.*, 2023, Beltrán *et al.*, 2019).

5.6 REGULATORY REQUIREMENTS FOR 3D PRINTING TECHNOLOGY: ENSURING SAFETY, QUALITY, AND COMPLIANCE

In the recent years, the EB3D technique has a wide acceptance in various industries such as healthcare and pharmaceuticals. This innovative manufacturing technique holds great promise for constructing personalized medicine, complex formulations, and devices of medical importance (Katakam *et al.*, 2015). However, the unique characteristics of 3D printing raise important regulatory considerations to ensure patient safety, product quality, and compliance with established regulations (Abo

El-Enin *et al.*, 2022). There are specific guidelines solely focused on 3D printing of pharmaceuticals that have not been issued by regulatory agencies. However, several existing regulatory frameworks and guidelines provide insights into how manufacturing pharmaceuticals utilizing 3D printing should approach regulatory compliance Reddy & Sharma, 2020). The regulatory requirement for pharmaceutical drugs is more stringent when compared to surgical procedures, medical devices, teaching, and training aids. While the ability to conduct studies on excipient compatibility, drug release, and other topics are more quick as a major benefit in the case of product development, the absence of clinical history and post-marketing data in comparison to established dosage forms and manufacturing processes and tools presents a number of challenges in terms of regulation and safety (Rowe *et al.*, 2000). *Technical Considerations for Additive Manufactured Devices* is a guidance document that the USFDA released in 2017 (FDA-2016-D-1210, 2017) to outline the FDA's early thoughts on technical issues related to additive manufacturing and to offer recommendations for testing and device characterization (West *et al.*, 2019).

However, the FDA is still developing rules, so there arenot any yet for 3D-printed pharmaceutical items. In *Technical considerations for additive manufacturing devices, 2017* (FDA-2016-D-1210, 2017), while not directly focused on pharmaceutical drugs, this FDA guidance document provides recommendations for manufacturers using additive manufacturing including 3D printing to produce medical devices. Specific guidelines solely focused on 3D printing of pharmaceuticals had not been issued by regulatory agencies. However, several existing regulatory frameworks and guidelines provide insights into howmanufacturing pharmaceuticals utilizing 3D printing should approach regulatory compliance (Nukala *et al.*, 2019).

5.6.1 Quality Control and Material Characterization

Thoroughly characterizing the materials use in 3D printing is crucial. The FDA recommends following established such as "Biological evaluation of medical devices-part 1: Evaluation and testing within a risk management framework, according to international standard ISO 10993-1". To assess material biocompatibility and safety the cGMP regulations are fundamental to ensuring that pharmaceutical products are consistently manufactured to meet quality standards. These principles apply to 3D printing as they do to traditional pharmaceutical manufacturing, emphasizing product quality, process control, and documentation (Yu *et al.*, 2008). The design control principles, which involve documenting and managing the design process, ensure that 3D-printed pharmaceutical products meet their intended specifications consistently. Transparency in design changes and validations is essential (FDA guidelines-2019). The existing regulatory pathways for drug approval, such as NDAs (new drug applications) or ANDA (abbreviated new drug applications), generally, apply to 3D-printed pharmaceuticals. Manufacturers need to provide comprehensive data demonstrating the safety, efficacy, and quality of their products. Depending on the specific application, 3D-printed pharmaceutical products might be classified as medical devices. In such cases, manufacturing should follow relevant device regulations, which could involve, premarket Notifications 510 (K) or premarket approval submission (Yu *et al.*, 2008). Various regulatory authorities have played a crucial role in overseeing the use of EB3D technologies in pharmaceuticals. USFDA have developed guidelines and regulations to handle the particular issues raised by the technology. The European Medicines Agency has also provided a set of guidelines to assure the effectiveness and safety of 3D-printed medicinal goods in the European Union (Goyanes *et al.*, 2015a, b). There are other regions and countries which have their own regulatory frameworks that govern the use of EB3D technologies in the pharma-industry (Alhnan *et al.*, 2016). To meet the regulatory requirements pharmaceutical companies and manufacturers utilizing 3D printing technologies must address several considerations (West *et al.*, 2019). The key considerations include the size of nozzle, wall thickness, and orientation, choice of material and design balance (Yu *et al.*, 2008).

5.6.2 Quality Assurance and Control

A conventional drug delivery system often results in underdosing or overdosing, lacking the ability to precisely tailor the dose regimen to an individual patient's requirement. In response to the challenges posed by existing drug delivery system methods, The American Society of Mechanical Engineers favors the term "additive manufacturing", which describes a process that has become very promising in the pharmaceutical industry, particularly in the area of customized medicine (Nukala *et al.*, 2019). The construction of products with complex 3D structures using three-dimensional 3D printing technology, which is acknowledged as a transformative process, is possible using computer-aided design (CAD) models. This innovation typically involves the deposition of materials layer by layer on a built platform, offering a novel and precise approach to drug-delivery customization. In the pacing pharmaceutical advancements, the traditional drug delivery system persists, often leading to the pitfalls of underdosing and overdosing, failing to hit the precision required to cater to individual patient needs (Katakam *et al.*, 2022). However, hope emerges on the horizon with transformative powder-additive manufacturing (Tian *et al.*, 2021, Yang *et al.*, 2017). Embracing its remarkable 3D printing prowess, it crafts intricate structures with an almost magical touch, all orchestrated by the melody of CAD models. With mesmerizing finesse, it lays down layer upon layer of materials on its build platform; bring forth a realm of customized drug-delivery possibilities with accuracy (Nukala *et al.*, 2019). In the world of advancing pharmaceutical breakthroughs, an enchanting spectacle has unfolded with the USFDA bestowing its dazzling approval upon the mesmerizing concept of EB3D printing technology. More than 100 3D-printed medical products, including orthopaedic, cranial implants, dental restorations such as crowns and external prosthesis, and surgical equipment, have received FDA approval. Additionally, it approved SPRITAM (levetiracetam), a 3D-printed medication that uses the Zip Dose technology to treat epilepsy (Katakam *et al.*, 2015).

5.7 CASESTUDY REPORTS ON EB3D PRINTING

5.7.1 Case Study 1

Personalized oral solid dosage forms fabricated using various polymers defining the ease of printing ability. The extrusion 3D is a progressive AM technique with flexibility and end-product customization. Material characteristics, process variables, printer-specific variables, and their interactions are complex. The mechanical, thermal, and rheological properties of several polymers and polymer-drug mixtures were evaluated after they were extruded (diameter 1.75–0.05 mm). These features, as well as the 3D printer's processing temperature, printing speed, and various nozzle diameters, were related to the final product's quality. Different (thermal and mechanical) failure causes were assessed. It was made evident the importance of the printer's design (nozzle diameter) and the significance of the material parameters that were crucial (such the cross-over point) for the optimal printing behavior. Filaments should have a high level of toughness and stiffness and a low level of brittleness in order to be able to be fed and compatible with the printers' gears. The effects of drug on a polymer matrix's solidification behavior, as well as the subsequent change in material extrusion additive manufacturing processibility and product quality (Reddy & Sharma, 2020).

5.7.2 CASE STUDY 2

Both orthopedic implants that are custom made for each patient and orthopedic implants that are produced in large quantities use additive manufacturing. In addition to being precisely suited to the patient's anatomical and surgical needs, AM implants can combine porous and solid components into a single mono-block with reduced implant rigidity, enhancing osseointegration. It is now possible to directly make functional parts because to the advancement of AM technology. The perfect balance of surface roughness, pore size, and porosity may be changed to produce an implant that lasts for a very long time by carefully selecting the machining parameters of the photolithography and material jetting processes. How 3D printing is useful from an economic standpoint has been determined from the analysis of a specific case study (Rowe *et al.*, 2000).

5.7.3 CASE STUDY 3

EB3D printing is used to create kid-friendly chocolate-based dosage forms for oral administration of both hydrophilic and lipophilic medications.A range of 10–90% of compliance-related issues in pediatric dosage forms is due to palatability, and characteristics of dosage forms. Due to the bitter taste of the majority of the active pharmaceutical ingredients (APIs), palatability, which is merely a measure of the general acceptance of oral pharmaceutical products, presents difficulties during formulation development. Effective therapy depends heavily on patient compliance with the therapeutic regimen, which is mostly determined by how well-tolerated the dosage form is by the patient. A patient's dislike of the medication's flavor was its main cause of rejection. Because they are more popular with children, cocoa-related goods like chocolate and chocolate milk have been utilized in the past as palatability enhancers (Karavasili *et al.*, 2021).

5.8 CONCLUSION

The revolutionary extrusion-based 3D printing has a progressive approach in design and development of complex geometries with ease and authenticity. Thus the utilization of EB3D printing is now the research interest of many drug development researchers. The tendency to mold the polymers (thermoplastic) and other materials into 3D shapes with required process and shape parameters has an optimized strategy based on the working principles of the EB3D process operated in various types of printers such as semi-solid-based extrusion, fusion deposition modeling, and pneumatic extrusion. Thus the advantages include the reduction in dose and also enhance targeted delivery thereby reducing the toxicity. Many orthopedic implants, tissue bioengineered implants were prepared and are working successfully at commercial gateways. Case studies on the successful extrusion models have suggested the optimization and advantages of extrusion printing in bioengineering of tissue models. Thus, extrusion-based 3D printing is widely acceptable with few limitations and is a novel research domain to address the challenges in drug development.

REFERENCES

Abo El-Enin HA, Elkomy MH, Naguib IA, Ahmed MF, Alsaidan OA, Alsalahat I, Ghoneim MM, and Eid HM. Lipid nanocarriers overlaid with chitosan for brain delivery of berberine via the nasal route. Pharmaceuticals. 2022; 15(3):281. https://doi.org/10.3390/ph15030281

Altıparmak SC, Yardley VA, Shi Z, Lin J. Extrusion-based additive manufacturing technologies: state of the art and future perspectives. *J Manuf Processes*. 2022; 83:607–36, ISSN 1526–6125, doi: 10.1016/j.jmapro.2022.09.032.

Alzahrani AM, Hakami A, AlHadi A, Al-Maflehi N, Aljawadi MH, Alotaibi RM, Alzahrani MM, Alammari SA, Batais MA, Almigbal TH. The effectiveness of mindfulness training in improving medical students' stress, depression, and anxiety. *PLoS One*. 2023 Oct 31;18(10):e0293539. doi: 10.1371/journal.pone.0293539. PMID: 37906599; PMCID: PMC10617730

Beltrán N, Blanco D, Álvarez BJ, Noriega Á, and Fernández P. Dimensional and geometrical quality enhancement in additively manufactured parts: Systematic framework and a case study. *Materials*. 2019;12(23): 3937.

Boehm RD, Miller PR, Daniels J, Stafslien S, Narayan RJ. Inkjet printing for pharmaceutical applications. *Mater Today*. 2014; 17(5):247–52. doi: 10.1016/j.mattod.2014.04.027.

Cao L, Xiao J, Kim JK, and Zhang X. Effect of post-process treatments on mechanical properties and surface characteristics of 3D printed short glass fiber reinforced PLA/TPU using the FDM process. *CIRP J Manuf Sci Technol*. 2023;41: 135–143.

Chakka LRJ, Chede S. 3D printing of pharmaceuticals for disease treatment. *Front Med Technol*. 2023 Jan 10;4:1040052. doi: 10.3389/fmedt.2022.1040052. PMID: 36704231; PMCID: PMC9871616.

Cui M, Pan H, Su Y, Fang D, Qiao S, Ding P, Pan W. Opportunities and challenges of three-dimensional printing technology in pharmaceutical formulation development. *Acta Pharm Sin B*. 2021 Aug;11(8):2488–2504. doi: 10.1016/j.apsb.2021.03.015. Epub 2021 Mar 12. PMID: 34567958; PMCID: PMC8447232.

Da Silva CG, Camps MGM, Li TMWY, Chan AB, Ossendorp F, Cruz LJ. Co-delivery of immunomodulators in biodegradable nanoparticles improves therapeutic efficacy of cancer vaccines. *Biomaterials*. 2019; 220: 119417. 10.1016/j.biomaterials.2019.119417

Derossi A, Caporizzi R, Azzollini D, Severini C. (2017). Application of 3D printing for customized food. A case on the development of a fruit-based snack for children. *J Food Eng*. 2017; 220:65–75. https://doi.org/10.1016/j.jfoodeng.2017.05.015

Ding S, Zou B, Wang P, Ding H. Effects of nozzle temperature and building orientation on mechanical properties and microstructure of PEEK and PEI printed by 3D-FDM. *Polymer Testing*. 2019; 78:105948. doi:10.1016/j.polymertesting.2019.105948

FDA-2016-D-1210, Technical Considerations for Additive Manufactured Medical Devices, 2017. Available from www.fda.gov/media/97633/download

Feilden E, Blanca EG-T, Giuliani F, Saiz E, Vandeperre L. Robocasting of structural ceramic parts with hydrogel inks. *J Eur Ceram Soc*. 2016; 36(10):2525–33. doi: 10.1016/j.jeurceramsoc.2016.03.001.

Firth J, Basit AW, Gaisford S. The role of semi-solid extrusion printing in clinical practice. In: AAPS Advances in the Pharmaceutical Sciences Series. Cham: Springer International Publishing; 2018. pp. 133–51.

Gonzalez-Gutierrez J, Cano S, Schuschnigg S, Kukla C, Sapkota J, Holzer C. Additive manufacturing of metallic and ceramic components by the material extrusion of highly-filled polymers: a review and future perspectives. *Materials (Basel)*. 2018; 11(5):840. doi: 10.3390/ma11050840, PMID 29783705.

Goyanes A, Chang H, Sedough D, Hatton GB, Wang J, Buanz A et al. Fabrication of controlled-release budesonide tablets via desktop (FDM) 3D printing. *Int J Pharm*. 2015a; 496(2):414–20. doi: 10.1016/j.ijpharm.2015.10.039, PMID 26481468.

Goyanes A, Robles Martinez P, Buanz A, Basit AW, Gaisford S. Effect of geometry on drug release from 3D printed tablets. *Int J Pharm*. 2015b; 494(2):657–63. doi: 10.1016/j.ijpharm.2015.04.069, PMID 25934428.

Haleem A, Javaid M, Singh RP, Suman R. Significant roles of 4D printing using smart materials in the field of manufacturing. Adv Ind Eng Polym Res. 2021; 4(4):301–11. doi: 10.1016/j.aiepr.2021.05.001.

Harrer W, Schwentenwein M, Lube T, Danzer R. Fractography of zirconia-specimens made using additive manufacturing (LCM) technology. J Eur Ceram Soc. 2017; 37(14):4331–8. doi: 10.1016/j.jeurceramsoc.2017.03.018.

He JS, Chen JZ, Hellwich KH, Hess M, Horie K, Jones RG et al.Abbreviations of polymer names and guidelines for abbreviating polymer names (IUPAC recommendations 2014). Pure ApplChem. 2014; 86(6):1003–15. doi: 10.1515/pac-2012-1203.

Hospodiuk M, Moncal KK, Dey M, Ozbolat IT. Extrusion-based biofabrication in tissue engineering and regenerative medicine. In: OvsianikovA, YooJ, MironovV, editors. 3D printing and biofabrication. Berlin: Springer International Publishing; 2018. pp. 255–81.

Huang S, Fu X. Naturally derived materials-based cell and drug delivery systems in skin regeneration. J Control Release. 2010; 142(2):149–59. doi: 10.1016/j.jconrel.2009.10.018, PMID 19850093.

Infanger S, Haemmerli A, Iliev S, Baier A, Stoyanov E, Quodbach J. Powder bed 3D-printing of highly loaded drug delivery devices with hydroxypropyl cellulose as solid binder. Int J Pharm. 2019; 555:198–206. doi: 10.1016/j.ijpharm.2018.11.048, PMID 30458260.

Jang MJ, Bae SK, Jung YS, Kim JC, Kim JS, Park SK, Suh JS, Yi SJ, Ahn SH, Lim JO. Enhanced wound healing using a 3D printed VEGF-mimicking peptide incorporated hydrogel patch in a pig model. Biomed Mater. 2021 Apr 9;16(4). doi: 10.1088/1748-605X/abf1a8. PMID: 33761488

Jung JW, Lee JS, Cho DW. Computer-aided multiple-head 3D printing system for printing of heterogeneous organ/tissue constructs. Sci Rep. 2016 Feb 22; 6:21685. doi: 10.1038/srep21685, PMID 26899876, PMCID PMC4761951.

Karavasili C, Gkaragkounis A, Moschakis T, Ritzoulis C, Fatouros DG. Pediatric-friendly chocolate-based dosage forms for the oral administration of both hydrophilic and lipophilic drugs fabricated with extrusion-based 3D printing. *Eur J Pharm Sci*. 2020 Apr 30; 147:105291. doi: 10.1016/j.ejps.2020.105291. Epub 2020 Mar 2. PMID: 32135271.

Karavasili C, Eleftheriadis GK, Gioumouxouzis C, Andriotis EG, and Fatouros DG. Mucosal drug delivery and 3D printing technologies: A focus on special patient populations. *Adv Drug Delivery Rev.* 2021; 176: 113858.

Katakam P, Dey B, Assaleh FH, Hwisa NT, Adiki SK, Chandu BR, Mitra A. Top-down and bottom-up approaches in 3D printing technologies for drug delivery challenges. *Crit Rev Ther Drug Carrier Syst.* 2015; 32(1):61–87. doi: 10.1615/critrevtherdrugcarriers yst.2014011157. PMID: 25746205.

Katakam P, Adiki SK, Satapathy SR. Recent advancements of additive manufacturing for patient-specific drug delivery. In Additive Manufacturing Processes in Biomedical Engineering, (pp. 1–26). CRC Press, 2022.

Lee BK, Yun YH, Choi JS, Choi YC, Kim JD, Cho YW. Fabrication of drug-loaded polymer microparticles with arbitrary geometries using a piezoelectric inkjet printing system. *Int J Pharm.* 2012; 427(2):305–10. doi: 10.1016/j.ijpharm.2012.02.011, PMID 22366486.

Lee J, Kim KE, Bang S, Noh I, Lee C. A desktop multi-material 3D bio-printing system with open-source hardware and software. *Int J Precis Eng Manuf.* 2017; 18(4):605–12. doi: 10.1007/s12541-017-0072-x.

Lee J-Y, An J, & Chua CK. Fundamentals and applications of 3D printing for novel materials. *Appl Mater Today.* 2017; 7:120–133. doi:10.1016/j.apmt.2017.02.004 10.1016/j.apmt.2017.02.004

Li J, Pumera M. 3D printing of functional microrobots. *Chem Soc Rev.* 2021 Feb 21; 50(4):2794–838. doi: 10.1039/d0cs01062f, PMID 33470252.

Li M, Zhang Z, Cao W, Liu Y, Du B, Chen C, … Wang X. Identifying novel factors associated with COVID-19 transmission and fatality using the machine learning approach. *Sci Total Environ.* 2020 142810. doi:10.1016/j.scitotenv.2020.142810 10.1016/j.scitotenv.2020.142810

Li Q, Guan X, Cui M, Zhu Z, Chen K, Wen H et al. Preparation and investigation of novel gastro-floating tablets with 3D extrusion-based printing. *Int J Pharm.* 2018 Jan 15; 535(1–2):325–32. doi: 10.1016/j.ijpharm.2017.10.037, PMID 29051121.

Liravi F, Darleux R, Toyserkani E. Nozzle dispensing additive manufacturing of polysiloxane: dimensional control. *IJRAPIDM.* 2015; 5(1):20–43. doi: 10.1504/IJRAPIDM.2015.073546.

Liu W, Zhang YS, Heinrich MA, De Ferrari F, Jang HL, Bakht SM et al. Rapid continuous multimaterial extrusion bioprinting. *Adv Mater.* 2017 Jan; 29(3). doi: 10.1002/adma.201604630, PMID 27859710, PMCID PMC5235978.

Liu Z, Zhang M, Bhandari B, Wang Y. 3D printing: Printing precision and application in food sector. *Trends Food Sci Technol.* 2017; 69: 83–94. doi:10.1016/j.tifs.2017.08.018 10.1016/j.tifs.2017.08.018

Long J, Etxeberria AE, Nand AV, Bunt CR, Ray S, Seyfoddin A. A 3D printed chitosan-pectin hydrogel wound dressing for lidocaine hydrochloride delivery. *Mater Sci Eng C Mater Biol Appl.* 2019 Nov; 104:109873. doi: 10.1016/j.msec.2019.109873. Epub 2019 Jun 8. PMID: 31500054.

Mahato RI, Narang AS. Pharmaceutical Dosage Forms and Drug Delivery: Revised and Expanded (3rd ed.). 2017. CRC Press. https://doi.org/10.1201/9781315156941

Mwema FM, Akinlabi ET. Basics of Fused Deposition Modelling (FDM). Fused Deposition Modeling. 2020 May 30:1–15. doi: 10.1007/978-3-030-48259-6_1. PMCID: PMC7257444.

Norman J, Madurawe RD, Moore CMV, Khan MA, Khairuzzaman A. A new chapter in pharmaceutical manufacturing: 3D-printed drug products. *Adv Drug Deliv Rev.* 2017; 108:39–50. doi: 10.1016/j.addr.2016.03.001, PMID 27001902.

Nukala PK, Palekar S, Solanki N, Fu Y, Patki M, Shohatee AA, Trombetta L, and Patel K. Investigating the application of FDM 3D printing pattern in preparation of patient-tailored dosage forms. J 3D Printing Med. 2019;3(1): 23–37.

Park S, Fu K (kelvin). Polymer-based filament feedstock for additive manufacturing. Compos Sci Technol [Internet]. 2021; 213(108876):108876. doi: 10.1016/j.compscitech.2021.108876.

Plott J, Shih A. The extrusion-based additive manufacturing of moisture-cured silicone elastomer with minimal void for pneumatic actuators. Addit Manuf. 2017; 17:1–14. doi: 10.1016/j.addma.2017.06.009.

Pugliese R, Beltrami B, Regondi S, Lunetta C. Polymeric biomaterials for 3D printing in medicine: An overview. Ann 3D Printed Med. 2021; 2: 100011. doi:10.1016/j.stlm.2021.100011

Rahmani Dabbagh S, Ozcan O, Tasoglu S. Machine learning-enabled optimization of extrusion-based 3D printing. *Methods [Internet]*. 2022;206:27–40. Available from: http://dx.doi.org/10.1016/j.ymeth.2022.08.002

Reddy DPR, Sharma V. Additive manufacturing in drug delivery applications: A review. *Int J Pharm*. 2020 Nov 15;589:119820. doi: 10.1016/j.ijpharm.2020.119820. Epub 2020 Sep 4. PMID: 32891718.

Rowe CW, Katstra WE, Palazzolo RD, Giritlioglu B, Teung P, Cima MJ. Multimechanism oral dosage forms fabricated by three dimensional printing™. *J Control Release*. 2000; 66(1):11–17.

Rutz AL, Hyland KE, Jakus AE, Burghardt WR, Shah RN. A multimaterial bioink method for 3D printing tunable, cell-compatible hydrogels. *Adv Mater*. 2015; 27(9):1607–14. doi: 10.1002/adma.201405076, PMID 25641220.

Sadia M, Sośnicka A, Arafat B, Isreb A, Ahmed W, Kelarakis A, and Alhnan MA. Adaptation of pharmaceutical excipients to FDM 3D printing for the fabrication of patient-tailored immediate release tablets. *Int J Pharma*. 2016;513(1–2): 659–668.

Sears N, Dhavalikar P, Whitely M, Cosgriff-Hernandez E. Fabrication of biomimetic bone grafts with multi-material 3D printing. *Biofabrication*. 2017 May 22; 9(2):025020. doi: 10.1088/1758-5090/aa7077, PMID 28530207.

Seiti M, Ginestra P. Additive Manufacturing for orthopedic applications: Case study on market impact. *Proc Comput Sci*. 2023; 217:737–745, ISSN 1877-0509, 10.1016/j.procs.2022.12.270.

Shahrjerdi A, Mojtaba K. Mahdi B. Enhancing mechanical properties of 3D-printed PLAs via optimization process and statistical modeling. J Comp Sci. 2023; 7(4):151. https://doi.org/10.3390/jcs7040151

Shim IK, Yi HJ, Yi HG, Lee CM, Lee YN, Choi YJ, Jeong SY, Jun E, Hoffman RM, Cho DW, Kim SC. Locally-applied 5-fluorouracil-loaded slow-release patch prevents pancreatic cancer growth in an orthotopic mouse model. Oncotarget. 2017 Jun 20;8(25):40140–40151. doi: 10.18632/oncotarget.17370

Singh S, Ramakrishna S, Berto F. 3D printing of polymer composites: a short review. *Mat Design Process Comms*. 2020; 2(2):e97. doi: 10.1002/mdp2.97.

Tagami T, Ando M, Nagata N, Goto E, Yoshimura N, Takeuchi T, et al. Fabrication of naftopidil-loaded tablets using a semisolid extrusion-type 3D printer and the characteristics of the printed hydrogel and resulting tablets. J Pharm Sci. 2019a; 108(2):907–13. doi: 10.1016/j.xphs.2018.08.026, PMID 30267782.

Tagami T, Hayashi N, Sakai N, Ozeki T. 3D printing of unique water-soluble polymer-based suppository shell for controlled drug release. Int J Pharm. 2019b; 118494. doi:10.1016/j.ijpharm.2019.118494 10.1016/j.ijpharm.2019.118494

Tagami T, Goto E, Kida R, Hirose K, Noda T, Ozeki T. Lyophilized ophthalmologic patches as novel corneal drug formulations using a semi-solid extrusion 3D printer. *Int J Pharm.* 2022 Apr 5; 617:121448. doi: 10.1016/j.ijpharm.2022.121448, PMID 35066116.

Tian Y, Chen CX, Xu X, Wang J, Hou X, Li K, Lu X, Shi HY, Lee E-S, and Heng Bo Jiang. A review of 3D printing in dentistry: Technologies, affecting factors, and applications. *Scanning.* 2021; 2021(1): 9950131.

Trenfield S, Madla C, Basit A, Gaisford S. The shape of things to come: emerging applications of 3D printing in healthcare; 2018. p. 1–19.

Wang Z, Han X, Chen R, Li J, Gao J, Zhang H, Liu N, Gao X, Zheng A. Innovative color jet 3D printing of levetiracetam personalized paediatric preparations. *Asian J Pharm Sci.* 2021 May; 16(3):374–386. doi: 10.1016/j.ajps.2021.02.003. Epub 2021 Mar 1. PMID: 34276825; PMCID: PMC8261256.

West TG, Bradbury TJ. 3D printing: a case of ZipDose® technology–world's first 3D printing platform to obtain FDA approval for a pharmaceutical product. *3D and 4D Printing in Biomedical Applications: Process Engineering and Additive Manufacturing.* 2019: 53–79.

West J, George K. The complementarity of openness: How MakerBot leveraged Thingiverse in 3D printing. *Technol Forecast Soc Change.* 2016; 102:169–181.

Wickramasinghe S, Truong D, Phuong T. FDM-based 3D printing of polymer and associated composite: a review on mechanical properties, defects and treatments. Polymers. 2020; 12(7): 1529. https://doi.org/10.3390/polym12071529

Yang C, Tian X, Liu T, Cao Y, and Li D. 3D printing for continuous fiber reinforced thermoplastic composites: mechanism and performance. Rapid Prototyp J. 2017; 23(1): 209–215.

Yu Z, Gao Y, Jiang J, Gu H, Lv S, Ni H, Wang X, and Jia C. Study on effects of FDM 3D printing parameters on mechanical properties of polylactic acid. In IOP Conference Series: Materials Science and Engineering, vol. 688, no. 3, p. 033026. IOP Publishing, 2019.

Section IV

Binder Jetting-Based 3D Printing in Pharmaceutics

6 Binder Jetting

A Versatile and Rapid Fast 3D Printing Phenomenon

Bhoopathi Deepika, P. Sunil Kumar Chaitanya, Naga Raju Kandukoori, Kiranmai Mandava, and Prakash Katakam

6.1 INTRODUCTION

3D printing (3DP) is a method to create three-dimensional samples (solid objects) of complex shapes with a (liquid) binder deposited to join powder from a digital file. It is based on ink-jet print technology. The American Society for Testing and Materials (ASTM) has divided the 3DP into seven process categories for producing 3D objects by successive layers of material and based on the required characteristics such as durability, surface finish, and applications. It produces parts directly or by combination of indirect processes with traditional manufacturing (TM) techniques. Direct process: the part of an object is directly produced with the machine. Indirect processes: it is a combination of AM and TM (Goole *et al.*, 2016). In order to advance pharmaceutical research, a number of printing techniques have been investigated. Aprecia Pharmaceuticals developed Spritam, the first 3DP tablet, authorized by the FDA in 2015 and recently approved Triastek, Inc.'s IND application for the 3DP dosage form T19 (Goole *et al.*, 2016). 3DP applications had reached a peak in the development of dosage forms. For the creation of solid dosage forms, other 3DP techniques are being looked into, but they are still in the research and development stage (Danae Karali *et al.*, 2012). The use of 3DP to create pharmaceutical dosage forms have a number of benefits, including the ability to customize medication, the development of complex dosage form geometries, the preparation of high drug loadings, and one 3D-printed product has been so far authorized for sale in the US (Chen *et al.*, 2022). It is widely employed in the biological, pharmaceutical, engineering, fashion, and cosmetics industries (Trenfield *et al.*, 2018a, b). It has become quite popular for dosage development, since FDA authorized SPRITAM®, the first 3DP dosage form (Chen *et al.*, 2022). A color-printing method "binder jetting" (BJ) uses ceramic, metal, and polymer-based materials. It is frequently quicker than alternative techniques, and by adding more material-depositing print head holes, the process can be sped up even further. Massive sand-casting cores and molds, full-color prototypes, and low-cost metal parts can all be produced with binder jetting. It is compatible with any powder materials, and rapid. Since the shaping process takes place at ambient temperature, oxidation, residual stress, elemental segregation, and phase shifts are not

DOI: 10.1201/9781003439509-10

a concern. Fusion-based AM technologies use heat to melt the powder layers, which causes residual tension in the finished product. Because the BJ method uses relatively little heat, heat-induced stress and distortion are quite rare. Various densities with controlled porosity are obtained on sintering temperature and time. It involves several steps and requires post-processing. Due to the relatively low relative density of the printed pieces, densification in this state typically causes severe geometric distortion. Compared to powder bed fusion, there is a higher surface roughness and lesser resolution. For the bulk materials, post-processing strategy development is still necessary (Danae Karali *et al.*, 2012).

6.2 PHARMACEUTICAL APPLICATIONS OF BINDING JETTING (PERSONALIZED MEDICINE AND DOSAGE FORMS)

6.2.1 CUSTOMIZED DRUG DOSING AND FORMULATIONS

Two methods exist for incorporating pure medications into the mixture (Goole *et al.*, 2016). According to one method, the solvent and binder are the only ingredients in the cartridge after the API and excipients are well combined into a printed powder. As an alternative, API can be sprayed onto the powder bed in the form of a suspension or solution. According to Goole *et al.* (2016), the final dispersible tablets created using 3D printing had a uniform drug content, improved mechanical qualities, and a highly porous structure that accelerated the rate of disintegration as shown in Figure 6.1. A children's formulation with an eye-catching appearance and instant release properties was created using color inkjet three-dimensional printing (CJ-3DP) and a binder. The tablet strength and model volume showed a consistently linear relationship (>0.999).

6.2.2 PATIENT-SPECIFIC IMPLANTS AND MEDICAL DEVICES

Drug implants created through 3D printing may have unique morphologies and intricate release schedules for every patient. Through the use of two potential water-soluble adhesives, technology was able to replace bone with hydroxyl apatite (HA) in the chemical composition phase and real bone in the inorganic phase. An implant made of bone tissue was coated with HA powder in order to improve the bond between the powdered HA and the HA in the implant. Micro-architecture, manufacturing precision and appropriate mechanical properties of the phosphoric acid implants was superior to those of the polyvinyl alcohol implants. The study also showed how varied HA and tricalcium phosphate (TCP) composition ratios affected

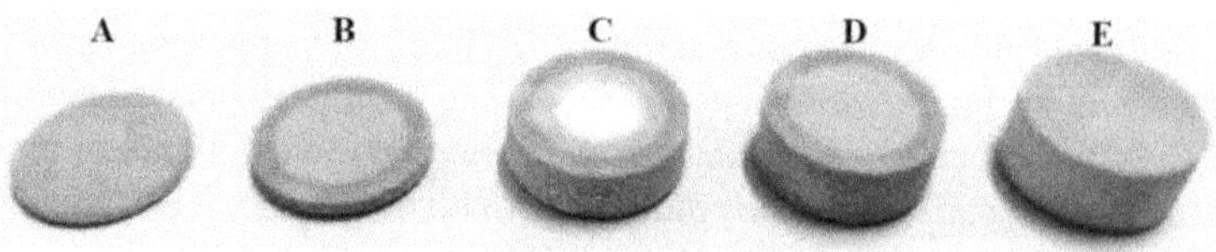

FIGURE 6.1	Structure diagram for the 3D-printed formulation. (Hong X et al., 2021)

TABLE 6.1
Examples of Rapid-Release Formulations used in BJ3DP

Dosage form	API	Powder	Binder	References
Dissolving tablets	Levetiracetam	Microcrystalline cellulose, mannitol, colloidal silicon dioxide (CSD), PVP	40% (v/v) isopropanol aqueous solution containing 0.05% (w/w) PVP and 4% (w/w) glycerin	Wang Z *et al.*, 2021
Dispersible tablets	Ketoprofen	Spray dried lactose monohydrate, spray-dried lactose, microcrystalline cellulose, mannitol, PVP grade K25, silica.	Ethanol solution with 10% polyethylene glycol 1500	Kreft K *et al.*, 2024
Fast dissolving tablets	Indomethacin	Lactose monohydrate Kollidon VA64 (KL)	5% (W/V) KL in water	Chang S-Y *et al.*, 2020
Oral disintegrating tablets	Warfarin sodium	D-sucrose, pregelatinizedstarch, Povidone K30, Microcrystalline cellulose, silicon dioxide	38% (v/v) ethanol solution	Tian P *et al.*, 2018
Dispersible tablets	Clozapine	Mannitol, lactose, microcrystalline cellulose, straw berry flavor, colloidal silicon dioxide	50% (v/v) ethanol solution containing 0, .3 (w/w) PVP and 4% (w/w) glycerin	Chen R *et al.*, 2021
Oral disintegrating tablets	Andrographolide	Sucrose, mannitol, PVP K30, microcrystalline cellulose, aspartame	30% (v/v) ethanol solution	Huang SY *et al.*, 2020

mechanical properties (Pandey *et al.*, 2020). Table 6.1 provides examples of rapid-release formulations used in BJ3DP.

6.3 NOVEL DRUG DELIVERY SYSTEMS

6.3.1 Sustained Release Formulations

To the first controlled-release 3D-printed tablet was created using alizarin yellow and methylene blue as model drugs. Second, acetaminophen served as the model drug for pie-shaped controlled-release. Third, lactose, HPMC, and PVP were combined to create an intermediate layer in an API gradient oral controlled-release drug-delivery system; BJ3DP and dissolved diclofenac sodium in the binder were used to create the top and bottom layers (Goole *et al.*, 2016).

6.3.2 Multi-Drug Combination Products

PN-containing solutions and blank printing solutions were the two categories into which the printing solutions were divided. Using BJ3DP technology, a PN printing solution was sprayed into the tablet to prevent medication deterioration caused by light and other factors. For this experiment, an LEV-PN compound with extraordinary mechanical properties was developed. This work involved precisely controlling the volume of a single-layer inkjet by varying the size and quantity of drug-containing droplets. Lisinopril and spironolactone were dissolved in light-curing biological inks before being injected into a two-chamber pharmaceutical carrier that was 3D printed with a binder-jet printer and a piezoelectric nozzle. During production, the subsequent treatment stopped the right drug solution from being absorbed into the carrier tablet, and each chamber held 250 L of drug solution (Goole *et al.*, 2016 and Chen *et al.*, 2022).

6.4 PROCESS PARAMETERS AND OPTIMIZATION FOR PHARMACEUTICAL APPLICATION

6.4.1 Rheological Properties and Flow Behavior of Pharmaceutical Binders

In BJ, viscosity is a deciding factor. It is determined by surface tension: Weber number (We) and Reynolds numbers (Re). These two factors decide the behavior of liquid binding with respect to drop formation during ink jetting. They are defined as follows:

$$\text{Re} = \rho dV/\eta$$

$$\text{We} = \rho dV^2/\gamma$$

where ρ = density of liquid, V = flow speed, d = droplet diameter, η = dynamic viscosity, γ = surface tension.

Normally binding jetting technology uses a drop-on demand inkjet deposition which acts by pushing liquid from a small nozzle with pressure as depicted in Figure 6.2. Jettability of a fluid can be determined by Ohnesorge number. It is a dimensionless variable. Liquid binders with Oh numbers 0.1 to 1 are used.

6.4.2 Binder Penetration and Bonding Strength Optimization for Drug Delivery Systems

Two types of print heads are as follows:

(1)   Drop-on demand (DoD) printheads; (2) continuous jet print heads.

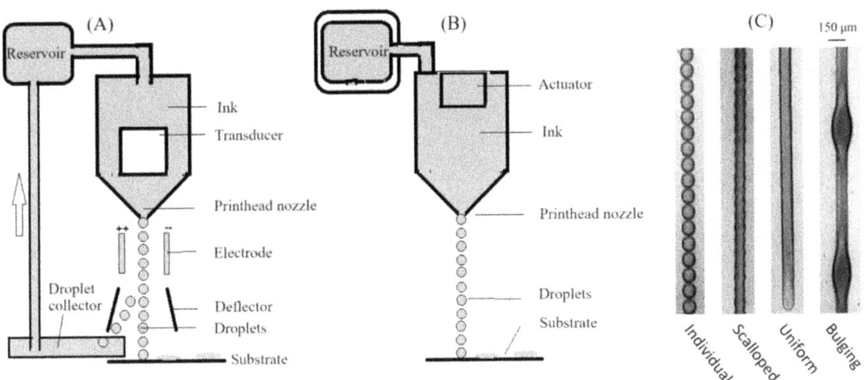

FIGURE 6.2   (A) Continuous jet print head, (B) Drop on demand print head. (C) Various modes of a droplet formation. (Soltman et al., 2008, Copyright 2008 American Chemical Society)

The DoD works by creating single drops on demand, DoD print heads are as follows: piezoelectric and thermal ink jet heads. Ink droplets are squeezed out in a specific shape using piezoelectric print heads. Liquid binder droplets are continuously produced in continuous-jet print heads (Goole *et al.*, 2016). Print head speed, binder diffusion rate, drop-to-drop distance, and line spacing are some of the variables that can affect pattern techniques and droplet deposition. Binder droplets migrate because of gravity or capillary pressure until equilibrium is reached. The factors that influence penetration depth (D) and binder spread (W) are powder morphology, particle surface chemistry, powder bed compactions, binder velocity and its chemistry, powder temperature, and binder bed compactions. Smaller line spacing increases the likelihood of oversaturation and bleeding while also slowing down printing. Too much space between the lines causes marginal stitching between them (Goole *et al.*, 2016). The shape, mean size, and dispersion of the powder can all affect its mobility. In an effort to minimize powder segregation in ink jet 3D printing, hybrid binder is developed. In recent times, scientists have been working with using a suspension of nanoparticles to bind the metal powder bed particles. Submicron particles in the polymeric binder help to increase the density of the green parts (Awad *et al*, 2019). The interaction between binder and powder bed during the process regulates the geometry, precision, strength of the green component, and final surface texture as described in Figure 6.3. The liquid binder wets the powder bed surface as soon as it enters into contact with the top surface of the powdered material. Due to the kinetic energy of the binder droplets, enabling the binder spread over the powder bed, a network of liquid bridges connecting the nearby particles forms in microseconds (Vithani *et al.*, 2018).

6.4.3   Print Parameters' Optimization

For printing purposes, it describes the height of the powder bed along the Z axis. The range is from 15 to 300 m. The powder bed's density decreases as layer thickness increases. Print speed is primarily determined by the combination of the recoat,

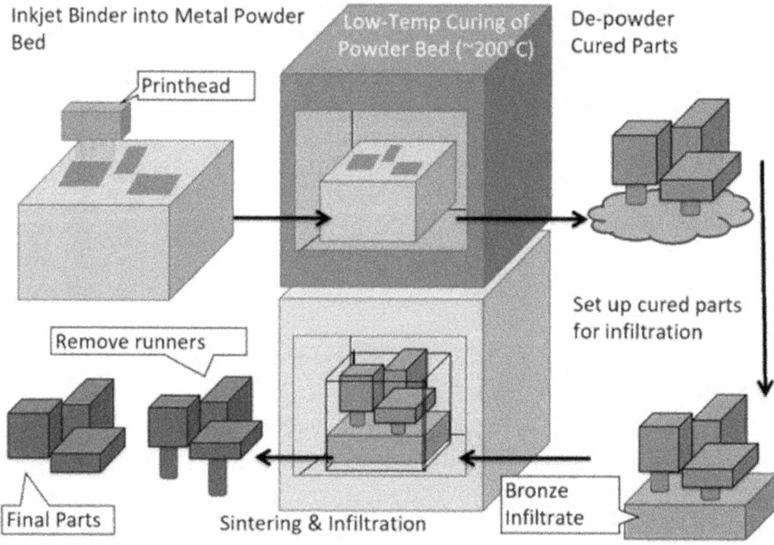

FIGURE 6.3 SLA technique showing a vat of liquid resin photopolymer from which the 3Dmodel is built layer by layer and cured by UV light. (Mostafaei et al., 2021)

oscillator, and roller traverse speeds. It is based on the system's ability to support print head drops when necessary as shown in Figure 6.4. Inadequate binder saturation can lead to a powder bed that does not maintain homogeneity as well as printed goods that are not precise in terms of dimensions. Following is an estimation of binder saturation: $S = 1000XV/(1- (PR/100))XY Z$.

Here, V-binder volume per drop, and PR packing pace. The layer thickness is Z, and the binder droplet spacing is X and Y.

Drying time is influenced by a number of variables, including the choice of binder saturation level, binder composition, and chemistry, layer thickness, powder wettability with binder, and packing density as mentioned in Figure 6.5. Thermal conductivity, surface area, permeability, and packing density are further considerations, controlled by heater power. Therefore, the green components' distortion, shrinkage, dimensional accuracy, and surface polish are affected by the liquid binder's drying period (Vithani *et al.*, 2018). The layer stacking orientation refers to the position of the object being printed with respect to the Z axis, which is the stacking direction of the roller. The build orientation describes how the printed parts are positioned in relation to the x, y, and z axes. The manufacturing parts' quality is significantly degraded (van den Heuvel *et al.*, 2021).

6.5 QUALITY CONTROL AND CHARACTERIZATION OF BINDER JETTED PHARMACEUTICAL PRODUCTS

6.5.1 MECHANICAL TESTING AND MATERIAL CHARACTERIZATION

The following are some of the crucial aspects of powder that BJ 3DP frequently considers: the powder spreading process is important because it influences the part's

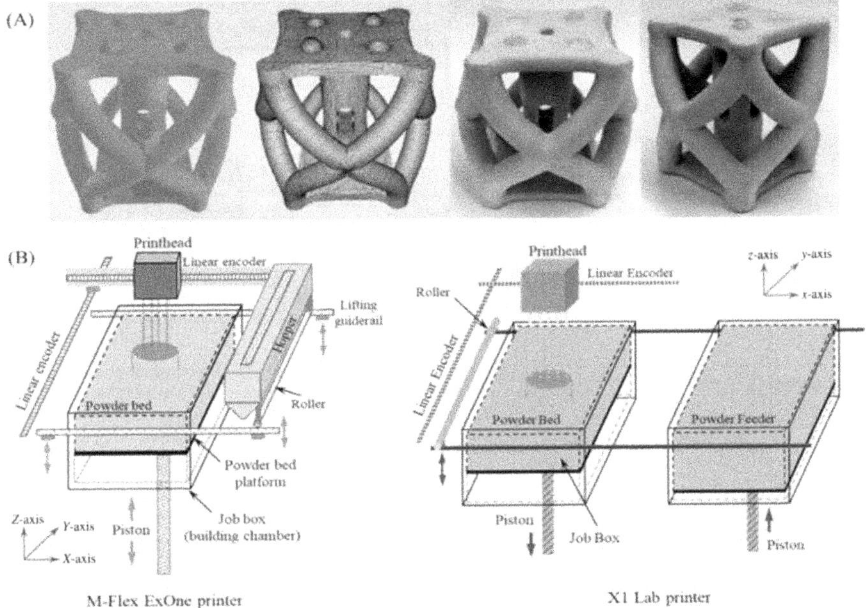

FIGURE 6.4 (A) CAD model, STL file, and binder jetted parts (Ingaglio et al., 2019), (B) Diagram illustrating various components of binder jet printers using two different powder feeding methods: (left) powders are supplied via a hopper that oscillates, distributing the powder on the powder bed and achieving powder compaction with a roller (the Innovent or M-Flex ExOne printer, for example); (right) powder supply as a feeder that uses a roller to swipe powder on the powder bed on the upper layer of the built area (the X1-Lab printer, for example). (Mostafaei et al., 2021)

homogeneity and density. Other factors to consider are the powder's flowability, packing density, and particle characteristics such as morphology, particle size, and size distribution as shown in Figure 6.6. Studies using powder beds have been done to investigate the results of powder distribution. Through experimental process optimization work in BJ with regard to the powder spreading parameters, such as layer thickness and spreading speed, the characteristics of the green component have been improved (Goole *et al.*, 2016).

6.5.2 Drug–Excipient Compatibility and Stability Studies

BJ is suitable with almost any powdered material because many powdered metals and ceramics are presently sintered to their complete densities. New binders must, however, satisfy a number of requirements in order to work with the process and increase green strength. Some of these requirements for binders include viscosity, surface tension, stability, reactivity with the components inside the inkjet print head, and compatibility with the printed material (Goole *et al.*, 2016).

The consistency and stability of the droplet formation process will be impacted by the viscosity, density, and surface tension of the binder, ultimately influencing the

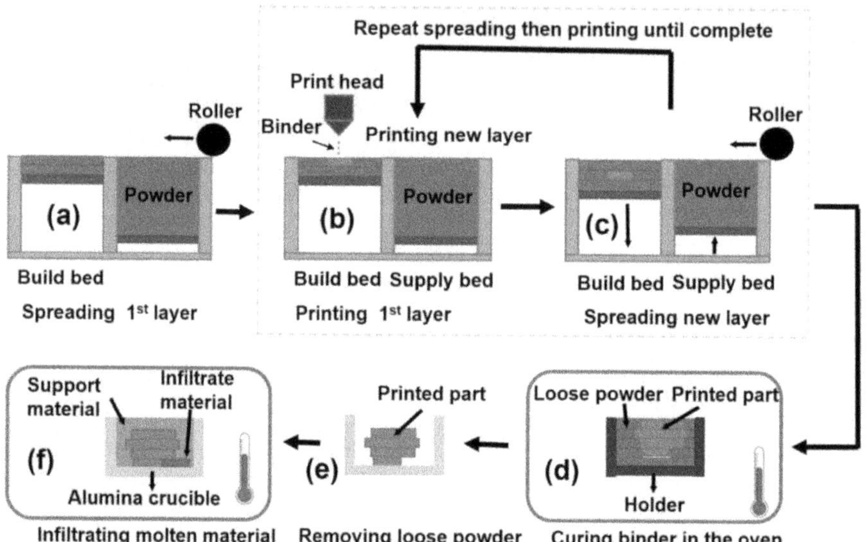

FIGURE 6.5   Schematic representation of BJ3DP followed by post processing. (Do et al., 2017)

printing result. Finally, for components with pre-designed channels, a 10% binder level was adequate to guarantee adequate handling stability, sintering, and particle packing (Goole *et al.*, 2016).

6.5.3   DISSOLUTION AND DRUG-RELEASE TESTING

Modern inkjet printing has made it possible for medications that are not very water soluble to dissolve more quickly. It is carried out using the USP (type I or type II) dissolving test instrument. Samples were collected at various periods, and the HPLC method was used to examine them (Gottschalk *et al.,* 2023).

6.5.4   *In Vitro* AND *In Vivo* PERFORMANCE ASSESSMENT

The relationship between an *in vivo* absorption profile and an *in vitro* drug dissolution curve is defined in large part by IVIVCs. The curves depend on the active pharmaceutical ingredient's (API) qualities and nature, which affect its solubility and rate of dissolution, the formulation's release profile, and the pH of the apparatus, dissolving medium, and procedure factors. The several elements influencing the drug's *in vivo* release, include pH, surfactant, bile, ionic strength, and mobility (Goole *et al.*, 2016).

6.6   CASE STUDIES AND EXAMPLES

6.6.1   CASE STUDY 1: BJ OF CUSTOMIZED ORAL DOSAGE FORMS

A thorough and systematic development process for drop-on powder 3D printing also referred to as binder jetting of tablets containing substantial quantities of an

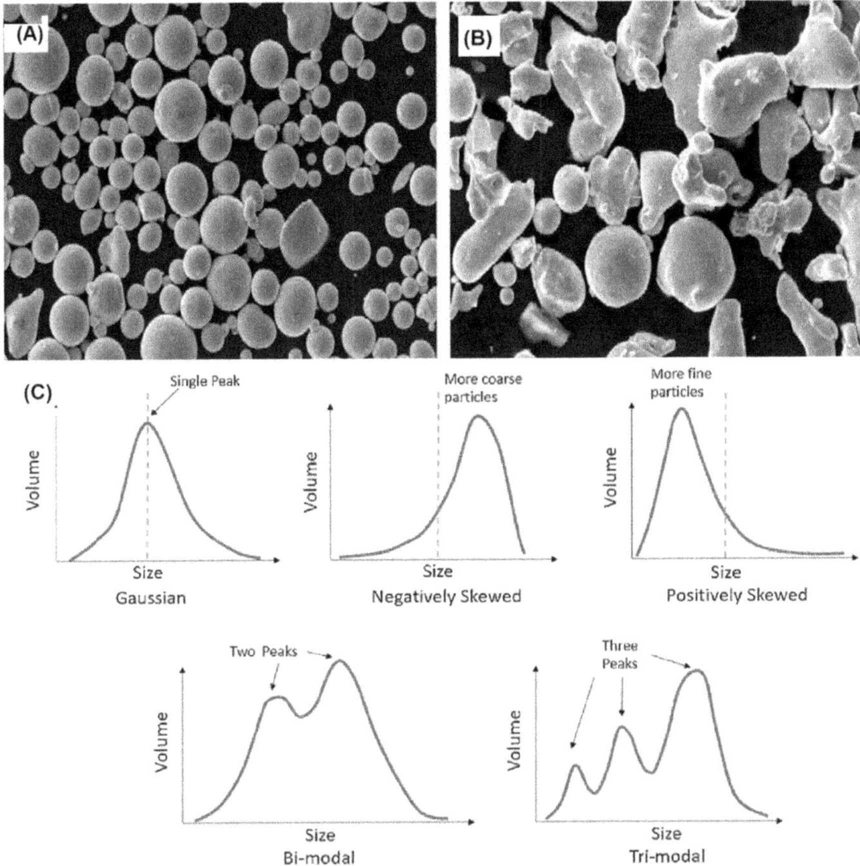

FIGURE 6.6   (A) Micrographs of powder materials prepared using (Li et al., 2010) (A) gas atomization, and (B) water atomization (Tan et al., 2017), and (C) Variations of size distribution in powder materials.

amorphized, poorly soluble drug is documented in this article. Using copovidone as the matrix polymer and ketoconazole as the model drug, the molecule was amorphized by hot melt extrusion with drug loadings of 20% and 40% (Goole *et al.*, 2016).

6.6.2   CASE STUDY 2: PATIENT-SPECIFIC IMPLANTS AND MEDICAL DEVICES

Phosphoric acid and polyvinyl alcohol (PVA) implants were created using the BJ3DP method. According to studies, the mechanical characteristics of the implants were barely affected by various HA and TCP composition ratios. A bone tissue implant containing HA powder was printed in order to enhance the bonding between the powdered HA and the HA within the implant. In terms of good printability, geometric precision, and compressive strength, the final testing results indicated that a combination of high molecular mass polyvinyl alcohol powder and HA performed better than commercial calcium sulfate bone implants. For bone tissue engineering applications, phosphoric acid implants with a HA/-TCP weight ratio of 60:40 would be the ideal choice due to their mechanical and biocompatible characteristics. Along with the weight ratio of HA to TCP, the implants' compressive strength increased. Using 3DP technology, they produced porous TCP phosphate and silica implants. Two substances that promote early bone development and mineralization upon implantation are iron and silicon. New blood vessels began to form after 12 weeks, which aided in the healing of the wound (Chen *et al.*, 2022).

6.6.3 Case Study 3: BJ for Controlled-Release Drug Delivery Systems

In 1996, the first controlled-release tablet developed utilizing binder-jet 3D printing with methylene blue and alizarin yellow as model medications and a pie-shaped controlled-release tablets were created by using acetaminophen as the model medication. A significant amount of a drug-release blocking substance was also present in high concentration in the annular region encircling the tablet. The drug-release area of the inner hole rises synchronously while the drug-release area of the outside cylindrical surface gradually declines. The height of the pill and the rate of medication release remained virtually unchanged throughout time. Another oral controlled-release medication delivery method was also created employing binder-jet 3D printing and diclofenac sodium that was dissolved in the binder. Lactose, HPMC, and PVP were combined to create the powder that made up the core layer, while the top and bottom layers were made to restrict release in an axial direction. Four lateral sections were created by dividing the model from inside to outside. Reducing the amount of binder spray at each location from inside to outside altered the drug gradient. The radial two-dimensional controlled release from the three-dimensional natural release was achieved by the drug-delivery method through the use of vertical up-and-down release inhibition. In order to compensate for the smaller drug release zone, the controlled release function might be achieved by raising the radial drug concentration (Goole *et al.*, 2016). Examples of porous implants for bone tissue regeneration on BJ3DP include various combinations of powders, binders, and layer thicknesses. One such example uses α-tricalcium phosphate, hydroxyapatite (HA), and polyvinyl alcohol with a 10% phosphoric acid solution as a binder, and a water-based binder, with layer thicknesses of 50 μm and 100 μm. Another example utilizes a mixture of calcium sulfate hemihydrate, HA, and tricalcium phosphate with a 2-pyrrolidinone solution and phosphate buffer with Tween 80, both having a layer thickness of 89 μm. A third example features α-tricalcium phosphate, HA microsphere binder, and a MgO/ZnO-TCP mixture with a 2% dihydrogen sodium phosphate solution, with a layer thickness of 90 μm.

6.7 REGULATORY CONSIDERATIONS AND CHALLENGES

Lack of a regulatory framework is another major barrier to producing pharmaceuticals using this technology. Despite the fact that the FDA has only approved one 3D-printed pharmaceutical product (Spritam), the agency did issue guidelines in 2017 outlining the legal prerequisites for producing medical devices. Regulating the use of

3D printing to create dosage forms has, regrettably, not yet been done by any regulatory body (Chen *et al.*, 2022). Furthermore, it is unclear at this time whether the regulatory approval will apply to the entire product or just to a set of specifications covering every component of the product as well as all phases of development and production (Goole *et al.*, 2016).

Binder jetting needs to be reliable and consistent throughout the entire process cycle in order to be used as a manufacturing method for large physical size and quantity end use parts. For all AM processes, achieving consistency in a process where each part is unique presents a significant challenge because geometry causes variation on a wide range of processes and part parameters. Parts that need to be sintered to full density as a single alloy can be handled by binder jetting with ease, but obtaining the desired final geometry requires multiple exploratory sintering attempts for parts that vary greatly in print. The main issues are erosion and slumping, even in cases of infiltration where shrinkage is only 1 to 2 percent (Chen *et al.*, 2022). However, depending on the final density that is established by the green density, holding temperature, and time, a binder jetted and sintered part may shrink by up to 25% after sintering. Swelling usually occurs more in the z-direction but more similarly in the x- and y-directions due to reduced packing density between layers and gravity. Because of differences in the density of the powder bed within or between layers, the green portion develops anisotropic properties that further distort the part during the sintering process. A change in packing density, powder displacement, or the z-dimension of the 3D-printed part may also result from the weight of the accumulating powder layers compressing the lower layers as the z-height increases. Therefore, further research into infiltration and complex geometry sintering is needed, if desired. While some research has been conducted on the creation of complex overhang structures, further investigation is needed to look at different feature types and the effects of powder properties, print process parameters, and furnace conditions on geometry distortion.

Differential shrinkage rates within the part as a result of thermal gradients are a significant cause of distortion during sintering. The final part will have incorrect geometry and undesirable properties if there is any unpredictable shrinkage rate or distortion. It takes gradual temperature ramping to get past this problem. Furthermore, the part may form in a semi-solid or even liquid phase at the sintering temperature due to its composition and hot spots in the sintering sample. This makes shape retention and prediction for binder-jet 3D printed parts even more difficult. Applying non-reactive powder (such as alumina powder) to the affected areas is a workable way to reduce the heat gradient. Additionally, the use of reactive binder is recommended, which improves part strength and shape retention by forming interparticle bridges between nano-crystalline structures during the initial stage of sintering. To simulate shrinkage and sintering, part distortion can be predicted theoretically through modeling. Additionally, adding nanoparticles has been found to reduce slumping and shrinkage.

A few studies looked at how printing parameters and powder affected the development of layering defects in binder-jetted parts. Because of the high-velocity binder and the potential for improper binder spreading, ultra-fine powder may be ejected from the powder bed's upper surface due to binder effects like impact and powder–binder interaction. Green part density can be impacted and the densification process delayed by powder effects such as satellite particles, varying packing densities throughout the powder bed, and printhead and recoater speeds with suspension of nanoparticles; this technique is known as "binderless jetting". There have been some recent attempts to use nanoparticle suspension in place of the organic binder; this technique is known as "binderless jetting". A few advantages of using nanoparticle suspensions could be the removal of the need for a debinding step, the removal of residual binder carbon that could change the final part's characteristics, and the need for exact and complex sintering profiles to ensure proper binder burn out and degassing. Nevertheless, there are still certain challenges, like inkjet nozzle clogging, particle sedimentation, and surface oxidation, even when nanoparticle suspensions are employed. Almost every step of the printing process has the potential to produce a final product that is defective, so it is important to look into these defect causes and take action to eliminate them.

6.8 INTELLECTUAL PROPERTY AND PATENT ISSUES IN PHARMACEUTICAL 3D PRINTING

When protected goods are manufactured at home, it becomes practically impossible to enforce patents. This portion of the paper examines the issues that 3D printing poses for India's patent system. The attractiveness of 3D printing is that it gives consumers the ability to "manufacture" at home, removing power from conventional corporations and supply chains. In terms of pinning liability and causing damages, this grab of authority, however, is bad for patent owners. Obtaining patents for 3D-printed goods and processes and reproducing patented goods are the two main categories of patent law concerns pertaining to 3D printers (Goole *et al.*, 2016). According to Section 48 of the Patents Act, 1970 (hereafter referred to as the "1970 Act"), a patent holder has the authority to bar others from developing, utilizing, or commercializing a patented good without their consent. As can be seen, patents go one step farther than copyright and forbid not just the sale of an item but also its mere use. The use of a 3D printer to produce copyrighted goods and then using those goods would thus unavoidably be regarded as infringement under the 1970 Act.

6.8.1 ADVANCEMENTS IN BJ TECHNOLOGY FOR PHARMACEUTICAL APPLICATIONS

3DP technologies, including ink jet systems, laser-assisted systems, and fused deposition for tablets, implants, and microneedles, are already accessible for producing suitable medicinal dosage forms. For the wider application of 3DP technology, oral solid dosage forms and transdermal administration techniques both of which appear to be making significantly more progress are preferable. It has also been claimed that 3DP technology may be used to fabricate DNA biosensors with higher selectivity against non-complementary DNA targets. In comparison to the conventional patch, transdermal delivery systems with very complex structures can be produced using 3DP technology. The creation of more effective and customized medicine patches has been made possible by recent methods that combine 3D scanning technology and 3DP techniques. The 3D scanning equipment makes it possible to gather pertinent data about a person's skin characteristics, which paves the way for the 3DP processes used to create customized patches. This approach can be utilized to improve patient compliance and is not just limited to patches; it can also be applied to other connected pharmacological dosage forms, such as buccal tablets. Using high-resolution 3DP, it is possible to create controlled-size nanoparticles (NPs) for use as anticancer drug-delivery systems. 3D tissue models offer stronger *in vitro* and *in vivo* correlation than traditional two-dimensional (2D) models during the drug screening stage because they more closely resemble the spatial and chemical features of real tissues. As a result, current advancements in 3DP technology have accelerated the production of biomimetic structures helpful at various stages of new drug discovery and development, possibly replacing preclinical animal models (Shahrubudin *et al.*, 2019).

6.8.2 Integration of BJ with other 3D Printing Techniques

Manufacturers of binder-jet 3D printers have been providing consumers with cutting-edge 3D printing solutions for more than 20 years. An AM technique called BJ printing involves the targeted application of binder fluids to bind powdered components together in layers. Instead of transferring ink to a sheet of paper to create a two-dimensional pattern, BJ 3D printing technologies work in a three-dimensional powder-bed technique by precisely and selectively adhering selected layers of powder together. BJ is based on digital CAD data sets, just like the majority of AM techniques. The print program "sliced" these into incredibly thin layers. The recoater and the print head are the next two crucial parts that cooperate in the printing system. The recoater applies a very thin layer of powder material that is intended to be printed onto a building platform. The platform is then passed over by the print head, which applies a binder, where the component will be printed in accordance with the sliced data set. A new layer is deposited by the recoater and once more selectively bonded by the print head after a precise one-layer thickness drop in the platform. Until the component is fully printed, these procedures are repeated. After being removed from the box, the component can be cleaned of any extra, non-bonded material (Trenfield *et al.*, 2018a, b).

6.9 POTENTIAL IMPACT ON PERSONALIZED MEDICINE AND PATIENT CARE

A major advantage of 3D printing for the pharmaceutical industry is the capacity to produce personalized dosage forms. To better meet the needs of the patients, appropriate dosage forms can be created, dosages can be changed or combined, or the release patterns of the dosage forms can be altered. The application of 3D printing presents one option for providing dosage flexibility in response to patient needs. Due to the fact that their therapeutic dose is dependent on their age and body weight, children are one of the main population groups that require dose flexibility. 3D printers can effectively alter the aforementioned dosage forms to give patients the maximum dosage feasible. The amount of liquid API that is applied to the film can be changed to achieve this simply. Dosage forms with individualized release profiles can be manufactured via 3D printing to suit each patient's requirements. By creating holes in the immediate-release tablets or decreasing their thickness, it was found that the drug released more quickly when low-dose medications were used sometimes in as little as five minutes. A researcher fashioned paracetamol tablets into rings and meshes, comparing them to alternative shapes and solid tablets. The quick release of the mesh tablets was contrasted with the prolonged release of the ring and solid tablets.

A polypill is a tablet that mixes multiple prescriptions and is especially made for people who take a lot of different medications. Additionally, each person's needs might influence how the medicine is released. This concept can reduce the amount of tablets used daily while simultaneously increasing patient compliance and medication adherence, which is especially beneficial for the geriatric population. Successfully combined three drugs into 3D-printed polypills, which may have produced a potential therapy alternative for diabetics with hypertension. These capsules include nifedipine, glipizide, and captopril osmotic compartments in sustained-release capsules. The same team also created a five-piece polypill that represented a course of cardiovascular medication including pravastatin, atenolol, and ramipril in three sustained-release chambers, along with aspirin and hydrochlorothiazide in two immediate release compartments (Norman*et al.*, 2017).

6.10 CONCLUSION

Materials that can be used to create parts in 3D printing include metal powders, polymers, ceramics, and sand. The process involves a few steps, though, like figuring out the powder's composition, morphology, and size distribution; making a liquid binder, selecting a binding method, and assessing how well it works with the particles; fine-tuning the binder-jet processing's parameters; and coming up with a densification plan. Further research is required to enhance understanding and forecast the impacts on wear resistance, mechanical, corrosion, magnetic, and biocompatibility properties, as well as final part density and green density. This includes deformation, theory, simulation, green density, and printing, curing, and post-processing parameters. *In situ* high-speed cameras and x-ray imaging systems are additional instruments that can be utilized to visually record the powder spreading and the binder–powder interaction during printing. Evaluate the performance of binder-jetted parts in various industrial applications and close any gaps in knowledge. In summary, BJ3DP will be able to take market share away from conventional manufacturing methods that are currently unable to take advantage of other well-established AM techniques, even though it will not entirely replace other AM production techniques.

REFERENCES

Awad F, Fina SJ, Trenfield P, Patel A, Goyanes S, Gaisfor, et al. 3D printed pellets (miniprintlets): a novel, multi-drug, controlled release platform technology. *Pharmaceutics*. 2019; 11:148.

Chang S-Y, Li SW, Kowsari K, Shetty A, Sorrells L, Sen K, et al. Binder-jet 3D printing of indomethacin-laden pharmaceutical dosage forms. J Pharm Sci [Internet]. 2020 [cited 2024 Aug 3];109(10):3054–63. Available from: https://pubmed.ncbi.nlm.nih.gov/32628950/

Chen RX, Han XL, Liu BS, Liu YB, Liu T, Wang ZM, Liu ZC, Zheng AP. Optimization of process parameters of 3D printed clozapine dispersive tablets and establishment of personalized dose model. Acta Pharmaceutica Sinica. 2021:1155–62.

Chen X, Wang S, Wu J, Duan S, Wang X, Hong X, et al. The application and challenge of binder jet 3D printing technology in pharmaceutical manufacturing. *Pharmaceutics* [Internet]. 2022; 14(12):2589. http://dx.doi.org/10.3390/pharmaceutics14122589

Danae Karalia, AS, Karalis V, Vlachou M. 3D-printed oral dosage forms: mechanical properties, computational approaches and applications. *Pharmaceutics*. 2021 Sep; 13 (9):1401. http://dx.doi.org/10.3390/pharmaceutics13091401.

Dürig T, Karan K. Binders in Pharmaceutical Granulation. In: *Handbook of Pharmaceutical Granulation Technology*. 4th Edition. Boca Raton, FL: CRC Press. Series: *Drugs and the pharmaceutical sciences*; 2021. p. 103–33.

Fitzpatrick S, McCabe JF, Petts CR, Booth SW. Effect of moisture on polyvinylpyrrolidone in accelerated stability testing. *International Journal of Pharmaceutics*. 2002; 246(1–2):143–151.

Goole J, Amighi K. 3D printing in pharmaceutics: a new tool for designing customized drug delivery systems. *International Journal of Pharmaceutics*. 2016; 499(1–2):376–394.

Gottschalk N, Burkard A, Quodbach J, Bogdahn M. Drop-on-powder 3D printing of amorphous high dose oral dosage forms: Process development, opportunities and printing limitations. *International Journal of Pharmaceutics X* [Internet]. 2023; 5(100151):100151. Available from: www.sciencedirect.com/science/article/pii/S2590156722000421.

Goyanes A, Allahham N, Trenfield SJ, Stoyanovd E, Gaisford S, Basit AW. Direct powder extrusion 3D printing: fabrication of drug products using a novel single-step process. *International Journal of Pharmaceutics*. 2019; 567:118471.

Hong X, Han X, Li X, Li J, Wang Z, Zheng A. Binder jet 3D printing of compound LEV-PN dispersible tablets: An innovative approach for fabricating drug systems with multicompartmental structures. *Pharmaceutics [Internet]*. 2021;13(11):1780. doi:10.3390/pharmaceutics13111780

Huang SY, Ye XC, Lv ZF, Chen YZ. Formulation optimization of andrographolide orally disintegrating tablets by 3D printing technology. Strait Pharm J. 2020;32:14–17.

Jamróz W, Kurek M, Łyszczarz E, Szafraniec J, Knapik-Kowalczuk J, Syrek K. 3D printed orodispersible films with aripiprazole. *International Journal of Pharmaceuticals*. 2017; 533:13–420.

Kreft K, Lavrič Z, Stanić T, Perhavec P, Dreu R. Influence of the binder jetting process parameters and binder liquid composition on the relevant attributes of 3D-printed tablets. Pharmaceutics [Internet]. 2022 [cited 2024 Aug 3];14(8):1568. Available from: http://dx.doi.org/10.3390/pharmaceutics14081568

Kiekens F, Zelko R, Remon JP. Effect of the storage conditions on the tensile strength of tablets in relation to the enthalpy relaxation of the binder. *Pharmaceutical Research*. 2000; 17(4):490–493.

Li R, Shi Y, Wang Z, Wang L, Liu J, Jiang W. Densification behavior of gas and water atomized 316L stainless steel powder during selective laser melting. *Appl Surf Sci [Internet]*. 2010;256(13):4350–4356. Available from: http://dx.doi.org/10.1016/j.apsusc.2010.02.030

Litster J, Ennis B. Wetting, Nucleation and Binder Distribution. In *The Science and Engineering of Granulation Processes*. Particle Technology Series, vol 15; 2004. pp. 37–74. Springer, Dordrecht. https://doi.org/10.1007/978-94-017-0546-2_3

Mostafaei A, Elliott AM, Barnes JE, Li F, Tan W, Cramer CL, Nandwana P, Chmielus M. Binder jet 3D printing—Process parameters, materials, properties, modeling, and challenges. *Progress in Material Science*. 2021; 119:1007071.

Musazzi UM, Selmin F, Ortenzi MA, Mohammed GK, Franzé SP. Minghetti et Personalized orodispersible films by hot melt ram extrusion 3D printing. *International Journal of Pharmaceuticals*. 2018; 551:52–59.

Naveen PK, Pugazendhi D, Santosh C, Dinesh SK. Design and fabrication of binder jetting 3D printer. *International Research Journal of Engineering and Technology*. 2021; 8(4):2598–2602.

Norman J, Madurawe RD, Moore CMV, Khan MA, Khairuzzaman A. A newchapter in pharmaceutical manufacturing: 3Dprinted drug products. *Advanced Drug Delivery Reviews*. 2017; 108:39–50.

Pandey M, Choudhury H, Fern JLC, Kee ATK, Kou J, Jing JLJ, et al. 3D printing for oral drug delivery: a new tool to customize drug delivery. *Drugs Delivery Translation Research*. 2020; 10:986–1001.

Pereira BC, Isreb A, Forbes RT, Dores F, Habashy R, Petit J-B, Alhnan MA, Oga EF. 'Temporary plasticiser': a novel solution to fabricate 3D printed patient-centred cardiovascular 'Polypill' architectures. *European Journal of Pharmaceuticals and Biopharmacy*. 2019; 135:94–103.

Sen K, Mukherjee R, Sansare S, Halder A, Kashi H, Ma AWK, Chaudhuri B. Impact of powder-binder interactions on 3D printability of pharmaceutical tablets using drop test methodology. *European Journal of Pharmaceutical Sciences*. 2021; 160:105755.

Shahrubudin NN, Lee TC, Ramlan R. An overview on 3D printing technology:technological, materials, and applications. *Procedia Manufacturing*. 2019; 35: 1286–1296.

Tan JH, Wong WLE, Dalgarno KW. An overview of powder granulometry on feedstock and part performance in the selective laser melting process. *Addit Manuf [Internet]*. 2017;18:228–55. Available from: http://dx.doi.org/10.1016/j.addma.2017.10.011

Tawfeek HM, Hassan YA, Aldawsari MF, Fayed MH. Enhancing the low oral bioavailability of sulpiride via fast orally disintegrating tablets: formulation, optimization and in vivo characterization. *Pharmaceuticals*. 2020; 13:446.

Tian P, Yang F, Xu Y, Lin M-M, Yu L-P, Lin W, *et al.* Oral disintegrating patient-tailored tablets of warfarin sodium produced by 3D printing. Drug Dev Ind Pharm [Internet]. 2018 [cited 2024 Aug 3];44(12):1918–23. Available from: https://pubmed.ncbi.nlm.nih.gov/30027774/

Trenfield SJ, Madla CM, Basit AW, Gaisford S. Binder Jet Printing in Pharmaceutical Manufacturing. In *3D Printing of Pharmaceuticals,* Vol. 31; Basit AW, Gaisford S Eds.; AAPS Advances in the Pharmaceutical Sciences Series; Springer International Publishing: Cham, Switzerland; 2018a. pp. 41–54. ISBN 978-3-319-90754-3.

Trenfield SJ, Awad A, Goyanes A, Gaisford S, Basit AW. 3D printing pharmaceuticals: drug development to frontline care. *Trends in Pharmacology Science*. 2018b; 39:440–451.

Van den Heuvel KA, de Wit MTW, Dickhoff BHJ. Evaluation of lactose based 3D powder bed printed pharmaceutical drug product tablets. *Powder Technology* [Internet]. 2021; 390:97–102. Available from: www.sciencedirect.com/science/article/pii/S0032591021004575

Vithani K, Goyanes A, Jannin V, Basit AW, Gaisford S, Boyd BJ. An overview of 3D printing technologies for soft materials and potential opportunities for lipid-based drug delivery systems. *Pharmacy Research*. 2018; 36: 4.

Wang Z, Li J, Hong X, Han X, Liu B, Li X, *et al.* Taste masking study based on an electronic tongue: The formulation design of 3D printed levetiracetam instant-dissolving tablets. Pharm Res [Internet]. 2021 [cited 2024 Aug 3];38(5):831–42. Available from: http://dx.doi.org/10.1007/s11095-021-03041-9

Yanden Heuvel KA, de Wit MTW, Dickhoff BHJ. Evaluation of lactose based 3D powder bed printed pharmaceutical drug product tablets. *Powder Technology*. 2021; 390:97–102. http://dx.doi.org/10.1016/j.powtec.2021.05.050

Zhou Z, Lennon A, Buchanan F, McCarthy HO, Dunne N. Binder jetting AM of hydroxyapatite powders: effects of adhesives on geometrical accuracy and green compressive strength. *Additive Manufacturing*. 2020; 36:101645

Ziaee M, Crane NB. Binder jetting: a review of process, materials, and methods. *Additive Manufacturing* [Internet]. 2019; 28:781–801. http://dx.doi.org/10.1016/j.addma.2019.05.031

7 Binder Jetting-Based 3D Printing in Pharmaceutics

Aakriti Patel, Mohit Agrawal, Aastha Singh, Kuldeep Singh, Swamita Arora, Swati Arya, and Sameer Rastogi

7.1 INTRODUCTION

The pharmaceutical industry consistently comes under pressure to improve the quality of its products. A continual desire exists to learn something new and improve manufacturing technology and material properties. Patient-centric medicine advancement has become an area of interest in the pharmaceutical industry with the objective of offering better patient care and increasing patient compliance. To overcome the challenges, the pharmaceutical industry has seen how novel drug delivery systems have overtaken traditional dosage forms. Three-dimensional printing (3DP) has been discovered that can revolutionize the drug manufacturing process. It is regarded as one of the most dynamically growing industries in science. From the production of organs to the creation of novel dosage forms, 3DP has proven its worth. ISO defines 3DP as "the process of creating objects via placing components with the aid of a print head, nozzle, or different printer technology". 3DP employs additive manufacturing (AM) technology, in which parts are constructed by successively adding layer after layer. In contrast to other frequently employed technologies such as subtractive or formative manufacturing, AM is potentially advantageous because it minimizes manufacturing duration and expense while also allowing for easy customization at the design level (Jose *et al.* 2018) (Figure 7.1).

Several technologies were discovered in the 40 years of 3DP. Each of these approaches has unique attributes; they can be extrusion-based, powder-based, or liquid-based (Jamroz *et al.*, 2018). Among all the other methods powder-based technology, particularly binder jet printing (BJP), was recognized long before any other technique. Sachs *et al.* (Sachs *et al.*, 1993) were the first group to discover and develop it. The design was patented (USOO5340656A) in the year 1993 at the MIT. It jets liquid or paste materials onto a powder bed to build up layer after layer, resulting in the development of a 3DP structure. BJP is regarded as one of the most advanced technologies in the discipline of pharmaceutical production to date. In 2015, BJP finally got approval from the Food and Drug Administration for large-scale manufacturing of "Spritam" (Aprecia Pharmaceuticals 2015).

DOI: 10.1201/9781003439509-11

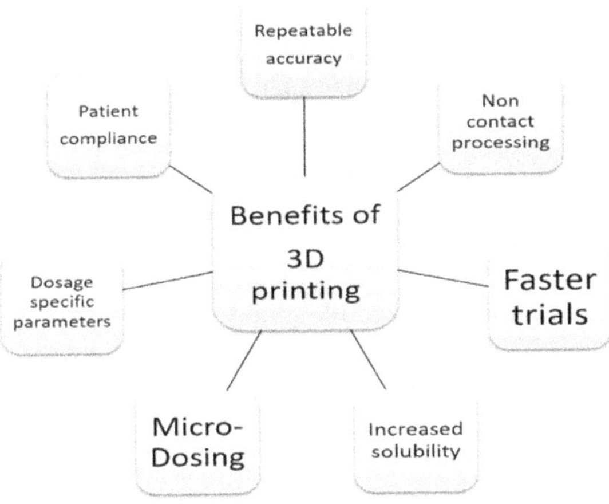

FIGURE 7.1   The figure illustrates the benefits of 3D printing in the pharmaceutical sector.

7.2   COMPONENTS OF BJP

BJP requires a variety of excipients based on its functionality. There are various factors that determine which excipients should be used. One of the most essential variables to consider prior to developing a drug is compatibility. Not only excipient be non-toxic, but it should also be stable in nature.

7.2.1   POWDER MIXTURE

It is an essential component of BJP that has a direct relationship to the printed dosage form's property. It must be noted that the powder utilized during this method should be printable, which is a feature of powders that is necessary for the 3D printing process (Zhou et *al.*, 2014). An excellent flowable powder is yet another requirement for convenient manufacturing using BJP. If enough powder flowability can be achieved, the roller can scatter the powder in a uniform as well as in a precisely thinner coating. Insufficient flowability reduces resolution and causes irregularity or quality impairments in printed dosage forms. In contrast, high flowability, results in powder bed instability (Rahman et *al.*, 2020). The rate of speed at which the powder is spread by the rotating roller is not only influenced by particle size/shape but also by the flow properties. Inadequate speed of spreading results in a non-uniform layer. Slower spreading speeds are advised at the expense of printing time (Miyanaji et *al.*, 2016). Due to high van der Waals forces, slow speeds are encouraged for smaller particle powder materials (>5 mm). In contrast, for coarse particles, a higher speed can be used (Yang et *al.*, 2013). To get the best results there are some critical parameters that should be considered before formulating. They are as follows:

7.2.1.1 Powder-specific properties

It is defined as the powder's ability to retain its firmness by being adhered to the subsequent layers sprayed on top. Additional features, such as flowability, particle dimension, homogeneity, and so on, have significance for upholding the integrity of the structural framework.

7.2.1.2 Powder–binding interaction

The powder should be competent to effortlessly associate with the ink solution; this relationship between the powder and the binder solution is referred to as powder–binder interaction. The interaction between these two phases is determined by the powder's surface area, wettability, and binding ability (Sen *et al.*, 2021) (Figure 7.2).

7.2.2 Binder Solution

It is essential to choose an efficient binder solution while producing an excellent 3D-printed dosage form. The consistency of the binder solution plays a vital role during formulation. An optimum binder solution possesses low viscosity, which allows smooth and uniform jetting of the solution (Bredt, 1995). For binder solution/suspension for BJP, the literature has reports showing viscosity and surface tension of 1.6e5.99 mPa.S and 25.7e52 mN/m, respectively (Genina *et al.*, 2013, Lee *et al.*, 2012, Sandler *et al.*, 2011). The binder must also be tolerant of the high shear stress induced during printing (Seto *et al.*, 2009). Additional considerations that are important while printing include long shelf life, clean burn-out features, and so on (Liu *et al.*, 2003). The overall composition of the binder solution affects binder system properties. In

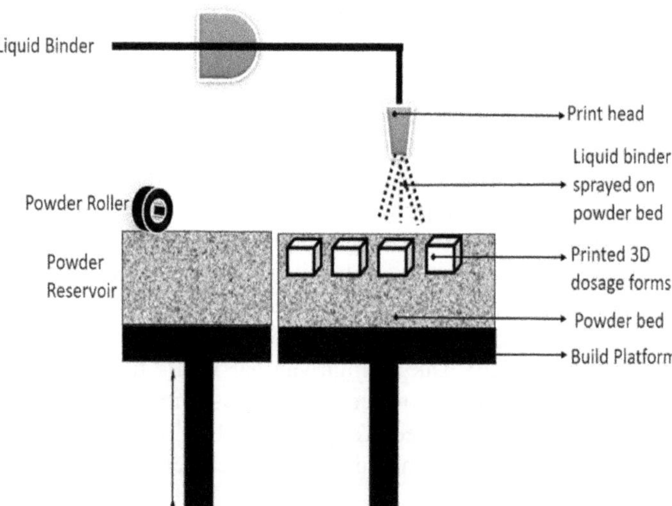

FIGURE 7.2 The figure illustrates the production of 3D-printed objects using binder jet printing.

the case of surface tension, it can be reduced by employing surfactants like Tween 80 (Rahman *et al.,* 2014). The binder viscosity can be controlled by controlling the overall viscosity, molecular weight grade and amount of the polymer. Most of the Polyols (PEG, glycerol) are employed as viscosity modifiers (Rahman *et al.,* 2020).

7.3 METHOD OF PREPARATION

BJP refers to an inkjet printing procedure in which the printer utilizes a binder solution to reprint an electronic file from a computer on a powder bed (Boland *et al.,* 2006). BJP has identical prerequisites to other 3DP methods, in which the digital file is generated via computer-based software or an imaging-based technique, like MRI or CAD, resulting in a 3D illustration of objects (Trenfeild *et al.,* 2018). BJP operates on traditional ink-jet printing methods and consists of five fundamental phases;

(i) A printer nozzle that contains binder liquid is configured in a way that it can oscillate an *x-y* axis and spray binder over the powder bed.

(ii) The droplet sprayed, wets the powder bed, resulting in the local hardness along with solidification of the powder layer. BJP typically uses two types of drop-on-demand (DoD) heads that regulate droplet deposition: piezoelectric and thermal heads (Day *et al.,* 2001). The thermal system consists of a print head with a compact liquid reservoir that contains a binder solution. Current is applied briefly through a resistive element on the print head, triggering the internal temperature rise followed by the vaporization, nucleation, and expansion of a single bubble to release a droplet (Buanz *et al.,* 2011, Vaddanda *et al.,* 2018).

(iii) The fabrication plate then travels lower on the vertical axis, while the powder delivery platform advances upward.

(iv) A thin powder layer is applied via a roller upon the previously formed layer, the procedure is performed repeatedly to construct printed objects.

(v) The 3DP object is extracted from the powder bed and the excess powder is removed. Thermal sintering is mostly utilized to achieve object permanence by removing any traces of volatile solvents (Daly *et al.,* 2015, Alomari *et al.,* 2015).

There are various factors that influence these steps, which can be divided into two categories:

7.3.1 Critical Raw Materials

As previously discussed binder solution and powder mixture play a major part in the manufacturing of the drugs using BJP. There are various critical parameters of the raw materials that can affect the product quality (Sen *et al.,* 2021).

(i) Size distribution: particle size distribution is an independent powder property, which affects the printed objects directly and controls powder flowability and pack density.

Particle size also significantly affects the physical strength as well as texture of the printed object. Lower particle size, measuring between 20–5 µm tends to offer a higher density of packing, while a low porosity particle-containing bed produces good physical strength and a smoother surface for the printed object (Lu *et al.*, 2009). Segregation of formulations leads to deterioration of the finished products due to non-uniformity of the content, which can happen in solid dosage development containing polydisperse and cohesive powder mixtures by manufacturing different printed dosage forms containing non-uniform API quantities (Gentzler *et al.*, 2015).

(ii) Packing density: maintaining the spread layer to achieve uniformity and good packing density is the most difficult challenge. The uniformity of the particle in the packed bed during printing is critical and is determined by packing characteristics, such as shape and size of powder particles (Ke *et al.*, 2018, Sen *et al.*, 2020). For smaller particles of 75 µm, the packing rate was significantly reduced because of the roller-spreading process (Lu *et al.*, 2009). The incorporation of bimodal powder blends enhances packing density up to 8.2% in comparison with a monosized fine powder mixture (75–5 mm) in which the ratio of the coarse to fine-sized particle remains between 1:3 and 1:6 (Bai *et al.*, 2017).

Powder packing density influences both mechanical strength and post-processing as well. Reduced porosity in the print bed is caused by higher bed packing density, which reduces thermal conductivity during the drying process.

(iii) Flowability of powder: powder flowability serves as one of the determining variables for BJP printing. Since the printing includes layering of multiple powder coats piled upon one another. A poor flow of powder in printing may compromise the printing bed by forming particle lump, lowering the print resolution and causing drug content non-uniformity in the produced product. Powder mixtures of larger particle sizes provide higher flow but cannot provide higher packing density when compared to the powder bed with smaller components. Inter-particle forces like van der Waal's, electrostatic forces dominate the flow of small particles (Sarkar *et al.*, 2017).

(iv) Jettability of binder solution: the printing efficacy during the inkjet procedure is determined by the resolution of print and drop location accuracy, in addition to the nature of the binder solution (Guo *et al.*, 2017). The spraying process while printing is accomplished through a drop formation process that holds repeatability in the formation of drops throughout the printing process. The binder solution must be jettable (McIlroy *et al.*, 2013). The fluid jet breakup behavior remains constant irrespective of nozzle size or type of acting on the jet (Blume *et al.*, 1997). Surface tension, viscosity, and droplet velocity are the factors that influence splitting behaviors. Depending on the fluid properties, the droplet generation/jet separation process may result in either stable or unstable droplets. When the smaller droplets combine into a single drop before it hits the print bed, a stable droplet is formed. In contrast, if there is unstable droplet formation, the satellite droplets may be incapable of combining or there will be no formation droplets, lowering the print resolution.

7.3.2 Critical Process Parameter

(i) Printing attributes: the speed of the roller, thickness of the powder bed, and binder concentration ratio are all important factors for achieving optimized printing during the BJP process. For example, in an excessively fed powder layer, the low roller height may result in roughness. Moreover, increased powder layer thickness reduces printing resolution and leads to less binder concentration resulting in low physical quality of printed parts (Bai *et al.*, 2015).

(ii) Binder concentration and layer thickness: the combination of binder concentration ratio and powder bed thickness has a major impact on the 3DP product manufactured via BJP method. The above variables can be adjusted during the BJP process to improve the physical durability of printed parts. The droplet might instantly penetrate into the deepest wet layer as thickness decreases. Even though the prior wet layer pushes back the binder droplet's vertical penetration, its spreading in the opposite direction is unhindered. This leads to a wider spreading of the layer while reducing the thickness. Lower binder saturation ratios while maintaining constant layer thickness result in limited binder spreading in the lateral directions.

(iii) Speed of roller: by applying a roller or spreader, powder is distributed upon a previously printed layer. The horizontal accuracy of the printed objects is influenced by roller speed. The time of contact of the roller with the powder bed decreases as its speed increases, which minimizes the roller's lateral bending of the powder bed.

(iv) Speed of printing: the total time of printing can be drastically reduced by improving the overall quantity of print cycles of the printer or by adjusting the pace at which printheads move on the print platform. An increase in the speed may have an effect on print resolution or shape preciseness. Because at faster printing rates, the binder might not evaporate completely from previously printed layers, resulting in increased texture, inferior precision in size, or uneven coating of the printed layer throughout the course of printing.

7.4 BENEFIT

BJP is a printing technique that can produce fast-dissolving tablets with minimal bulk density and high drug loadings, such as Spritam, used in epilepsy medicine manufacturing (Yu *et al.*, 2008). It can also develop sophisticated formulations due to its powder bed, eliminating the need for supports or rafts. BJP incorporates API in dosage forms, making precision drug loading easier and more achievable at higher loading percentages (Sen *et al.*, 2020). This makes it suitable for low drug-loaded formulations where content uniformity is a concern (Shi *et al.*, 2019). BJP also offers personalized API dosing of drugs, allowing differentiation between geriatric and pediatric patients and avoiding drug interaction and overdosing complications (Jose *et al.*, 2018, Norman *et al.*, 2017). Compared to traditional manufacturing processes, BJP allows easy scale-up, allowing for increased printed object manufacturing by

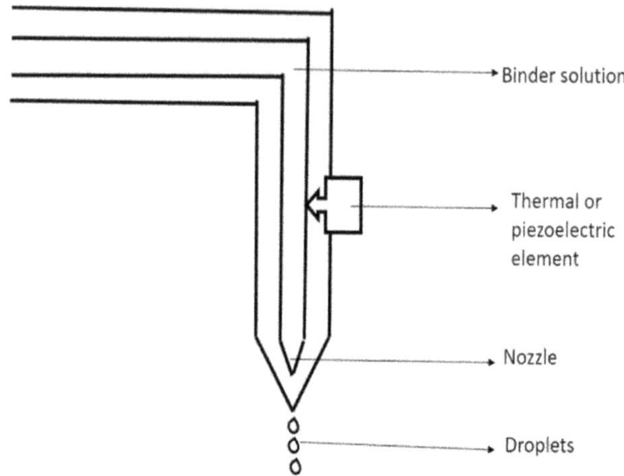

FIGURE 7.3 The figure illustrates drop-on-demand (DoD) heads that regulate droplet deposition.

increasing the number of printhead inkjet nozzles and building envelope (Levy *et al.*, 2017) (Figure 7.3).

7.5 DRAWBACKS/CHALLENGES

The process of developing BJP involves expanding capabilities and enhancing material properties. However, transitioning from prototyping to industrial use requires enhancing average properties, improving geometric accuracy, and minimizing fluctuation. Variations in powder bed density can cause property variations, porosity, and distortion (Miyanji *et al.*, 2018). Large arrays of jets can be vulnerable to saturation errors and local imperfections (Fan 1996). Droplets may merge to create "balling", which occurs when powder wetting is poor and binder dispensing rate is high (Fan 1996). BJP provides distinct characteristics that are difficult to assess with standard or quality control procedures. Deformities like warping, delamination, or cracking require extensive knowledge of the technique and material properties.

7.6 APPLICATION OF BJP IN PHARMACEUTICAL MANUFACTURING

Early studies in the mid-1990s utilized BJP for quickly creating tools with metal powder and ceramics, as the approach was originally developed for this sort of use (Sachs *et al.*, 1990). BJP provides unprecedented versatility. In terms of materials, almost any powder bed can be utilized to make objects, given that it can be blended with an approved binder. Furthermore, the BJP can be expanded to produce large-sized items (in the metre range) as well as tiny ones (in the millimetre range) (Lu *et al.*, 2008). This technology provides outstanding precision, allowing the development of items with exceptionally complicated designs that would be challenging, or unattainable to manufacture using traditional manufacturing processes. Because of its ability to fabricate complex structures, there has been rising attention to using this approach in pharmaceuticals for the production of scaffolds. Several research papers, for example, have described the development of scaffolds made of the natural material hydroxyapatite (Cox *et al.*, 2015, Duan *et al.*, 2010, Leulers *et al.*, 2005), in addition to polylactic acid (PLA) mixed together with bioactive calcium phosphate (Serra *et al.*, 2013).

7.6.1 DRUGS IN INK METHOD

(i)   Rapid dispersible tablets (RDT): Lee *et al.* developed an RDT of Captopril, with the help of ink with PVP 25, and a buffer throughout the process (Lee *et al.*, 2003). Maltitol, maltodextrin, and polyvinyl pyrrolidone were used as powder excipients in this experiment. Sen *et al.* (Sen *et al.*, 2020, Lee *et al.*, 2003) used BJP to formulate an RDT containing Amitriptyline HCL in the binder solution and PVP K30 in the excipient mixture.

(ii) Delayed-release tablets: several other scientists have formulated a delayed-release tablet in which they used different types of polymers (Eudragit 100, Eudragit RLPO) with a range of different concentrations from 8.9 to 17.9%. The powder beds used for the process are microcrystalline cellulose and dried lactose (Katstra *et al.*, 2000).

(iii) Zero-order release: one of the many approaches of BJP was applied by Wang *et al.* (Wang *et al.*, 2021). When they fabricated a zero-order release tablet in which they incorporated pseudoephedrine hydrochloride as API in the binder solution and Kollidon SR, HPMC was used as a powder bed.

(iv) Controlled-release tablet: in the year 1996, a debut pharmaceutical tablet fabricated using BJ-3DP was produced. (Wu *et al.*, 1996) used methylene blue and alizarin yellow as prototype API in order to formulate a control-released tablet. Aside from the drug, the dosage form also included powder excipients polyethylene oxide and poly-caprolactone, as well as a binder solution of dichloromethane and chloroform. It was deemed unsafe due to its toxic nature and issues in the removal of binder traces found in the formulation. Nevertheless, this work was regarded as an important break-through because 3DP in the pharmaceutical industry began to rise following this study.

7.6.2 DRUGS IN POWDER METHOD

(i)   Orodispersible tablets (ODT): the BJP was utilized to develop the first publicly sold "FDA-approved 3DP tablet, Spritam" (Jacob *et al.*, 2016). Aprecia Pharmaceuticals acquired the patent for the manufacturing of an ODT in which levetiracetam, was combined in a powder approach.
      ODT tend to be restricted by two factors:
      • Little drug loading.
      • Slow disintegration.

- "Spritam" surpassed both of the major obstacles by achieving higher drug loading (up to 1000 mg) that is greater than a traditional production method, and rapid disintegration. When compared to traditional ODT (3 minutes), Spritam disintegrates in 11 seconds, shortening the time it takes for an action to begin.

(ii) Oral disintegrating tablets (ODIT): ODIT of Warfarin sodium were developed in the year 2018, by Tian *et al.* (Tian *et al.*, 2018). The drug was contained in a powder blend of microcrystalline cellulose, pregelatinized starch, D sucrose, povidone K30, and silicon dioxide. In the investigation, ethanol was used as a moistening agent which was added to the ink container. They then tested the tablets for things like dose uniformity, hardness, friability, as well as dissolution. The mean disintegration time for tablets containing 3, 2, and 1 mg was 50.0, 35.7, and 11.0 seconds, respectively. Furthermore, hardness and friability were found to be within acceptable limits, and tablets have a uniformly rigid structure and uniform visuals.

(iii) Fast disintegrating tablets (FDT): using 3D printing, it is possible to fabricate tablets of varying types. Yu *et al.* (Yu *et al.*, 2009) employed thermal printheads that had four jet nozzles. PVPK30, Acetaminophen, lactose, mannitol, and colloidal silica were used as the powder bed, and the binder contained methylene blue and PVPK30 in 75% ethanol in water. When compared to traditional tablets made with the punch method, the 3D-printed tablets had a suitable hardness of 54.5 ± 4.2 N/cm^2 and a total mass loss of $0.92 \pm 0.14\%$ during the friability test.

(iv) Novel donut-shaped tablets (NDS): 3DP allows for manufacturing tablets of different forms and releases. To achieve linear release profiles, Yu *et al.* built an NDS dosage that contained lipophilic drugs and release retardant substances (Yu *et al.*, 2009). Acetaminophen was used as the prototype drug, with HPMC serving as the matrix and ethyl cellulose working as the release retardant.

7.7 CONCLUSION AND FUTURE PERSPECTIVE

The global market size of 3D printing is enormous and growing at an accelerating pace year after year. From 2019 to 2026, the global 3D printing medical industry is expected to be worth US$3692 million, expanding at a compound annual growth rate (CAGR) of 18.2%. The authorization of Spritam1 sparked intense interest from global pharmaceutical manufacturers, particularly those in North America, Europe, China, and Japan. To expedite product approval, regulatory agencies must also be prepared with a thorough understanding of technical details and product review pathways. This also necessitates reducing the distance among every party involved, including scientists, drug producers, and regulators, in order to convert theory into achievable and revolutionary solutions. Above all, real-time evaluation of the safety and effectiveness of 3DP items in clinical practice is required to produce extremely versatile and personalized dosage forms on request (Wu *et al.*, 1996).

In conclusion, 3DP using BJP is revolutionizing the pharmaceutical industry by offering a novel approach to drug manufacturing. BJP, an AM technology, deposits liquid binders onto a powder bed layer by layer, providing advantages such as customization, reduced manufacturing time, and scalability. Key components of BJP, including the powder mixture and binder solution, are crucial for ensuring quality in printed dosage forms. Considerations such as powder flowability, binding interactions, and critical formulation parameters play pivotal roles in the success of BJP applications. The method involves inkjet printing, where a binder solution is sprayed onto a powder bed to create layers and construct 3D-printed objects. Despite its benefits, BJP faces challenges such as variations in raw material parameters and deformities during the transition to industrial use. In pharmaceutical manufacturing, BJP has been applied to produce various formulations, from rapid dispersible tablets to controlled-release tablets, showcasing advantages like high drug loadings and precision drug loading. While acknowledging BJP's drawbacks such as property variations, its potential extends beyond tablets to include scaffolds for tissue engineering. As the industry continues to explore 3DP techniques like BJP, there is the promise of revolutionizing drug manufacturing processes, offering personalized dosing, improved drug delivery, and increased production efficiency.

REFERENCES

Alomari M, Mohamed FH, Basit AW, Gaisford S. Personalised dosing: printing a dose of one's own medicine. Int J Pharm. 2015; 494(2):568–77.

Aprecia Pharmaceuticals. 3D printing - ZipDose technology. 2015. Available from: www.aprecia.com/zipdose-platform/3d-printing.php.

Bai Y, Wagner G, Williams CB. Effect of bimodal powder mixture on powder packing density and sintered density in binder jetting of metals. In 2015 International Solid Freeform Fabrication Symposium. University of Texas at Austin. 2015.

Bai Y, Wagner G, Williams CB. Effect of particle size distribution on powder packing and sintering in binder jetting additive manufacturing of metals. ASME J Manufact Sci Eng. 2017 Aug; 139(8): 081019. https://doi.org/10.1115/1.4036640

Blume A. Codex indulgence: Leonardo's Codex Leicester and the issue of value. On Paper. 1997 Nov 1; 2(2):16–9.

Boland T, Xu T, Damon B, Cui X. Application of inkjet printing to tissue engineering. Biotechnol J: Healthc Nutri Technol. 2006 Sep; 1(9):910–7.

Bredt JF. Binder stability and powder/binder interaction in three-dimensional printing. Thesis (Ph. D.)--Massachusetts Institute of Technology, Dept. of Mechanical Engineering, 1995. Includes bibliographical references (378–382).

Buanz AB, Saunders MH, Basit AW, Gaisford S. Preparation of personalized-dose salbutamol sulphate oral films with thermal ink-jet printing. Pharm Res. 2011; 28(10):2386–92.

Cox SC, Thornby JA, Gibbons GJ, Williams MA, Mallick KK. 3D printing of porous hydroxyapatite scaffolds intended for use in bone tissue engineering applications. Mater Sci Eng C. 2015; 47(Supplement C):237–47.

Daly R, Harrington TS, Martin GD, Hutchings IM. Inkjet printing for pharmaceutics– a review of research and manufacturing. Int J Pharm. 2015; 494(2):554–67.

Day SP, Shufflebottom L. Evidential value from inkjet printers. Probl Forensic Sci. 2001; XLVI: 356–74.

Duan B, Wang M, Zhou WY, Cheung WL, Li ZY, Lu WW. Three-dimensional nanocomposite scaffolds fabricated via selective laser sintering for bone tissue engineering. Acta Biomater. 2010; 6(12):4495–505.

Genina N, Fors D, Palo M, Peltonen J, Sandler N. Behavior of printable formulations of loperamide and caffeine on different substrates-effect of print density in inkjet printing. Int J Pharm. 2013; 453:488e97.

Genina N, Fors D, Vakili H, Ihalainen P, Pohjala L, Ehlers H, Kassamakov I, Haeggstrom E, Vuorela P, Peltonen J, Sandler N. Tailoring controlled release oral dosage forms by combining inkjet and flexographic printing techniques. Eur J Pharm Sci. 2012; 47:615e23.

Gentzler M, Michaels JN, Tardos GI. Quantification of segregation potential for polydisperse, cohesive, multi-component powders and prediction of tablet die-filling performance-a methodology for practical testing, re-formulation and process design. Powder Technol. 2015 Nov 1; 285:96–102.

Guo Y, Patanwala HS, Bognet B, Ma AW. Inkjet and inkjet-based 3D printing: connecting fluid properties and printing performance. Rapid Prototyping J. 2017 Apr 18; 23(3):562–76.

Fan T. Droplet-powder impact interaction in three-dimensional printing (Doctoral dissertation, Massachusetts Institute of Technology).1996.

Jacob J, Coyle N, West TG, Surprenant HL, Jain NB, US9669009B2. United States: US Patent, 2016.

Jamróz W, Szafraniec J, Kurek M, Jachowicz R. 3D printing in pharmaceutical and medical applications–recent achievements and challenges. Pharm Res. 2018 Sep; 35:1–22.

Jose PA, GV PC. 3D printing of pharmaceuticals–a potential technology in developing personalized medicine. Asian J Pharm Res Develop. 2018 Jul 10; 6(3):46–54.

Katstra WE, Palazzolo RD, Rowe CW, Giritlioglu B, Teung P, Cima MJ. Oral dosage forms fabricated by three dimensional printing™. J Controlled Release. 2000 May 3;66(1):1–9.

Ke D, Bose S. Effects of pore distribution and chemistry on physical, mechanical, and biological properties of tricalcium phosphate scaffolds by binder-jet 3D printing. Additive Manufact. 2018 Aug 1; 22:111–7.

Lee BK, Yun YH, Choi JS, Choi YC, Kim JD, Cho YW. Fabrication of drug loaded polymer microparticles with arbitrary geometries using a piezoelectric inkjet printing system. Int J Pharm. 2012; 427:305310.

Lee KJ, Kang A, Delfino JJ, West TG, Chetty D, Monkhouse DC, Yoo J. Evaluation of critical formulation factors in the development of a rapidly dispersing captopril oral dosage form. Drug Develop Ind Pharm. 2003 Jan 1;29(9):967–79.

Leukers B, Gülkan H, Irsen SH, Milz S, Tille C, Schieker M, et al. Hydroxyapatite scaffolds for bone tissue engineering made by 3D printing. J Mater Sci Mater Med. 2005; 16(12):1121–4.

Levy A, Miriyev A, Elliott A, Babu SS, Frage N. Additive manufacturing of complex-shaped graded TiC/steel composites. Mater Design. 2017 Mar 15; 118:198–203.

Liu J, Rynerson M, inventors; Extrude Hone Corp, assignee. Method for article fabrication using carbohydrate binder. United States patent US 6585930. 2003 Jul 1.

Lu K, Hiser M, Wu W. Effect of particle size on three dimensional printed mesh structures. Powder Technol. 2009 Jun 5; 192(2):178–83.

Lu K, Reynolds WT. 3DP process for fine mesh structure printing. Powder Technol. 2008; 187(1):11–8.

McIlroy C, Harlen OG, Morrison NF. Modelling the jetting of dilute polymer solutions in drop-on-demand inkjet printing. J Non-Newtonian Fluid Mech. 2013 Nov 1; 201:17–28.

Meier C, Weissbach R, Weinberg J, Wall WA, Hart AJ. Critical influences of particle size and adhesion on the powder layer uniformity in metal additive manufacturing. *J Mater Proc Technol*. 2019 Apr 1; 266:484–501.

Miyanaji H, Momenzadeh N, Yang L. Effect of printing speed on the quality of printed parts in binder Jetting process. *Additive Manufact.* 2018 Mar 1; 20:1–0.

Miyanaji H, Zhang S, Lassell A, Zandinejad A, Yang L. Process development of porcelain ceramic material with binder jetting process for dental applications. *JOM* 2016; 68(3):831e41.

Norman J, Madurawe RD, Moore CM, Khan MA, Khairuzzaman A. A new chapter in pharmaceutical manufacturing: 3D-printed drug products. *Adv Drug Delivery Rev.* 2017 Jan 1; 108:39–50.

Rahman Z, Charoo NA, Kuttolamadom M, Asadi A, Khan MA. Printing of personalized medication using binder jetting 3D printer. *Precision Medicine for Investigators, Practitioners and Providers.* 2020: 473–481.

Rahman Z, Xu X, Katragadda U, Krishnaiah YS, Yu L, Khan MA. Quality by design approach for understanding the critical quality attributes of cyclosporine ophthalmic emulsion. *Mol Pharm.* 2014; 11(3):787e99.

Raijada D, Genina N, Fors D, Wisaeus E, Peltonen J, Rantanen J, Sandler N. A step toward development of printable dosage forms for poorly soluble drugs. *J Pharm Sci.* 2013; 102:3694e704. 11.

Roopavath UK, Kalaskar DM. Introduction to 3D printing in medicine. In 3D printing in medicine. Woodhead Publishing. 2017 Jan 1. pp. 1–20.

Sachs E, Brancazio D, Bredt JF, Tuerck H, Curodeau A, Khanuja S, Cima M, Fan T, Michaels SP, Lauder A, inventors; Massachusetts Institute Of Technology, assignee. Three-dimensional printing techniques. 1993 Dec 23.

Sachs E, Cima M, Cornie J. Three-dimensional printing: rapid tooling and prototypes directly from a CAD model. *CIRP Ann.* 1990; 39(1):201–4.

Sandler N, Maattanen A, Ihalainen P, Kronberg L, Meierjohann A, Viitala T, Peltonen J. Inkjet printing of drug substances and use of porous substrates-towards individualized dosing. *J Pharm Sci.* 2011; 100:3386e95.

Sarkar S, Mukherjee R, Chaudhuri B. A review of the role of forces governing particulate interactions in pharmaceutical systems. *Int J Pharm.* 2017 Jun 30; 526(1–2):516–37.

Sen K. A mechanistic understanding of binder-jet based 3D printing process. *Doctoral Dissertations*, 2455. 2020. https://digitalcommons.lib.uconn.edu/dissertations/2455

Sen K, Manchanda A, Mehta T, Ma AW, Chaudhuri B. Formulation design for inkjet-based 3D printed tablets. *Int J Pharm.* 2020 Jun 30; 584:119430.

Sen K, Mehta T, Ma AW, Chaudhuri B. DEM based investigation of powder packing in 3D printing of pharmaceutical tablets In EPJ Web of Conferences (Vol. 249). EDP Sciences. 2021. p. 14012.

Sen K, Mehta T, Sansare S, Sharifi L, Ma AW, Chaudhuri B. Pharmaceutical applications of powder-based binder jet 3D printing process–a review. *Adv Drug Delivery Rev.* 2021 Oct 1;177:113943.

Sen K, Mukherjee R, Sansare S, Halder A, Kashi H, Ma AW, Chaudhuri B. Impact of powder-binder interactions on 3D printability of pharmaceutical tablets using drop test methodology. *Euro J Pharm Sci.* 2021 May 1; 160:105755.

Serra T, Planell JA, Navarro M. High-resolution PLA-based composite scaffolds via 3-D printing technology. *Acta Biomater.* 2013; 9(3):5521–30.

Seto S, Yagi T, Okuda M, Umehara S, Kataoka M. Lifetime improvement for full-width-array Piezo Ink Jet print head using matrix nozzle arrangement. *J Imaging Sci Technol.* 2009 Sep 1; 53(5):50305–1.

Shi K, Tan DK, Nokhodchi A, Maniruzzaman M. Drop-on-powder 3D printing of tablets with an anti-cancer drug, 5-fluorouracil. *Pharmaceutics.* 2019 Apr 1; 11(4):150.

Tian P, Yang F, Xu Y, Lin MM, Yu LP, Lin W, Lin QF, Lv ZF, Huang SY, Chen YZ. Oral disintegrating patient-tailored tablets of warfarin sodium produced by 3D printing. *Drug Develop Ind Pharm*. 2018 Dec 2; 44(12):1918–23.

Trenfield SJ, Madla CM, Basit AW, Gaisford S. Binder jet printing in pharmaceutical manufacturing. *3D Printing Pharm*. 2018; 31:41–54.

Voura C, Gruber M, Schroedl N, Strohmeier D, Eltzinger B, Bauer W, Brenn G, Khinast J, Zimmer A. Printable medicines: a microdosing device for producing personalised medicines. *Pharm Technol Eur*. 2011; 5(1):32e6.

Vuddanda PR, Alomari M, Dodoo CC, Trenfield SJ, Velga S, Basit AW, Gaisford S. Personalisation of warfarin therapy using thermal ink-jet printing. *Eur J Pharm Sci*. 2018; 117:80–7.

Wang Z, Han X, Chen R, Li J, Gao J, Zhang H, Liu N, Gao X, Zheng A. Innovative color jet 3D printing of levetiracetam personalized paediatric preparations. *Asian J Pharm Sci*. 2021 May 1;16(3):374–86.

Wu BM, Borland SW, Giordano RA, Cima LG, Sachs EM, Cima MJ. Solid free-form fabrication of drug delivery devices. *J Control Release*. 1996; 40(1):77–87.

Yang L, Zhang S, Oliveira G, Stucker B. Development of a 3D printing method for production of dental application. In 2013 International Solid Freeform Fabrication Symposium. University of Texas at Austin. 2013.

Yu DG, Shen XX, Branford-White C, Zhu LM, White K, Yang XL. Novel oral fast-disintegrating drug delivery devices with predefined inner structure fabricated by three-dimensional printing. *J Pharm Pharmacol*. 2009 Mar; 61(3):323–9.

Yu DG, Zhu L-M, Branford-White CJ, Yang XL. Three-dimensional printing in pharmaceutics: promises and problems. *J Pharm Sci*. 2008; 97(9):3666–90.

Zhou Z, Buchanan F, Mitchell C, Dunne N. Printability of calcium phosphate: calcium sulfate powders for the application of tissue-engineered bone scaffolds using the 3D printing technique. *Mater Sci Eng: C*. 2014 May 1; 38:1–10.

Section V

SLS and SLA-Based 3D Printing in Pharmaceutics

8 SLS and SLA Techniques in 3D Printing for Better Pharmaceutical Applicability of Soft Materials

Venu Madhav Katla, Naga Haritha Pamujula, Somnath De, and Manoj Shahare

8.1 INTRODUCTION

A three-dimensional (3D) subject is developed via 3 dimensional printing (3DP) or by additive manufacturing (AM) from a Computer-Aided Design (CAD) or 3D digital model (Ngo *et al.*, 2018). Materials (such as polymers, liquids, or fused powder grains) are usually added layer-by-layer using different procedures, which are connected, deposited, or solidified using computer (Excell, 2010). Rapid prototyping was the word fitting at the time of 3DP processes, which were then useful primarily in producing of functional and aesthetic prototypes (Katakam *et al.*, 2015). As of 2019, the accuracy, repeatability and the use of a variety of 3DP materials have improved to where some of 3DP procedures are thought to be viable as an industrial-production technique. Hence, the phrase "3DP" has become more widespread (Lam *et al.*, 2019). Technologies like 3DP have several advantages for the pharmaceutical sector, particularly in the early stages of medication research. 3DP could be utilized as a quick prototyping method to test individual drug product iterations or small batches throughout the development of pre-clinical and clinical formulations (Martinez *et al.*, 2017). Through fast prototyping, it may be possible to assess more quickly how various formulation compositions affect important quality criteria, such as medication performance in *in vitro* and *in vivo* models.

8.1.1 IMPORTANCE OF SOFT MATERIALS IN 3DP

Pharmaceutical companies have used 3DP to develop complex dosage forms with a variety of sizes, shapes, structures, dose combinations, dose changes, and release characteristics because it is impractical to produce them using traditional production methods (Gross *et al.*, 2014). Binder jetting, FDM, inkjet printing, SLA, SLS,

TABLE 8.1

Pharmaceutical Applications of Soft Materials Using 3DP Technologies

3DP method	Ingredients	Findings	References
MJ - Inkjet	Fenofibrate along beeswax	Fabricated structure with flexible shape for controlled drug-release	(Kyobula *et al.*, 2017)
SLA	Naproxen with PEG 3350 and PlF 38	The HPMC polymer-based films with printed dosage forms	(Icten *et al.*, 2015)
	Riboflavin, Ibuprofen with PEG	Hydrogels produced from cross-linked resins that contain a drug	(Martinez *et al.*, 2017)
SSE	Captopril, glipizide and nifedipine along with HPMC	SR profiles for nifedipine, glipizide, as well as captopril's osmotic pump	(Khaled *et al.*, 2015a, b)
	Hydrochlorothiazide, atenolol, aspirin along PEG 6000 and D-mannitol	Developed combined drug tablets	(Khaled *et al.*, 2015a, b)

and semi-solid extrusion are the most popular 3DP methods for soft materials (Decard, 1989; Sachs *et al.*, 1993). SLS and SLA approaches are the main topics in this chapter. The goods that are structurally transformed or deformed by the application of stress by mechanical or thermal variations at ambient temperature are known as soft materials, or more simply, soft matter. These soft substances, include lipids, gels, colloids, biological substances (such as collagen and gelatine), and culinary substances (such as chocolate, liquid bread, and jams). A different type of material, i.e., polymers, polyesters, ceramic powders, metals, glass and maybe high melting point lipids, can be used with SLS and SLA processes (Wendel *et al.*, 2008). The technology has also been applied to soft materials of the food sector and tissue engineering via bioprinting.

Table 8.1 gives the information about how different soft materials are used in various 3DP techniques in getting the desired dosage forms with relevant pharmacological effect.

8.1.2　SIGNIFICANCE OF SLS AND SLA TECHNIQUES IN PHARMACEUTICALS

3DP can create printlets with various geometries and compositions, it is anticipated to revolutionize personalized treatment. How process variables and the formulation characteristics affect drug solubility and porosity has been discovered; SLS also holds the potential for personalized medicine (Trenfield *et al.*, 2018). It also contributes significantly to the creation of controlled-release printlets (CRPs) and orally disintegrating printlets (ODPs) (Mohamed *et al.*, 2020; Davis *et al.*, 2021; Mancisidor *et al.*, 2016). Personalized medicine is also interested in dose combinations, which have various release characteristics depending on the polymeric carrier. Finally, SLS may greatly increase therapy adherence in vulnerable populations like children, the elderly, and patients with disabilities, etc. For patients who are blind or visually challenged, these forms may help to increase drug adherence and decrease medical errors (Mancisidor *et al.*, 2016). SLA technology can result in high-quality, accuracy and standard products. It is also a cost-effective technology.

8.2 PURPOSE AND SCOPE OF THE CHAPTER

In the past, 3DP has increased attraction and interest in the pharmaceutical industry, it was used to create various dosage forms and drug delivery systems that have been referred to as printlets in recent studies. Layer-by-layer construction is the foundation of 3DP, which is used to create digitally designed items. When compared to conventional methods, such as powder preparation, mixing, milling, granulation and finally compression, 3DP offers innovative advantages. These processes lack production flexibility and process capabilities. It also opens up a wide range of opportunities for pharmaceutics, including the creation of complicated, customized, and made-to-order goods. There is a lot of information in this chapter about the usage of 3DP technologies, particularly SLS and SLA methods. Here, the overall idea, guiding principles, benefits, drawbacks, use of soft materials, potentials, and difficulties of two 3D approaches are covered.

8.3 FUNDAMENTALS OF SLS AND SLA TECHNIQUES

In the middle of the 1980s, with funding from DARPA, Dr. Carl Deckard and Dr. Joe Beaman created and patented SLS in the University of Texas, Austin, U.S. SLS uses a powerful laser such as carbon dioxide to melt powdered pieces of plastic, ceramic, metal or glass into a mass with the desired 3D shape. When cross-sections are scanned from a 3D digital on to the powder bed surface, the laser fuses the powdered material. Each cross-section is scanned, and then the powder bed is drained of one layer, a new layer of material is put on top, and the process is repeated (Deckard, 1986). The earliest and most popular 3DP technology is stereolithography, or "SLA" printing. Hideo Kodama, a Japanese researcher, developed the present layered method of SLA in the early 1980s by curing photosensitive polymers with ultraviolet radiation (Gibson *et al.*, 2011). In 1984, Alain Le Mehaute applied a patent on SLA procedure, immediately Chuck Hull did the same (Crivello *et al.*, 2014). In SLS an ultraviolet laser is used for concentration on photopolymer resin (Moon *et al.*, 2005). Using CAD software, the UV laser is utilized on the surface of the photopolymer to work on a previously programmed design or pattern. When photopolymers are exposed to UV light it solidifies and creates a layer desired 3D object, this process is called photochemical solidification. A blade then applies glue to the tank's top once the build platform has descended one layer (Charoo *et al.*, 2020). The 3D item is created by repeating this procedure for each layer of the design.

8.4 EXPLANATION OF SLS TECHNIQUE

SLS is a fusion technique of powder bed, which utilizes laser energy to target heat-specific powder materials, causing melting of the powder, particle fusion and finally solidification in order to produce a 3D structure in accordance with CAD (Fina *et al.*, 2018). It can use various excipients, solvents and also has the benefit of recycling feed stock needed for various excipients and solvents, and it also has the added benefit of reprocessing and recycling feedstock. It can produce different sizes and shapes of oral solid dosage forms in single step with great precision. Different process parameters, such as feed bed and print bed temperatures, laser power usage, etc., must be taken into account in order to manufacture products with different release characteristics, porosity, and structures (Yang *et al.*, 2021). There are numerous SLS 3D printers in the market right now, and they all have a variety of laser sources. Several researchers have already investigated in the field of pharmaceuticals (Jinke Trading: blue diode laser, 3.5 W, 450 nm; Sintratec Kit with blue diode laser, 2.3 W, 445 nm; Sharebot: CO_2 laser, 14 W, 10.6 mm) (Gueche *et al.*, 2021a, b; Goodridge *et al.*, 2012).

An SLS 3D printer has two main components: the powder bed (building platform) and the reservoir platform (Figure 8.1), both are heated to below melting point or glass transition temperature of the material being utilized. A high-power laser beam (*X-Y* axis) is used to for the object design onto the powder's top surface layer inside the preheated printing chamber. A subsequent, thin coating of powder is spread out once each layer is finished. Up until the printing of the last layer, this procedure is repeated (Jain *et al.*, 2008).

- **Materials**

Powder is the foundation of SLS feedstock, which is typical of traditional pharmaceutical production techniques, including tableting and granulation. Various formulation components are first combined in this method, and the resulting mixture is then put directly into the printer (Yuan *et al.*, 2019). Thermoplastic polymers must be used as drug-delivery matrices according to SLS. When polymers are subjected

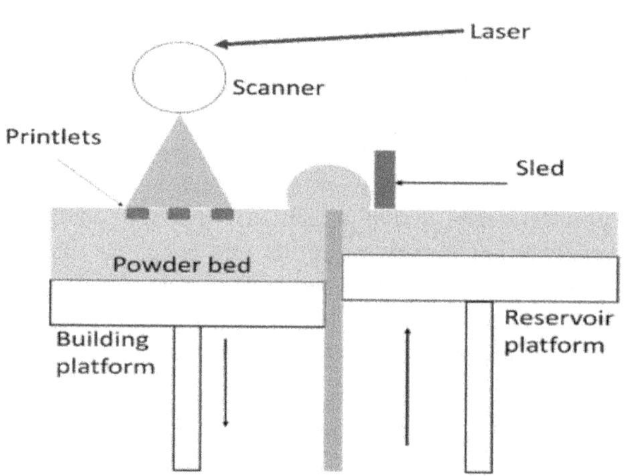

FIGURE 8.1   Selective laser sintering process.

to temperature fluctuations (heating and cooling), it will change its physical property (Goodridge *et al.*, 2012). Prior to sintering, the heating temperature is set below the glass transition temperature for amorphous polymers and below the melting point temperature for semi-crystalline polymers (Fina *et al.*, 2018). Hydroxypropyl methylcellulose (HPMC), copovidone (Kollidon VA64), PEG-PVA (Kollicoat IR) and ethyl cellulose are a few common medicinal thermoplastic polymers.

8.5 EXPLANATION OF SLA TECHNIQUE

An ultraviolet laser is used in SLA to cure photo polymeric cross-sections, turning them solid from the liquid. From CAD data, components are created in layers to create prototypes, tools, casting patterns, and end parts (Halioran *et al.*, 1997). SLA is frequently employed when form, fit, and assembly are crucial because it is all about precision and accuracy. SLA the best AM technique for surface finish, with tolerances on products often less than 0.05 mm. SLA is very helpful for producing highly accurate casting patterns, presentation models, prototypes (Bloomquist *et al.*, 2018). SLA is adaptable and can be utilized in a variety of settings where accuracy is crucial. SLA offers parts with properties similar to those typically produced in low- to medium-volume manufacturing from polypropylene or ABS (Martinez *et al.*, 2017). The laser falls on the liquid resin above the platform when the laser source board. Therefore, the laser's effect causes the liquid resin layer above the platform to solidify (Figure 8.2). Platform descends as a result, a fresh layer containing liquid solidify on the previous layer until the total product is developed.

- **Materials**

Resins are also known as thermoset polymers the liquid components utilized for SLA printing. According to formulation configurations, different materials have different

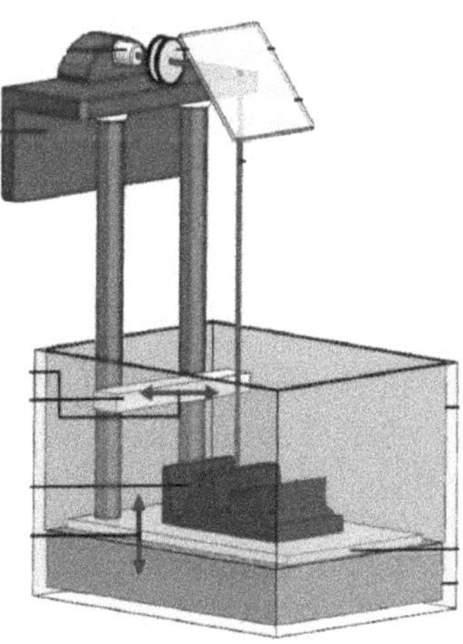

FIGURE 8.2 Stereolithography equipment.

TABLE 8.2
Advantages and Disadvantages of Some Resins

Material	Characteristics	
	Advantages	**Disadvantages**
Standard resin	Smooth surface	Brittle
High detail resin	High accuracy	High price
Castable resin	Used for producing mold patterns	Less ash
Tough or durable resin	Good mechanical properties	Less thermal resistance
Dental resin	Biocompatible	More cost
Flexible resin	Flexible	Low accuracy

physical characteristics. Recent research has looked into the viability of using recycled or green materials to make "sustainable" resins. The resins can be categorized into the following:

- Engineering resins with mechanical and thermal characteristics.
- Standard resins used for prototyping.
- Castable resins for zero-ash products are used.
- Dental and medical resins used for biocompatibility.
- Biomaterial resins.

The other way, hydrogels with a 3D network and high-water content have been successfully used in tissue engineering and regeneration. They are perfect for drug-delivery applications because of tunable mechanical and diffusive properties, which are regulated by the degree of crosslinking (Martinez *et al.*, 2017). Nevertheless, the creation of drug delivery systems with controlled release has shown hydrogels to be particularly useful.

Advantages and disadvantages of some commonly used resins are shown in Table 8.2. It gives information on different resins which in turn can be better used in relevant 3DP.

8.6   SOFT MATERIALS IN PHARMACEUTICAL APPLICATION

3DP is has been utilized to build complicated products of various sizes, shapes and structures, dose variations and combinations with different release characteristics that were previously impossible to make using traditional manufacturing methods (Chen *et al.*, 2021). Soft biomaterials include hydrogels as well as a wide range of hydrophilic macromolecules use different techniques such as the layer-by-layer methodology. Soft materials process various uses in that they enable the altered release of protein compounds (Chen *et al.*, 2020). Furthermore, these materials with hydrophilic properties enable the regulation of protein binding and cell adhesion which prevents blood coagulation and alters immune response, and encourages tissue regeneration (Ng *et al.*, 2022). Soft materials are a transformational tool that crosses research fields and industries, with applications in chemistry, engineering, physics, and life sciences. Scaffoldable and moldable, soft materials frequently include water. They may recover on their own, react to stimuli, and act as the starting point for the development of coatings and other components (Zhan *et al.*, 2022).

Young's modulus is the major parameter that differentiates the soft and rigid materials where the range of soft polymers made of biological materials to range from 103 to 109 Pa (Truby *et al.*, 2016). In SLS printing, the PCL and HC have got wide application in the synthesis of bone scaffolds with microspheres involving multiscale porous structure and good biocompatibility (Pugliese *et al.*, 2021). Further the use of gelatin and PCL or collagen/gelatin combination in fabricated structures with scaffolds have high mechanical and tensile strength (Hofmann, 2014). Many of the tissue engineering scaffolds employ the use of HC and PCL (Ren *et al.*, 2021). In the SLA printing the use of PEG-based hydrogel scaffolds have resulted in open channels in the scaffolds with photo polymer PEGDA inner structures as complex shells with hydrogels. The oligomeric PCL structures such as Irgacure 369 biodegradable resins when employed resulted in gain macromer with photo initiator application (Stano *et al.*, 2021).

8.6.1 DEVELOPING PERSONALIZED MEDICINE, CONTROLLED AND SUSTAINED RELEASE FORMULATIONS USING SOFT MATERIALS

The controlled rug loading capacity of Fenofibrate was enhanced using bees wax MJ - Inkjet Fenofibrate with beeswax in honey comb like structures using 3D SLS (*Kim et al.*, 2013). The drugs such as hydrochlorthiazide, aspirin, pravastatin, HPMC, PAA and MCC along with PEG 6000 as multi-active ingredients functional as one to have increased release profile compared to commercial tablet was successful with SLE soft material printing. Further dexamethasone-2-phosphate disodium coated with PLGA and PVA were encapsulated in between printing layers for controlled drug delivery in treating chronic inflammation (Seok *et al.*, 2013). Many NSAIDs such as paracetamol along with soft material such as HPMC, dipyramidole, PVP and sodium phosphate were developed as high drug loading forms with the concept of personalized medicine. Further NSAIDs like ibuprofen was transformed into high drug loaded hydrogel formulation using SLS soft material printing involving PEG and riboflavin with cross-linking resins (Pikul *et al.*, 2017). The SSE soft printing technique could generate multiple drug-loaded sustained-release formulations with captopril, nifedipine, and glipzide APIs (Wang *et al.*, 2021).

8.6.2 SOFT MATERIALS APPLICATIONS WITH 3DP IN GENERATING TISSUE SCAFFOLDS

Biological materials (collagen and gelatine) as well as liquids, lubricants, adhesives, foams, paints, gels, liquid crystals, lipids, and colloids are examples of soft materials with a high internal freedom and weak interactions in between the molecules (Pikul *et al.*, 2017). The advantage includes production 3D tissue scaffolds with controlled cell pattern that attains the cellular function and capacity to reproduce. In brief, the technique has mass application in layered deposition of soft biomaterials such as bioinks to develop high porous structures of living biological tissue and other biomaterials in desired form and shape (Wang *et al.*, 2021). These bioinks may contain cellular mixtures matrix and other nutrients, which when placed in an incubator with cell-based matriz transforms into a tissue. These materials are used more frequently in the biological, pharmaceutical, and industries. 3DP is a commonly used in tissue engineering for developing new organs and tissues for replacing injured or defective organ. The biological scaffolds should comprise of 3D structure of porous nature for achieving desired outcomes (Terryn *et al.*, 2021). A 3D structure comprising of living tissue and biomaterials is formed with relevant shape 3D bioprinting, which create layer-by-layer deposition of biomaterials known as bioinks (Studart *et al.*, 2016). The bioinks are produced using a printer cartridge while containing cells and nutrients, and they are then stored in an incubator to develop a tissue's cell-based matrix (Choi *et al.*, 2021).

8.7   OPTIMIZATION OF SLS AND SLA PARAMETERS FOR SOFT MATERIAL

Layers of powder material are successively solidified throughout the SLS process to create complicated three-dimensional components (Mahendiran *et al.*, 2021). CAD is required to begin SLS process and also solidification of powder material layers. The model actively takes part in the process after being divided into cross-sections by specialist software (Kruth *et al.*, 2003). SLS is commonly used to make functional and end-use parts from thermoplastic polyurethane elastomer (TPU), a soft polymer that can bear moderate amounts of stress and is durable, wear resistant, and chemical resistant. TPU is the most popular polymer because it has the best tensile strength, flexibility, hydrolytic stability, longevity, corrosion resistance, and resistance to abrasion. TPU materials are a potential material for laser sintering because of their unique and adaptive characteristics, including the good flowing powders, low melting, and little shrink of material during drying process (Yadroitsev *et al.*, 2007). The registered trademark SLS is also known as laser beam PBF. In the SLS technique, laser-sintered powdered polymer materials are used to produce complex 3D things by layering multiple materials on top of one another.

The ultimate section is fully constructed after the layers have been consistently produced. Micro-SLS stands for SLS with a greater resolution at the micron scale. This method can result in features with a resolution of less than 5 µm (Desai *et al.*, 2023). Its primary uses include the production of microscale sensors, actuators, micro-optoelectronic parts, etc. SLA, out of all the commercially available rapid prototyping (RP) techniques, has continuously positioned itself as the top RP process over the years. In comparison to all other commercially available Prible RP techniques, SLA has consistently proven to be the most effective RP approach. It can be used to build prototype models and tooling quickly, accurately, and at a reasonable cost. Layers of material are added as part of the basic construction process; therefore, it naturally has some benefits and drawbacks. The most significant benefit is the capacity to construct virtually any complex geometric three-dimensional shape, which may be challenging to make using traditional techniques.

TABLE 8.3
Case Studies and Examples of SLS and SLA Printing

3DP	Dosage form	Ingredients	Summary	References
SLS	Shell core	Polyamide and Microbinder	The work has demonstrated that SLS is a versatile and practical 3D printing technology which can be applied to the pharmaceutical field for the manufacture of modern medicines.	(Fina *et al.*, 2017)
	Tablet dosage forms with various drug loading and shapes	Acetaminophen, Kollicoat IR, Eudragit L100–55,	SLS-fabricated devices have been explored for their potential application in controlling the release of drugs in a simulated body environment.	(Cheah *et al.*, 2002)
	ODT	Acetaminophen, Hydroxy Propyl Methyl Cellulose E5, and 4% Canndurin gold sheen	The versatility of the SLS technology was demonstrated by drastically accelerating the drug dissolution profiles of printlets prepared with two pharmaceutical grade polymers that have not been explored previously with SLS 3DP	(Fina *et al.*, 2018)
SLA	Anti-acne transdermal patch	Salicylic acid, Poly Ethylene Glycol and PEG-DA	Acne patches with salicylic acid have been created using SLA technique with good invitro release performance	(Trenfield *et al.*, 2016)
	Tablet	Acetaminophen, di-phenyl (2,4,6–trimethyl benzoyl) phosphine oxide and PEG 300	Tablets prepared using SLA technique have resulted in better drug release characteristics	(Trenfield *et al.*, 2016)

8.8 CASE STUDIES AND EXAMPLES OF SLS AND SLA PRINTING

Table 8.3 represents some of the examples which utilized SLS and SLA techniques in the development of some dosage forms, which improved drug release and therapeutic activity of some drugs.

- **SLS and SLA Bioprinting Using Soft Materials**

Examples of soft materials for biological applications using SLS-SLA techniques are discussed in Table 8.4.

TABLE 8.4
SLS and SLA Bioprinting using Soft Materials for Biological Applications

3DP	Soft Materials	Summary	References
SLS	Polycaprolactone and hydroxyapatite	A new manufacturing method for multi-scaled, microsphere-based bone scaffolds with good biocompatibility has been developed.	(Wang et al., 2016)
	Polycaprolactone and gelatine or collagen	Constructed scaffolds out of collagen or gelatin, and examined their biological and mechanical qualities	(Du et al., 2015)
	Polycaprolactone and hydroxyapatite	Tissue engineering scaffolds are manufactured	(Chen et al., 2014)
SLA	Hydrogel scaffolds based on photopolymerizable PEG	Hydrogel scaffolds were created within the open channels of 3D scaffold designs	(Wiria et al., 2007)
	Photo-polymerizable Poly (ethylene glycol) diacrylate	The complicated interior designs of cell-encapsulating hydrogels were created	(Neiman et al., 2015)
	Polycaprolactone oligomers, resins, Irgacure, photo-initiator and dye	Developed porous three-dimensional scaffolds	(Chan et al., 2010)

Table 8.4 shows the use of soft materials in SLS and SLA techniques for improving biological performance of some drugs.

8.9 FUTURE PERSPECTIVES AND CHALLENGES

8.9.1 CHALLENGES AND LIMITATIONS

Although SLS technology offers several advantages, users should be aware of several difficulties and limitations. These factors can affect the overall efficiency, cost, and quality of the completed product (Elomaa *et al.*, 2011).

8.9.2 POST-PROCESSING

The post-processing required after the component parts are manufactured is one of the key issues connected with SLS printing. While the method normally does not necessitate the use of support structures, the parts are immersed in unsintered powder inside the print bed. It will be necessary to remove this powder, which could be a tedious and time-consuming task. Moreover, unsintered powder cannot be continually reused due to its degradation over time, which raises the cost of materials. Products that are SLS printed have rough surface texture, which is not ideal for all purposes. In certain situations, further post-processing steps like sanding or polishing could be needed to get the desired smoother surface. These additional steps could raise the overall production time and cost by both money and time.

8.9.3 MATERIAL LIMITATIONS

The sintering process requires materials with certain properties, like a suitable melting temperature, thermal stability, and the capacity to fuse together without undue bending or deformation. Consequently, compared to other 3DP techniques, the selection of materials for SLS printing is more constrained. Metals, ceramics, and many thermoplastic polymer types are all suitable with SLS. The available materials for SLS printing may be restricted by the need for powder form. Some materials can be expensive and difficult to turn into small, uniform powders, which reduces the range of options available to SLS users. The quality and size distribution of the powder particles greatly impacts the final component quality, hence restricting the available possibilities for selection. Elevated temperatures have the potential to degrade or alter the properties of some materials, leading to components that do not meet the required criteria.

8.9.4 SIZE CONSTRAINTS

Minimum component dimensions are influenced by variables like laser spot size, which determines the smallest feature size that can be successfully duplicated during the sintering process. The average range of the laser spot size in SLS printers is between 50 and 200 μm, contingent upon the printer model and specifications. The size of features that can be successfully created is limited by the possibility of smaller details being partially resolved or undergoing warping or distortion due to the heat required during the sintering process (Deshmukh *et al.*, 2020). On the other hand, the build volume of the SLS printer largely determines the maximum part dimensions. The volume ought to be small enough to fit inside the printer's chamber. While industrial SLS printers may provide build sizes of 1000 × 1000 × 1000 mm or beyond, smaller desktop variants may have substantially reduced build volumes, thus restricting the sorts of projects that can be completed with these machines. The time required to produce an SLS print is proportional to the size and complexity of the item. Larger components take longer to print, affecting production schedules and resource allocation.

8.10 REGULATORY CONSIDERATIONS FOR 3DP SOFT MATERIALS IN PHARMACEUTICALS

Sufficient rules must be in place to ensure the safety of 3D-printed medications for patients, but not so many that producers are discouraged, their inventive efforts are frustrated, and patients' access to therapy is hampered. Testing of 3D products: after production, QC tests were performed on the samples selected from each batch by randomization method, which includes inspections and measurements. While comparable procedures may be used for mass-produced 3D-printed medications, it is not the same for personalized pharmaceuticals created for particular patients. Because personalized drugs would be manufactured on a pilot scale, few non-invasive tests may be performed. Trenfield *et al.* (2018), used process analytical technology (PAT) to examine the utilization of paracetamol-loaded 3D-printed tablets. The researchers also employed Raman confocal microscopy to show that the medication was distributed evenly throughout the tablet. Similarly, Vakili *et al.* (2015) used hyperspectral imaging to verify non-destructive quality control on theophylline dosage form prepared by an ink-jet method. When non-destructive testing procedures are unavailable or impractical, additional goods can be prepared by printing, and QC tests can be done. Otherwise, regulatory measures must place a greater focus on other QA and management procedures that lead up to product development, such as developing techniques to assure quality throughout the manufacturing process (Bergonzi *et al.*, 2023).

8.11 CONCLUSION

3DP technologies, particularly SLS and SLA, have significantly impacted the pharmaceutical industry by enabling the production of complex dosage forms and drug delivery systems, referred to as printlets. Soft materials, including hydrogels, lipids, and biological substances, play a crucial role in expanding the applications of 3DP in pharmaceuticals. Moreover, the use of soft materials in 3DP has opened avenues for tissue engineering, creating scaffolds and structures with controlled cell patterns. While both SLS and SLA have their respective advantages and limitations, ongoing research aims to optimize parameters and address challenges. The future of 3DP in pharmaceuticals holds potential for personalized medicine, efficient drug development, and the creation of innovative drug delivery systems. However, regulatory considerations, post-processing challenges, and material limitations must be carefully addressed to ensure the safety and quality of 3D-printed pharmaceuticals in the evolving landscape of AM.

REFERENCES

Bergonzi, C., Bianchera, A., Remaggi, G., Ossiprandi, M. C., Bettini, R., & Elviri, L. (2023). 3D printed chitosan/alginate hydrogels for the controlled release of silver sulfadiazine in wound healing applications: Design, characterization and antimicrobial activity. *Micromachines*, 14, 137–139.

Bloomquist, C. J., Mecham, M. B., Paradzinsky, M. D., Janusziewicz, R., Warner, S. B., Luft, J. C., & DeSimone, J. M. (2018). Controlling release from 3D printed medical devices using CLIP and drug-loaded liquid resins. *Journal of Controlled Release*, 278, 9–23.

Chan, V., Zorlutuna, P., Jeong, J. H., Kong, H., & Bashir, R. (2010). Three-dimensional photopatterning of hydrogels using stereolithography for long-term cell encapsulation. *Lab on a Chip*, 10, 2062–2070.

Charoo, N. A., Barakh Ali, S. F., Mohamed, E. M., Kuttolamadom, M. A., Ozkan, T., Khan, M. A., & Rahman, Z. (2020). Selective laser sintering 3D printing–An overview of the technology and pharmaceutical applications. *Drug Development and Industrial Pharmacy*, 46, 869–877.

Cheah, C. M., Leong, K. F., Chua, C. K., Low, K. H., & Quek, H. S. (2002). Characterization of microfeatures in selective laser sintered drug delivery devices. *Proceedings of the Institution of Mechanical Engineers. Part H, Journal of Engineering in Medicine*, 216, 369–383.

Chen, C. H., Lee, M. Y., Shyu, V. B.-H., Chen, Y. C., Chen, C. T., & Chen, J. P. (2014). Surface modification of polycaprolactone scaffolds fabricated via selective laser sintering for cartilage tissue engineering. *Materials Science and Engineering. C, Materials for Biological Applications*, 40, 389–397.

Chen, C. H., Lee, M. Y., Shyu, V. B.-H., Chen, Y. C., Chen, C. T., & Chen, J. P. (2014). Surface modification of polycaprolactone scaffolds fabricated via selective laser sintering for cartilage tissue engineering. *Materials Science and Engineering. C, Materials for Biological Applications*, 40, 389–397.

Chen, L. H., Cheng, L. C., & Doyle, P. S. (2020). Nanoemulsion-loaded capsules for controlled delivery of lipophilic active ingredients. *Advanced Science*, 7, 2001677.

Chen, L. H., & Doyle, P. S. (2021). Design and use of a thermogelling methylcellulose nanoemulsion to formulate nanocrystalline oral dosage forms. *Advanced Materials*, 33, e2008618.

Choi, Y., Kim, C., Kim, H. S., Moon, C., & Lee, K. Y. (2021). 3D Printing of dynamic tissue scaffold by combining self-healing hydrogel and self-healing ferrogel. *Colloids and Surfaces. B, Biointerfaces*, 208, 112108.

Crivello, J. V., & Reichmanis, E. (2014). Photopolymer materials and processes for advanced technologies. *Chemistry of Materials*, 26, 533–548.

Davis, D. A., Thakkar, R., Su, Y., Williams, R. O., & Maniruzzaman, M. (2021). Selective laser sintering 3-dimensional printing as a single step process to prepare amorphous solid dispersion dosage forms for improved solubility and dissolution rate. *Journal of Pharmaceutical Sciences*, 110, 1432–1443.

Deckard, C. R. (1989). Method and apparatus for producing parts by selective sintering. In *Google* Patents.

Deckard. (1986). Method and apparatus for producing parts by selective sintering. U.S. Patent 4 863 538.

Desai, S. M., Sonawane, R. Y., & More, A. P. (2023). Thermoplastic polyurethane for three-dimensional printing applications: A review. *Polymers for Advanced Technologies*, 34, 2061–2082.

Deshmukh K., Muzaffar A., Kovářík T., Křenek T., & Ahamed M. B. (2020). Fundamentals and applications of 3D and 4D printing of polymers: Challenges in polymer processing and prospects of future research. In *3D and 4D Printing of Polymer Nanocomposite Materials*, 527–560.

Du, Y., Liu, H., Shuang, J., Wang, J., Ma, J., & Zhang, S. (2015). Microsphere-based selective laser sintering for building macroporous bone scaffolds with controlled microstructure and excellent biocompatibility. *Colloids and Surfaces. B, Biointerfaces*, 135, 81–89.

Elomaa, L., Teixeira, S., Hakala, R., Korhonen, H., Grijpma, D. W., & Seppälä, J. V. (2011). Preparation of poly(ε-caprolactone)-based tissue engineering scaffolds by stereolithography. *Acta Biomaterialia*, 7, 3850–3856.

Excell, J. (2010). The rise of additive manufacturing. *Engineer*.

Fina, F., Goyanes, A., Madla, C. M., Awad, A., Trenfield, S. J., Kuek, J. M., & Basit, A. W. (2018). 3D printing of drug-loaded gyroid lattices using selective laser sintering. *International Journal of Pharmaceutics*, 547, 44–52.

Fina, F., Goyanes, A., Gaisford, S., & Basit, A. W. (2017). Selective laser sintering (SLS) 3D printing of medicines. *International Journal of Pharmaceutics*, 529, 285–293.

Fina, F., Madla, C. M., Goyanes, A., Zhang, J., Gaisford, S., & Basit, A. W. (2018). Fabricating 3D printed orally disintegrating printlets using selective laser sintering. *International Journal of Pharmaceutics*, 541, 101–107.

Gibson, I., & Bártolo, P. J. (2011). History of stereolithography processes. In P. J. Bártolo *Stereolithography Materials Processes Application* (pp. 37–56). New York: Springer

Goodridge, R. D., Tuck, C. J., & Hague, R. J. M. (2012). Laser sintering of polyamides and other polymers. *Progress in Materials Science*, 57, 229–267.

Gross, B. C., Erkal, J. L., Lockwood, S. Y., Chen, C., & Spence, D. M. (2014). Evaluation of 3D printing and its potential impact on biotechnology and the chemical sciences. *Analytical Chemistry*, 86, 3240–3253.

Gueche, Y. A., Sanchez-Ballester, N. M., Bataille, B., Aubert, A., Rossi, J. C., & Soulairol, I. A. (2021a). QbD approach for evaluating the effect of selective laser sintering parameters on printability and properties of solid oral forms. *Pharmaceutics*, 13, 1701.

Gueche, Y. A., Sanchez-Ballester, N. M., Cailleaux, S., Bataille, B., & Soulairol, I. (2021b). Selective laser sintering (SLS), a new chapter in the production of Solid Oral Forms (SOFs) by 3D Printing. *Pharmaceutics*, 13, 1–26.

Halloran, J. W., Grith, M., & Chu, T. M. (1997). Stereolithography resin for rapid prototyping of ceramics and metals. U.S. Patent 6 117 612.

Hofmann, M. (2014). 3D printing gets a boost and opportunities with polymer materials. *ACS Macro Letters*, 3, 382–386.

Içten, E., Giridhar, A., Taylor, L. S., Nagy, Z. K., & Reklaitis, G. V. (2015). Dropwise additive manufacturing of pharmaceutical products for melt-based dosage forms. *Journal of Pharmaceutical Sciences*, 104, 1641–1649.

Jain, P. K., Pandey, P. M., & P. V. M., Rao. (2008). Experimental investigations for improving part strength in selective laser sintering. *Virtual Physical Prototype*, 3, 177–188.

Kassem, T., Sarkar, T., Nguyen, T., Saha, D., & Ahsan, F. (2022). 3D printing in solid dosage forms and organ-on-chip applications. *Biosensors*, 12, 186.

Katakam, P., Dey, B., Assaleh, F. H., Hwisa, N. T., Adiki, S. K., Chandu, B. R., & Mitra, A. (2015). Top-down and bottom-up approaches in 3D printing technologies for drug delivery challenges. *Critical Reviews in Therapeutic Drug Carrier Systems*, 32, 61–87.

Khaled, S. A., Burley, J. C., Alexander, M. R., Yang, J., & Roberts, C. J. (2015a). 3D printing of tablets containing multiple drugs with defined release profiles. *International Journal of Pharmaceutics*, 494, 643–650.

Khaled, S. A., Burley, J. C., Alexander, M. R., Yang, J., & Roberts, C. J. (2015b). 3D printing of five-in-one dose combination polypill with defined immediate and sustained release profiles. *Journal of Controlled Release*, 217, 308–314.

Kim, S., Laschi, C., & Trimmer, B. (2013). Soft robotics: A bioinspired evolution in robotics. *Trends in Biotechnology*, 31, 287–294.

Kruth, J. P., Wang, X., Laoui, T., & Froyen, L. (2003). Lasers and materials in selective laser sintering. *Assembly Automation*, 23, 357–371.

Kyobula, M., Adedeji, A., Alexander, M. R., Saleh, E., Wildman, R., Ashcroft, I., Roberts, C. J. (2017). 3D inkjet printing of tablets exploiting bespoke complex geometries for controlled and tuneable drug release. *Journal of Controlled Release*, 261, 207–215.

Lam, H. K. S., Ding, L., Cheng, T. C. E., & Zhou, H. (2019). The impact of 3D printing implementation on stock returns: A contingent dynamic capabilities perspective. *International Journal of Operations and Production Management*, 39, 935–961.

Mahendiran, B., Muthusamy, S., Sampath, S., Jaisankar, S. N., Popat, K. C., Selvakumar, R., & Krishnakumar, G. S. (2021). Recent trends in natural polysaccharide based bioinks for multiscale 3D printing in tissue regeneration: A review. *International Journal of Biological Macromolecules*, 183, 564–588.

Mancisidor, A. M., Garciandia, F., Sebastian, M. S., Álvarez, P., Díaz, J., & Unanue, I. (2016). Reduction of the residual porosity in parts manufactured by selective laser melting using skywriting and high focus offset strategies. *Physics Procedia*, 83, 864–873.

Martinez, P. R., Goyanes, A., Basit, A. W., & Gaisford, S. (2017). Fabrication of drug-loaded hydrogels with stereolithographic 3D printing. *International Journal of Pharmaceutics*, 532, 313–317.

Mohamed, E. M., Barakh Ali, S. F., Rahman, Z., Dharani, T., & Ozkan, M. A. (2020). Formulation optimization of selective laser sintering 3D-printed tablets of clindamycin palmitate hydrochloride by response surface methodology, *AAPS PharmSciTech*, 21, 232.

Moon, F. C., Hai, J., & Paventi, C. (2005, Sept). 3-D printing the history of mechanisms. *Journal of Mechanical Design*, 127(5), 1029–1033.

Neiman, J. A., Raman, R., Chan, V., Rhoads, M. G., Raredon, M. S. B., Velazquez, J. J., & Griffith, L. G. (2015). Photopatterning of hydrogel scaffolds coupled to filter materials using stereolithography for perfused 3D culture of hepatocytes. *Biotechnology and Bioengineering*, 112, 777–787.

Ng, D. Z. L., Nelson, A. Z., Ward, G., Lai, D., Doyle, P. S., & Khan, S. A. (2022). Control of drug-excipient particle attributes with droplet microfluidic-based extractive solidification enables improved powder rheology. *Pharmaceutical Research*, 39, 411–421.

Ngo, T. D., Kashani, A., Imbalzano, G., Nguyen, K. T. Q., & Hui, D. (2018). Additive manufacturing (3D printing): A review of materials, methods, applications and challenges. *Composites Part B Engineering*, 143, 172–196.

Pikul, J. H., Li, S., Bai, H., Hanlon, R. T., Cohen, I., & Shepherd, R. F. (2017). Stretchable surfaces with programmable 3D texture morphing for synthetic camouflaging skins. *Science*, 358, 210–214.

Pugliese, R., Beltrami, B., Regondi, S., & Lunetta, C. (2021). Polymeric biomaterials for 3D printing in medicine: An overview. *Annals of 3D Printed Medicine*, 2, 100011.

Ren, L., Li, B., Wei, G., Wang, K., Song, Z., Wei, Y., Qingping, (2021). Biology and bioinspiration of soft robotics: Actuation, sensing, and system integration. *iScience*, 24, 103075.

Roy, N. K., Behera, D., Dibua, O. G., Foong, C. S., & Cullinan, M. A. (2019). A novel microscale selective laser sintering (μ-SLS) process for the fabrication of microelectronic parts. *Microsystems and Nanoengineering*, 5, 64.

Sachs, E. M., Haggerty, J. S. C., Williams, M. J., & P. A. (1993). Three-dimensional printing techniques. U.S. Patent 5, 204 055, issued April 20, 1993.

Seok, S., Onal, C. D., Cho, K., Wood, R. J., Rus, D., & Kim, S. (2013). Meshworm: A peristaltic soft robot with antagonistic nickel titanium coil actuators. *IEEE/ASME Transactions on Mechatronics*, 18, 1485–1497.

Stano, G., & Percoco, G. (2021). Additive manufacturing aimed to soft robots' fabrication: A review. *Extreme Mechanics Letters*, 42, 1211–1222.

Studart, A. R. (2016). Additive manufacturing of biologically inspired materials. *Chemical Society Reviews*, 45, 359–376.

Terryn, S., Langenbach, J., Roels, E., Brancart, J., Bakkali-Hassani, C., & Poutrel, Q. A. (2021). A review on self-healing polymers for soft robotics. *Materials Today*, 47, 187–205.

Trenfield, S. J., Goyanes, A., Telford, R., Wilsdon, D., Rowland, M., Gaisford, S., & Basit, A. W. (2016). Printing as innovative technologies for fabricating personalized topical drug delivery systems. *Journal of Controlled Release*, 234, 41–48.

Trenfield, S. J., Goyanes, A., Telford, R., Wilsdon, D., Rowland, M., Gaisford, S., & Basit, A. W. (2018). 3D printed drug products: Non-destructive dose verification using a rapid point-and-shoot approach. *International Journal of Pharmaceutics*, 549, 283–292.

Truby, R. L., & Lewis, J. A. (2016). Printing soft matter in three dimensions. *Nature*, 540, 371–378.

Vakil, H., Kolakovic, R., Genina, N., Marmion, M., Salo, H., & Ihalainen, P. (2015). Hyperspectral imaging in quality control of inkjet printer personalized dosage forms. *International Journal of Pharmacy*, 483, 244–249.

Wang, J., Goyanes, A., Gaisford, S., & Basit, A. W. (2016). Basit, stereolithographic (SLA) 3D printing of oral modified-release dosage forms. *International Journal of Pharmacy*, 503, 207–212.

Wang, Q., Wu, Z., Huang, J., Du, Z., Yue, Y., Chen, D., & Su, B. (2021). Integration of sensing and shape-deforming capabilities for a bioinspired soft robot. *Composites Part B Engineering*, 223, 109–116.

Wendel, B., Rietzel, D., Kühnlein, F., Feulner, R., Hülder, G., & Schmachtenberg, E. (2008). Additive processing of polymers. *Macromolecular Materials and Engineering*, 293, 799–809.

Wiria, F. E., Leong, K. F., Chua, C. K., & Liu, Y. (2007). Poly-ε-caprolactone/hydroxyapatite for tissue engineering scaffold fabrication via selective laser sintering. *Acta Biomaterialia*, 3, 1–12.

Yadroitsev, I., Bertrand, P., & Smurov, I. (2007). Parametric analysis of the selective laser melting process. *Applied Surface Science*, 253, 8064–8069.

Yang, Y., Xu, Y., Wei, S., & Shan, W. (2021). Oral preparations with tunable dissolution behavior based on selective laser sintering technique. *International Journal of Pharmaceutics*, 593, 120127.

Yuan, S., Shen, F., Chua, C. K., & Zhou, K. (2019). Polymeric composites for powder-based additive manufacturing: Materials and applications. *Progress in Polymer Science*, 91, 141–168.

Zhan, S., Guo, A. X. Y., Cao, S. C., & Liu, N. (2022). 3D printing soft matters and applications: A review. *International Journal of Molecular Sciences*, 23, 3790–3799.

Section VI

Hybrid 3D Printing Techniques in Pharmaceutical Applications

9 Next-Generation Computational Automation-Based Additive Manufacturing of Pharmaceuticals

An Approach to Fabricate Precise Medicine

Jigar Vyas, Nensi Raytthatha, Sudarshan Singh, and Bhupendra Prajapati

9.1 INTRODUCTION

With the advent of 3D printing (3DP) and 4D printing, the development of drugs and biomedical devices has undergone an evolutionary change. Such novel manufacturing processes have opened new avenues for developing personalized drugs and biomedical devices with greater precision and practicality. Unlike traditional manufacturing processes, 3D/4D printing enables the layer-by-layer fabrication of complex structures, allowing for greater customization and optimization of drug formulations and medical devices. 3D printing is one of the most rapidly developing innovations of the last 30 years; however, given its enormous potential, it should be explored more. The possibility of cost-effective and time-efficient 3D printing is an enticing prospect; additionally, the latest breakthrough in 3D printing is the focus of interest for creating products having the potential to alter shape after being taken out of the 3D printer (Sadasivuni *et al.*, 2019). This technical development has been accompanied by a new age of printing known as 4D printing. The fundamental goal of 4D printing is to make 3D-printed products suitable for self-assembling when exposed to particular stimuli, such as pressure, heat, humidity, chemical processes, etc. In basic terms, 4D printing is a breakthrough technology similar to 3D printing with the addition of a time dimension; that is, by adding a time frame to 3D printing (Wei *et al.*, 2015). The inclusion of an additional dimension to 3D printing allows for the pre-programming of materials in terms of their responsiveness to diverse stimuli (Ambrosi & Pumera,

2016; Deshmukh *et al.*, 2017). 4D printing is an approach to printing technology with enormous possibilities as 4D allows creating and transforming shapes from a range of materials with shape-changing properties. The development of dynamic self-assembling and morphing objects via 4D printing can be applied in various industries for various applications (Guo & Leu, 2013).

9.2   PROCESSES FOR 3D PRINTING

There are four processes for 3D printing, mainly radiation-based processes, fusion-based process, lamination-based processes, and extrusion-based processes; a laser or electron beam is used in the radiation process that bonds powder particles together layer-by-layer, and the powdered material is spread out on a platform before being melted in a precise pattern; examples of printers include material jetting (MJ), digital light processing (DLP), stereolithography (SLA), and continuous liquid interface production. The fusion process uses heat to fuse materials layer-by-layer, wherein the material usually is spread out on a platform in powder form; examples include powder bed fusion printers (PBF), selective laser sintering (SLS) printers, and binder jetting (BJ). The lamination process adds material by depositing layers of material on top of one other, such as paper or plastic and the layers are fused with pressure, heat, or adhesive; an example includes laminated object manufacturing (LOM). The extrusion process includes melting a material filament followed by extruding it via a nozzle to add materials, and the molten material is subsequently poured layer-by-layer on a platform; examples include fused deposition modeling (FDM) and direct inkjet printers (Kuebler *et al.*, 1999).

9.3   COMPUTATIONAL AUTOMATION INVOLVED COMPUTER-AIDED DESIGNS AND AI-BASED SOFTWARE IN 3D PRINTING

The Tinkercad is a helpful learning tool for individuals that can create and code Arduino Uno-based devices and is used for developing and testing early-stage Arduino Uno firmware systems (Ellul & Debono, 2022). It has an easy web interface. If support is added for communication with external web devices and services, this could meet the necessities for a platform that is easy to use, web-based, and allows using external connections without physical hardware. The extension offers the following advantages for the Internet of Things (IoT) device experimentation, it allows IoT device code, which interacts with external web services and devices, to be built as well as investigated; and (ii) it allows a network of internet-connected modeled IoT devices to be scaled up without physical IoT devices, which saves money and time. Tinkercad already allows various Arduino simulators but does not support communication with other web services (Ellul & Debono, 2022). Tinkercad makes it easy to integrate simulated Arduino Uno devices with other Tinkercad simulated devices in different tabs, basic Arduino external web services, or any other hardware or software. The routing software might be written in any language/framework necessary (as long as it can process HTTP requests), and it could also contain network-/event-based management software (e.g., Node-RED4) (Dominic *et al.*, 2010).

Multi-gene genetic programming (MGGP) is a strategy in which the approximate function is a weighted sum of the genes. MGGP includes a high-level crossover function in which individual genes can be swapped with another gene of another individual as long as the permitted number of genes is not exceeded. Computational regression is often used to grow a population of trees using traditional (standard) genetic programming (GP).

An autonomous materials discovery and manufacturing system allows for the continuous as well as adaptable execution of the active learning of PSP relationships and also sequential experimentation to search a materials design space via a closed-loop relationship among a hardware (body) and software (brain) component, with less human interference. The software brain comprises two parts: forward mapping, which tries to learn the PSP correlations by combining data from several sources and to forecast the properties-of-interest and structure of a material at a given process and design configuration. It seeks answers to the question: "Given a set of material descriptors that can be manipulated through materials synthesis and processing, what are the corresponding properties and performance characteristics?" On the other hand, inversion mapping contains modules for experimental conditions or improves the search of materials design space to identify material and production stages based on the PSP connection model (Bukkapatnam, 2023).

M3D intelligent design and engineering trains AI models to predict vital manufacturing parameters, such as mechanical properties, filaments, printing temperature, extrusion temperature, and printability using a dataset of over 600 drug-loaded formulations. The programme can also forecast the disintegration of 3D-printed drugs, which is critical for ensuring their efficacy. It is designed to enable users to develop 3D-printed drug-loaded formulations as well as predict different process parameters in an offsite setting, namely extrusion and printing temperature, printability and, filament mechanical characteristics thereby accelerating the manufacturing of 3D-printed drug-loaded products (Pokala & Samatham, 2016).

The tested machine-learning techniques are incorporated into a web-based app platform and can be accessed from any internet-connected smart devices. The application is hosted in an elastic compute cloud, for example, Amazon Web Services, which uses the open-source programme Apache HTTP Server to serve an internet application written in Python3 and built using the Django web framework and uses the scikit-learn package for integration. It enables the user to validate the training models offshore before comparing the projected findings to FDM studies, speeding up the 3DP process (Pokala & Samatham, 2016).

9.4 MATERIALS USED IN THE 3D PRINTING PROCESS

The materials used in 3D printing vary depending on the specific technology and desired outcome. Some commonly used materials in 3D printing are discussed in Table 9.1.

TABLE 9.1
Additive Materials with a Guide to Properties, Advantages, and Applications

Additive Materials	Process of 3D Printing/ Instruments	Properties	Advantages	Applications	Ref.
Polymers					
HDPE	FDM	Impact resistant: +++ Corrosion resistant: +++; Durability: ++; Thermoplastic: ++; Temp. resistant: ++; Inert: +++; Optic: ++; Electric: ++; Hydrophobicity: ++	Versatile, low cost, recyclable, ease of fabrication, biocompatible, UV Resistance	Auricle reconstruction, medical devices (such as blood bags and IV tubing).	(Karian, 2003)
Poly propylene	FDM	Impact resistant: ++; Corrosion resistant: ++; Durability: ++; Thermoplastic: +++; Temp. resistant: +; Inert: ++; Optic: +; Electric: ++; Hydrophobicity: ++	Low cost, recyclable, light weight, ease of fabrication, biocompatible, transparent, and dimensional stability.	Implants, Medical devices such as syringes, catheters, and surgical instruments, packaging for pharmaceutical products.	(Hata *et al.*, 2021)
PA	FDM, SLS	Impact resistant: ++; Corrosion resistant: +++; Durability: +++; Thermoplastic: ++; Temp. resistant: +++; Inert: ++; Optic: ++; Electric: +++; Hydrophobicity: +	Versatile, recyclable, ease of fabrication, dimensional stability, low friction self-lubrication.	Medical devices, such as sutures and artificial heart valves.	(Casalini *et al.*, 2019)
Metals					
Aluminum Alloys	PBF, SLM	Impact resistant: ++; Corrosion resistant: ++; Durability: ++; Thermoplastic: +; Temp. resistant: ++; Inert: +; Optic: +; Electric: +; Hydrophobicity: ++	Versatile, low cost, recyclable, ease of fabrication, lightweight	Crowns and dentures, Pseudo Organs Although the size of a penny, this "lung" shows the feasibility of 3D printing living cells	(Ali *et al.*, 2019), (Uddin *et al.*, 2015)

Material	Technique	Properties	Advantages	Applications	Reference
Magnesium Alloys	PBF, Radiation based techniques	Impact resistant: +; Corrosion resistant: +; Durability: +; Thermoplastic: +; Temp. resistant: +;; Inert: +; Optic: +; Electric: +; Hydrophobicity: +	Recyclable, ease of fabrication, biocompatible, lightweight, high damping capacity	Orthopaedics, urology, cardiology, respirology	(Peeters *et al.*, 2005) (Luffy *et al.*, 2014)
Ceramics					
Glass powders	SLA, DLP, SL, SLS	Impact resistant: ++; Corrosion resistant: ++; Durability: +++; Thermoplastic: NA; Temp. resistant: +++; Inert: +++; Optic: +++; Electric: NA; Hydrophobicity: ++	Versatile, recyclable, biocompatible	Optoelectronics	(Chen *et al.*, 2019)
Ceramic powders eg. Zirconia, Alumina, Hydroxyapatite	MJ, BJ, PBF	Impact resistant: +++; Corrosion resistant: +++; Durability: +++; Thermoplastic: NA; Temp. resistant: +++; Inert: +++; Optic: ++; Electric: NA Hydrophobicity: ++	Recyclable, biocompatible, dimensional stability	Tissue engineering, scaffolds, dental implants, prosthetic limbs	(Ly et al., 2022)
Composites					
Metal matrix composites	Laser melting	Impact resistant: ++; Corrosion resistant: +; Durability: +++; Thermoplastic: +; Temp. resistant: +++; Inert: ++ Optic: +; Electric: ++ Hydrophobicity: ++	Ease of fabrication, lightweight, ease of fabrication, high dimensional stability	Electronic packaging, medical devices	(Wong, 2012), (Hamidi & Altan, 2017)
Ceramic matrix composites	FDM, SLS, LOM	Impact resistant: +; Corrosion resistant: +++; Durability: +; Thermoplastic: NA; Temp. resistant: +++; Inert: +++; Optic: NA; Electric: NA; Hydrophobicity: +	Versatile, Light weight, dimensional stability, high resistance to oxidation	Artificial joints and bone implants.	(Lee & Cha, 2020)

9.5 MATERIAL REQUIREMENTS FOR PREPARATION OF BIOPRINTING INK

Biological inks or bioinks are an essential element in all bioprinting procedures, which are crosslinked or stabilized during or immediately after bioprinting to form the final shapes of the required tissues. The choice of bioinks is influenced by the particular use (such as the target tissue), the kind of cells being employed, and the bioprinter used in the process.

9.5.1 Natural Bioinks

Agarose is a natural polymer produced by red seaweed consisting of repeated D-galactose and 3,6-anhydro-L-galactopyranose disaccharide units (Bertassoni *et al.*, 2014). It is primarily employed in the printing of vascularized tissue constructions to aid in shape formation (Norotte *et al.*, 2009) (Aydın *et al.*, 2020). When generating tubular vascular grafts, two printheads, one for printing agarose filaments and the second is employed for depositing different cell types such as smooth muscle cells and fibroblasts into multicellular cylinders (Aydın *et al.*, 2020). Agarose can also be employed as a component of a bioink that self-erodes to generate microchannels (Daly *et al.*, 2016). A bioink for printing 3D neural mini-tissue structures is developed using agarose especially for supporting structures and to assure the appropriate viscosity bioink for printing (Bouhadir *et al.*, 2001). Agarose hydrogels can be employed for bioprinting cartilage tissue for, e.g., mesenchymal stem-cell-laden agarose hydrogels are reinforced with two percent polycaprolactone to increase stiffness and this mixture promotes hyaline cartilage formation, which results in 80 % cell viability upon printing (Bouhadir *et al.*, 2001). Alginate is a biocompatible anionic polymer derived from brown algae and can be used to develop hydrogels with characteristics the same as extracellular matrix. Mammals lack enzymes, alginase hence it is non-biodegradable, and it remains in the biosystem for a longer time. Periodate-oxidized alginate is susceptible to hydrolytic breakdown, and ionically crosslinked alginate gels dissolve *in vivo* due to divalent ions leaking into the surrounding medium (Müller *et al.*, 2017). It is unique when compared to other natural bioinks because it has extremely low bioactivity, as it does not stimulate cell growth (Janarthanan *et al.*, 2020). The challenges related to employing bioink can be overcome by altering it or combining it with different materials for, e.g., the addition of nanocellulose shows that there is an increase in rheological as well as mechanical characteristics of alginate-based bioinks, and consequently their printability (Jiang *et al.*, 2020). Another material for, e.g., decellularized extracellular matrix can be added to an alginate-based bioink to increase bioactivity (Janarthanan *et al.*, 2020). Carboxymethyl cellulose, a water-soluble polymer, can be used to change the viscosity of other polymers and also allows cells to be incorporated in the bioink to print effectively. Carboxymethyl cellulose stabilizes the hydrogels, enhancing the final stability of structure and form integrity (Ahmadi *et al.*, 2015). Cellulose and its nanocrystals can be added into many different bioinks, boosting their elasticity, endurance, and porosity, and when combined with other materials, they can also increase bioink viscosity. A bioink can be combined using cellulose nanocrystals with oxidized dextran and gelatin hydrogels, and this aids in increasing the permeability of the created structures (He *et al.*, 2020). Chitosan is a gel-forming substance produced via partial deacetylation of chitin and has potential uses for applications in tissue engineering (Lee *et al.*, 2019). When chitosan is modified with ethylenediaminetetraacetic acid (EDTA) and Ca^{2+}, the modified chitosan possesses enhanced mechanical properties and stability for chondrocyte support. Varying concentrations modified chitosan and chitosan, give rise to altering the printability and gelation capabilities, and more proportions of modified chitosan give rise to loss of moduli and higher storage. Modified chitosan is the only element which is responsible for increasing the strength (Osidak *et al.*, 2019). Collagens are the most found proteins in mammals and account for 30 % protein in mammals. Alone collagen as a bioink is often used to improve mechanical characteristics by modifying the properties of bioink, such as crosslinking process or concentration, or by using sacrificial supports (Turner *et al.*, 2020; Yang *et al.*, 2018). Collagen is often blended with different biomaterials to improve the natural printability of the bioink, structural integrity, and bioactive properties. When printing cartilage structures, collagen (type I) with an alginate ink increases mechanical strength, helped maintain chondrocyte morphology, and reduced unwanted variation. Dextran is a natural, hydrophilic homopolysaccharide, composed primarily of α-1,6-linked D-glucopyranose residues and as dextran includes just hydroxy groups, which do not allow the attachment of cell, it is usual to alter dextran to provide for functional affinities' binding site. Dextran is beneficial being biodegradable due to its breakdown by dextranase but it has low mechanical strength, dextran is frequently mixed with other natural biomaterials as a bioink (de Melo *et al.*, 2020). It has been proven that oxidized dextran acts as crosslinkers for gelatin-based bioinks, which results in augmented structural fidelity, e.g., hydroxyethyl-methacrylate-derivatized dextran, (photocrosslinkable polymer) is added to increase the toughness of 3D-printed hyaluronic acid-based hydrogel formulations (De la Vega *et al.*, 2018). Fibrin is a biocompatible, insoluble, and biodegradable biopolymer whose characteristics can adjust by varying the amounts of fibrinogen and thrombin. It can also be combined with other materials, for, e.g., polycaprolactone, to make it versatile and this allows both hard and soft tissues to be imitated. As a result, fibrin characteristics can mimic hard and soft tissues. It is also a prominent bioink material because its nonlinear elasticity enables cell communication (Sharma *et al.*, 2020). It is also used for creating a variety of tissues, including vascularized, cardiac, neuronal, cutaneous, and tissues. Fibrin-based bioink produced using innovative RX1 bioprinter manufactured by Aspect Biosystems demonstrated brain progenitor cell survival levels (Monslow *et al.*, 2015). It can also be combined with microspheres that comprises guggulsterone to develop human initiated pluripotent stem cell (hiPSC)-derived NPCs into dopaminergic neurons (Monslow *et al.*, 2015). Hyaluronic acid (HA) is a glycosaminoglycan that is present in the natural extra cellular matrix but is not sulfated. It is vital in synovial fluid, aqueous humour, and hyaline cartilage (Cowman *et al.*, 2015). When suspended in water, HA solutions possess a thick viscous solution, making it a suitable material for tissue engineering applications (Zhu & Marchant, 2011). It is also ideal for bioprinting which requires good rheological characteristics (Schuurman *et al.*, 2013). A HA-based 3D-printed product that used secondary crosslinking is developed and found that the HA-based bioink forms dual crosslinked structures for

3D bioprinting, and there was no loss in mechanical properties after printing. Gelatin, produced by denaturation of collagen or can be extracted from skins, tendons, animal bones, or by basic or acidic hydrolysis (Gungor-Ozkerim *et al.*, 2018). Gelatin has several benefits, including biodegradability, biocompatibility, low antigenicity, the inclusion of intrinsic Arg-Gly-Asp structures, accessible active groups, the lack of toxic by-products, simplicity of processing, and less expensive (Lee *et al.*, 2015). All of the properties particularly its cellular affinity makes it a versatile material for bioprinting and tissue engineering applications. Myoblasts were enveloped in gelatin-alginate composite bioinks, and mechanical properties were improved through structure design (Xin *et al.*, 2019). Figure 9.1 demonstrates chemical structure of natural and synthetic bioinks used in the 3DP process.

9.5.2 Synthetic Bioinks

These bioinks provide a supportive matrix for the cells, allowing them to maintain their viability, proliferate, and differentiate into desired tissue types. Synthetic bioinks offer several advantages, such as reproducibility, tunable properties, and the ability to control the bioink composition precisely. There are various types of synthetic bioinks used in 3D bioprinting, including the following.

Polyethylene glycol has low-cost synthetic polyether with great biocompatibility that is soluble in aqueous solutions or organic solvents. Improving cell adhesion can be done by including cell-binding groups such as arginyl-glycyl-aspartic acid (Arg-Gly-Asp) peptides into a PEG hydrogel network. A novel polyethylene glycol microgel using off-stoichiometry thiolene click chemistry, was readily extruded and shows great stability after printing due to intra-particle adhesion forces (Haaf *et al.*, 1985). Polycaprolactone is a bioresorbable biodegradable, and semicrystalline polyalphahydroxy ester and it can be used to fabricate novel osteochondral tissue constructs for improved bone marrow (human mesenchymal stem cell functions) using casting technique (Izgordu *et al.*, 2021). Polyvinylpyrrolidone is a water-soluble, nontoxic, non-ionic amorphous polymer having a good solubility in polar solvents. Polyvinylpyrrolidone is often used in medications, tissue engineering, cosmetics, etc. (Naseri *et al.*, 2020). Polycaprolactone as well as polyvinylpyrrolidone were combined with HA, chitosan, and sodium alginate with the goal to find the optimal correlations among improving biological substitutes that can restore damaged tissue and are able to be included with the polymer matrix. Polylactic acid (PLA) is a biodegradable and aliphatic polyester created from renewable sugarcane or maize starch that contains lactic acid. PLA is a biocompatible polymer that is frequently used in biomedical applications since it is not carcinogenic or does not cause toxic effects in the surrounding tissue. 3D-printed l-arginine/graphite nanoplatelets and polylactic acid nanocomposites are created using fused deposition modeling and have high heat stability and mechanical properties using a solvent-based mixing process before being extruded via fused deposition modeling. Adding l-arginine/GNPs to the PLA nanocomposite increased its tensile and flexural strengths, and thermal stability can also be enhanced (Lan *et al.*, 2021). Polylactic-co-glycolic acid is a polymer widely employed in tissue engineering and drug administration due to its

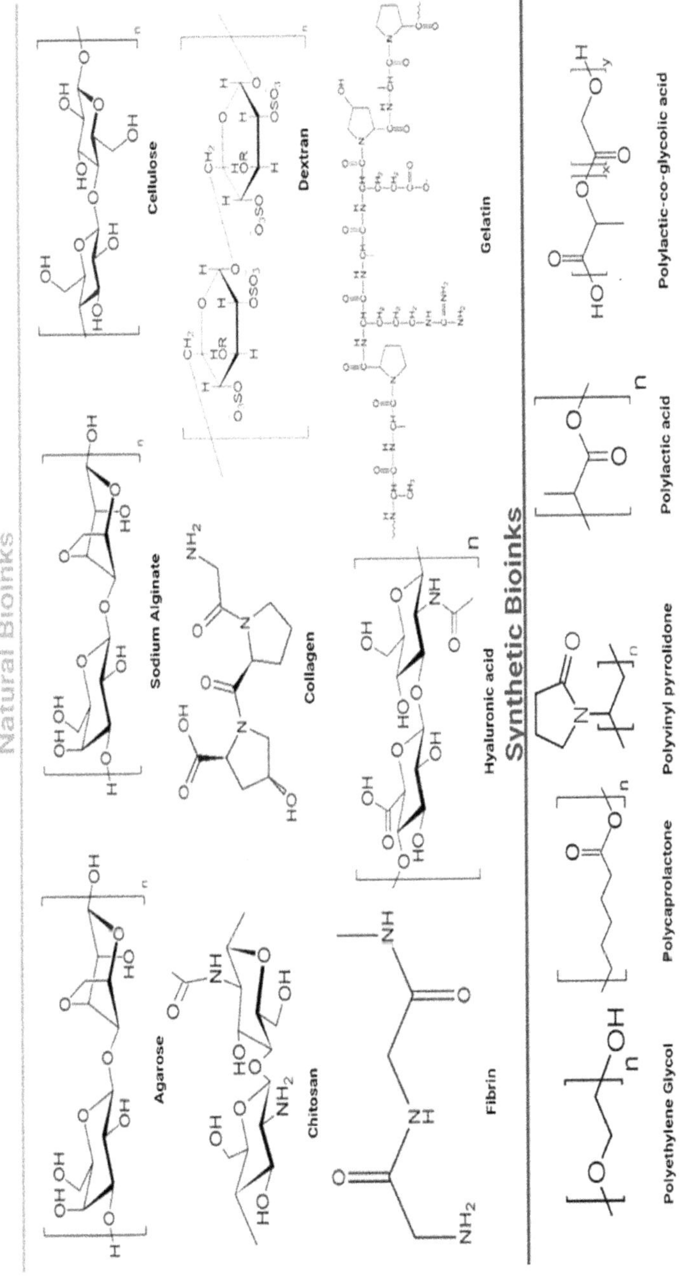

FIGURE 9.1 Chemical structure of natural and synthetic bioinks used in the 3DP process.

biocompatibility, biodegradability, broad erosion times, and flexible mechanical characteristics (Tagami *et al.*, 2017). Summarize additive materials for 3DP with mechanical properties and drug delivery presented in Table 9.2.

9.6 CHALLENGES AND OPPORTUNITIES IN BIOINK

Challenges: while 3D printing has made significant advancements in recent years, there are still several challenges that researchers and industry professionals are working to overcome. Here are some of the key challenges in 3D printing.

Printability: the correctness of the structure and size of the 3D-printed object has a direct relationship to the performance. The requirement for printability of materials will change depending on the printing technology used, e.g., highly viscous materials can be used to retain the first 3D shape after printing in micro-extrusion bioprinting, and the final structure is created by crosslinking. As a result, the material must have shear thinning qualities or specific crosslinking process (Lv *et al.*, 2010). Many novel materials for 3D bioprinting are reported; however, these materials are limited to particular basic printing processes, reducing their practical application values.

Biocompatibility: as research has progressed, the knowledge and recognition of biocompatibility has progressed from the initial need of the materials that can coexist with organs and tissues and does not have any adverse effects and the implanted materials possess beneficial relationships with the immune systems and/or host tissues, and regulating the activity and function of host cells, tissues, and organs (Courtney *et al.*, 2006). The materials must be biocompatible when using 3D bioprinting to create implantable (such as teeth, artificial eyes, 3D-printed joints, and other implants), tissue engineering scaffolds, organ substitutes and cell-laden tissue). The structural morphology, surface features, chemical composition, surface charge, and mechanical characteristics of the material primarily influence biocompatibility. The most difficult challenge is to identify a biocompatible material.

Appropriate mechanical properties: materials with a definite mechanical strength, which can withstand external forces, maintains the printed initial shape and structure play a significant role in implementing the functionalities of printed structures (Alonzo *et al.*, 2019). For instance, when using 3D bioprinting to develop tissues and organs, materials with the appropriate mechanical characteristics should be chosen based on the different mechanical surroundings that the intended tissues and organs require. Furthermore, materials with superior mechanical characteristics should be used as a support in the process of printing, especially for natural polymer materials with weak mechanical characteristics (Martina & Hutmacher, 2007).

Biodegradability: after the implant is placed inside the body, 3D bioprinted materials should progressively decay due to cell proliferation and synthesis of extracellular matrix (Martina & Hutmacher, 2007; Zhang *et al.*, 2021). The rate of degradation should correlate to the pace at which the cell manufactures an extracellular matrix to replace implanted materials, as well as the rate at which new tissue is formed. At the same time, the breakdown substances should readily breakdown, be non-toxic, and be promptly eliminated. The primary challenge currently is to find a suitable material that degrades over time.

TABLE 9.2

Additive Materials for 3DP with Mechanical Properties and Drug Delivery

Additive Materials	Process of 3D Printing	Mechanical Property	Drug Delivery	Ref.
PVA	Fused-deposition modeling-type 3D printer	Elasticity: +++; Plasticity: ++; Ductability: +; Toughness: +; Machinability: ++; Malleability: +	Polyvinyl alcohol (PVA)-based tablets	(Boetker *et al.*, 2016)
PLA and HPMC	Hot melt extrusion	Elasticity: ++; Plasticity: +++; Ductability: +; Toughness: +++; Machinability: +; Malleability: ++	Model disk geometries	(Goyanes *et al.*, 2016)
Silk Fibroin/PEG	Extrusion based 3D- printing	Elasticity: ++; Plasticity: ++; Ductability: +; Toughness: ++; Machinability: NA; Malleability: ++	Disk/meniscus-shaped scaffold	(Avila *et al.*, 2021)
PLLA and PCL	SLM	Elasticity: ++; Plasticity: +++; Ductability: ++; Toughness: ++; Machinability: +; Malleability: +	coronary stent prototype with customized geometries	(Sharma *et al.*, 2021)
Polyether ether ketone (PEEK)	SLM, EBP	Elasticity: +++; Plasticity: ++; Ductability: + ; Toughness: ++; Machinability: NA; Malleability: +	Dental, orthopedic, trauma, and spinal implants	(Arif *et al.*, 2023)
PLA/PGA and PCL/HA	FDM	Elasticity: ++; Plasticity: ++; Ductability: +; Toughness: +++; Machinability: +; Malleability: +	Native stiff bone-like constructs	(Jain *et al.*, 2020)
Chitosan-based polymers-polyacrylamide	3D-Printing	Elasticity: ++; Plasticity: ++; Ductability: + ; Toughness: +; Machinability: NA; Malleability: ++	Hydrogel for bone regenerative therapies	(Saroia *et al.*, 2018)

Sterilisation stability: it is an important step in biomaterials' application and typically, biomaterials are sterilized using physical or chemical methods such as e-beam, autoclaving, or gamma irradiation, incubation with ethanol, ethylene oxide treatment, etc., to inactivate every type of microbial life. Each sterilization method has its own set of benefits and drawbacks, as well as a specific spectrum of use. As a result, 3D bioprinting materials should be suitable with at minimum one type of sterilization treatment.

Opportunities: because of many standards, selecting the suitable biomaterial for 3D printing bioinks for skin replacements and the main objective is achieving the optimum balance of mechanical properties and biocompatibility (Brassard *et al.*, 2021). Biomaterials which provide strong mechanical characteristics to the printed structure is not considered as ideal for cell housing, while materials that mimic a tissue-like environment for live cell protection do not have sufficient physical properties that are required for effective printability and stability (Lee *et al.*, 2019). As a result, the opportunity lies in developing the best and most suitable bioinks for 3D printing.

Traditional organoid production is less repeatable and suffers from fluctuation across culture batches and therefore, the production of the associated organoids is limited. To some extent, bioprinting overcomes these issues. Bioprinting has been described for creating centimeter-level intestinal organoids as a breakthrough in resolving standard culture-scale restrictions (Humphreys, 2021). Bioprinting may also create sophisticated circulatory networks for organoids, increase organoid yield by a factor of 9, and reduce organoid size variability by only 1–4% (Lin *et al.*, 2020). Another challenge in bioprinting organoids is the formation of macroscopic tissues, although bioprinting technology can efficiently regulate cell deposition in 3D space, it is difficult to generate macroscopic tissues by self-organization. To solve the existing challenges of size of organoids, future opportunity lies on how to print small functional units of the organoids, deposit and assemble these functional units into larger organoids. By using various bioprinting methods and bioprinting material strategies, 3D bioprinting may develop bioprinting products that fulfil a variety of purposes. These printing techniques have been used to restore skin, particularly skin wounds. A novel bioink composed of Silica-GelMa (Gelatin methacrylamide and collagen doped with tyrosinase), was developed by integrating Silica with GelMA, that has a lower rate of degradation and increases the activity of human skin fibroblasts without lowering its own printability point (Lin *et al.*, 2020). 3D printing has shown promising potential in the field of tissue engineering, including the development of nasal cartilage. For, e.g., using type I COL hydrogels loaded with human nasal chondrocytes, 3D bioprinting for nasal cartilage structures has shown promising effects and is a feasible rhinoplasty approach (Khaled *et al.*, 2014). 3DP is a promising approach that decreases the surgical complexity of rhinoplasty by allowing the customization of unique nasal cartilage components for, e.g., craniofacial bones.

The biocompatibility of 3D bioprinting materials may be improved in a number of ways such as surface modification methods, modifying the topology of the materials, controlling surface hydrophobicity and hydrophilicity, increasing surface charge strength, and encompassing the surface with bioactive substances. Another strategy is to combine various types of materials in order to enhance the mechanical characteristics and biocompatibility of 3D bioprinting materials. Furthermore, the biomimicry approach may be used to create materials which mimic both the structure and function of those that exist in *in vivo*. These methods present great prospects to increase the biocompatibility of 3D bioprinting materials, potentially leading to the creation of more effective and safe biomedical devices and therapies. More study is needed to fully explore the potential and develop them for practical use. A single breakthrough in 3D bioprinting technology signifies the endless potential of life sciences.

9.7 BIO-MEDICAL APPLICATION OF 3D PRINTING

3D printing is a rapidly developing technology that has the potential to revolutionize the pharmaceutical, biomedical, and tissue engineering industries. Here are some of the ways that 3D printing is being used in these fields.

9.7.1 APPLICATION OF 3D PRINTING IN FABRICATING PHARMACEUTICALS

As standard manufacturing techniques are ineffective for producing personalized medicines and cannot manufacture individualized dosage forms with modified release profiles and highly complicated geometries, 3D printing technology has a promising future in personalized medicine. The advancements in personalized medicine have led to an urge for tablets that can be digitally handled by healthcare workers that are rapid, precise, and reliable. Through a software command, size of 3D manufactured tablet can be to modify the dosage. A variable dosage of theophylline tablet for immediate and prolonged release is developed with precise drug-loading capabilities and an easy-to-swallow tablet form. The manufacturing technique is inexpensive, digitally controllable, and compatible with polymers such as hydroxypropyl cellulose, Eudragit RS, RL, and E. Up to 95% dosage accuracy was found with the necessary *in vitro* release pattern and weight accuracy. Because of the high flexibility of the printer, as well as its compact size and ease of use, the approach provides the possibility for future individualized treatment (Li *et al.*, 2022).

One of the most researched applications is the formulation of drugs with *complex drug release profiles.* 3D printing technology is used to create sustained release tablets of guaifenesin that have the same release profile as normal commercial tablets and can pass regulatory testing. The matrix was made of hydroxypropyl methylcellulose and polyacrylic acid, with hypromellose as a binder and sodium starch glycolate as a disintegrant. A medication release profile similar to that of a commercial guaifenesin bilayer tablet and the printed formulations were examined for physical and mechanical characteristics and determined to be within an acceptable range according to US Pharmacopoeia (Gregor *et al.*, 2017). Implantable with customized drug-release profiles can be created using 3D printing technology. A 3D-printed implant was formed that takes use of the benefits of osseous regeneration as well as a local combination therapy to prevent medication resistance and adverse effects, while using this approach macro/mesoporous scaffolds are developed that was loaded with large doses of isoniazid and rifampicin. The scaffolds have longer release profiles as well as the desired drug level in peripheral tissue and low levels in blood (Liaskoni *et al.*, 2021).

Conventional chemotherapy limits in terms of reaching therapeutic concentrations at the tumor site, as well as build up in important organs such as the liver and heart, both of which produce major adverse effects. To address the challenges of traditional chemotherapy, a local, highly effective delivery mechanism is required. A biodegradable patch biodegradable patch containing 5-fluorouracil is developed and can be applied to a specific tumor location, which has a variable form and this method can achieve the required therapeutic drug concentration with a sustained and controlled release with fewer adverse effects, the patch was able to inhibit the proliferation of subcutaneous pancreatic cancer xenografts in mice. This approach can be used for other bioabsorbable implants containing anti-cancer medications developed using 3D printing technology could represent an excellent strategy for local administration of anti-cancer agents (Ulery *et al.*, 2011).

9.7.2 Application of 3D Printing in Biodegradable Biomedicals

Aliphatic polyesters such as polylactic acid and polycaprolactone are frequently used in first-generation tissue engineering. Polycaprolactone exhibited a prolonged release mechanism which is determined by the Korsmeyer-Peppas model, and proves slow degradation kinetics. Thus, a combination of 3D printing and precise biomaterial selection can produce patient-specific tissue structures with required mechanical strength while also allowing sustained release of particular molecules at the target site thereby speeding up the healing process. Polylactic acid is another polymer that has received a lot of attention in the field of bone tissue engineering. An extrusion-based 3D printing procedure used to create polylactic acid scaffolds with an approx. pore size of 350 microns with 30% porosity, which were then assessed using osteosarcoma cells. Cells proliferated rapidly on porous scaffolds with 50 % and 30 % porosity while retaining the mechanical characteristics required for load-bearing bone development (Zanini *et al.*, 2021).

Polylactic-co-glycolic acid has been used in commercial sutures since the 1970s manufacturing of pharmaceutical product. For load-bearing applications, polylactic acid is the most-used polyester due to its intrinsic high mechanical strength and is used in internal fixation devices, such as screws, plates, pins, and rods to support the repair of broken bones and hold them together.

9.7.3 Application of 3D Printing in Tissue and Bone Engineering

Depending on the use, the porous scaffolds have cytotoxicity, great biocompatibility, porosity, appropriate interconnectivity, and pore size. Furthermore, these scaffolds play an important role in drug delivery systems, manufacturing surgical equipment and, devices and the encapsulation of animal and human cells (Goh *et al.*, 2015). A multi-drug eluting 3D-printed stent was developed by extruding graphene nanoplatelets into a biodegradable polycaprolactone-based polymer. The increased mechanical characteristics, as well as the *in vitro* data, demonstrated that these innovative biodegradable stents can be used to treat cardiac patients with blocked coronary arteries. Bone is a naturally restoring tissue, but accidents can inflict severe harm to the tissue, impeding normal regeneration and leading to bone abnormalities.

A 3D printing technology (SLA bioprinters) used to create biodegradable implants for bone regeneration. A 3D-printed scaffolds is developed by adding 51 wt.% β-tricalcium phosphate into poly trimethylene carbonate and this scaffold exhibits good printability and mechanical properties (Praveen & Kim, 2018). Similarly, a polycaprolactone-based biodegradable material used to make scaffolds for repairing the socket of a human tooth. A 3DP was employed to create the polycaprolactone scaffold that might be used in bone repair of the human tooth for this purpose and this scaffold is designed to mimic the natural architecture of the alveolar ridge and provide a framework for tissue ingrowth and regeneration (Liu *et al.*, 2020).

To print scaffolds for tissue engineering applications, several natural biopolymers (alpha keratin, chitosan, HA, alginate, and collagen) and synthetic biopolymers (polycaprolactone, polyethylene glycol, and their copolymers) can be used (Huang *et al.*, 2021). For example, poly l-lactide-co-ε-caprolactone copolymer scaffolds controlled the elastic modulus and stiffness of the poly l-lactide-co-ε-caprolactone by adding polycaprolactone-based biopolymer and shown excellent biocompatibility and mechanical characteristics. Thus, copolymerized poly l-lactide-co-ε-caprolactone based scaffolds show great promise for muscle, cardiac, tendon, and skin tissue regeneration and repair (Huang *et al.*, 2021).

For 3D printing of lung tissue scaffolds, a unique bioink composed of regenerated silk fibroin (SF) and 2,2,6,6-tetramethylpiperidine-1-oxyl-oxidized bacterial cellulose (OBC) nanofibrils are developed and this bioink demonstrates to be printable with the ability of forming 3D structures and high shape fidelity. The SF-OBC (silk fibroin and oxidized bacterial cellulose) composite inks demonstrated good shear thinning and reversible stress softening, resulting in a unique silk-based ink for 3DP. 3D bioprinted cell-loaded GelMA hydrogels have been demonstrated to be a viable new technique for corneal stroma engineering. Human corneal keratocytes were loaded into GelMA hydrogels, and these hydrogels are found to be transparent, with optical characteristics equivalent to native cornea and also showed sufficient mechanical strength (Robles-Martinez *et al.*, 2019). Systemic illustration of various types of implants fabricated using 3D/4D printing using artificial-intelligence-based additive manufacturing is presented in Figure 9.2. Moreover, the use of additive materials, designing software, printing parameters with biomedical applications is presented in Table 9.3.

9.8 CONCLUSIONS

Although computational-automation-based additive manufacturing is a relatively recent idea, 4D printing technology combined with smart material is utilized to build a shape-changing mechanism over time, however 3D printing has evolved significantly since beginning of automation and has spread its influence in numerous industrial areas. More adaptability and diversity are possible with additive manufacturing since a single structure that may be used for several purpose. In addition, 4D printing materials hold great promise for the future since they can eliminate the basic vulnerabilities of mechanical systems. Additionally, potential application of 4D-printed smart materials include the fabrication of innovative systems that are not constrained by a certain degree of freedom. Hence novel smart fabrication of pharmaceuticals via the use of computational automation can have more effective ways to develop precise

TABLE 9.3
Additive Materials, Designing Software, Printing Parameters with Biomedical Applications

Additive Materials	Process of 3D Printing/ Instruments	Designing Software/ Printing Parameters	Biomedical Applications	Ref.
HPMC, PEG	Extrusion-based 3D Printing	**Solidworks,** Printing temperature: 190 °C; Nozzle temperature: 200°C; Nozzle diameter: 0.4 mm; Bed temperature: 60 °C; Printing speed: 20 mm/s; Layer thickness: 0.1mm	Controlled drug delivery and pharmaceutical product development.	(Boniatti *et al.,* 2021)
Polyethylene glycol diacrylate	SLA	**AutoCAD,** Printing temperature: 210 °C; Nozzle temperature: 220 °C; Nozzle diameter: 0.2 mm; Bed temperature: 60 °C; Printing speed: 30 mm/s; Layer thickness: 0.1 mm	Polypill	(Chew *et al.,* 2019)
Kollidon	Extrusion-based 3D Printing	**AutoCAD,** Printing temperature: 210 °C; Nozzle temperature: 230 °C; Nozzle diameter: 0.4 mm; Bed temperature: 45°C; Printing speed: 20 mm/s Layer thickness: 0.1 mm	Pediatric formulation of praziquantel to treat schistosomiasis	(Ioannou *et al.,* 2023)
PVA	FDM	**TinkerCAD,** Printing temperature: 190°C; Nozzle temperature: 220 °C; Nozzle diameter: 0.43mm; Bed temperature: 50 °C; Printing speed: 10 mm/s; Layer thickness: 0.1mm	3D-printed product of fluorescein sodium and 5-aminosalicyclic acid.	(Boniatti *et al.,* 2021; Sadia *et al.,* 2016)
Polycaprolactone and chitosan	Extrusion-based 3D Printing	**TinkerCAD,** Printing temperature: 180°C; Nozzle temperature: 200 °C; Nozzle diameter: 0.41 mm; Bed temperature: 60 °C; Printing speed: 2 mm/s; Layer thickness: 0.1mm	Sustained release drug implant replacing the need for repeated 5-FU injections	(Ioannou *et al.,* 2023)
Eudragit EPO	FDM, Extrusion-based 3D Printing	**Autodesk® 3ds Max,** Printing temperature: 135°C; Nozzle temperature: 200°C; Bed temperature: 100°C; Printing speed: 10 mm/s; Layer thickness: 0.2 mm	Theophylline, Captopril and Prednisolone	(Sadia *et al.,* 2016)

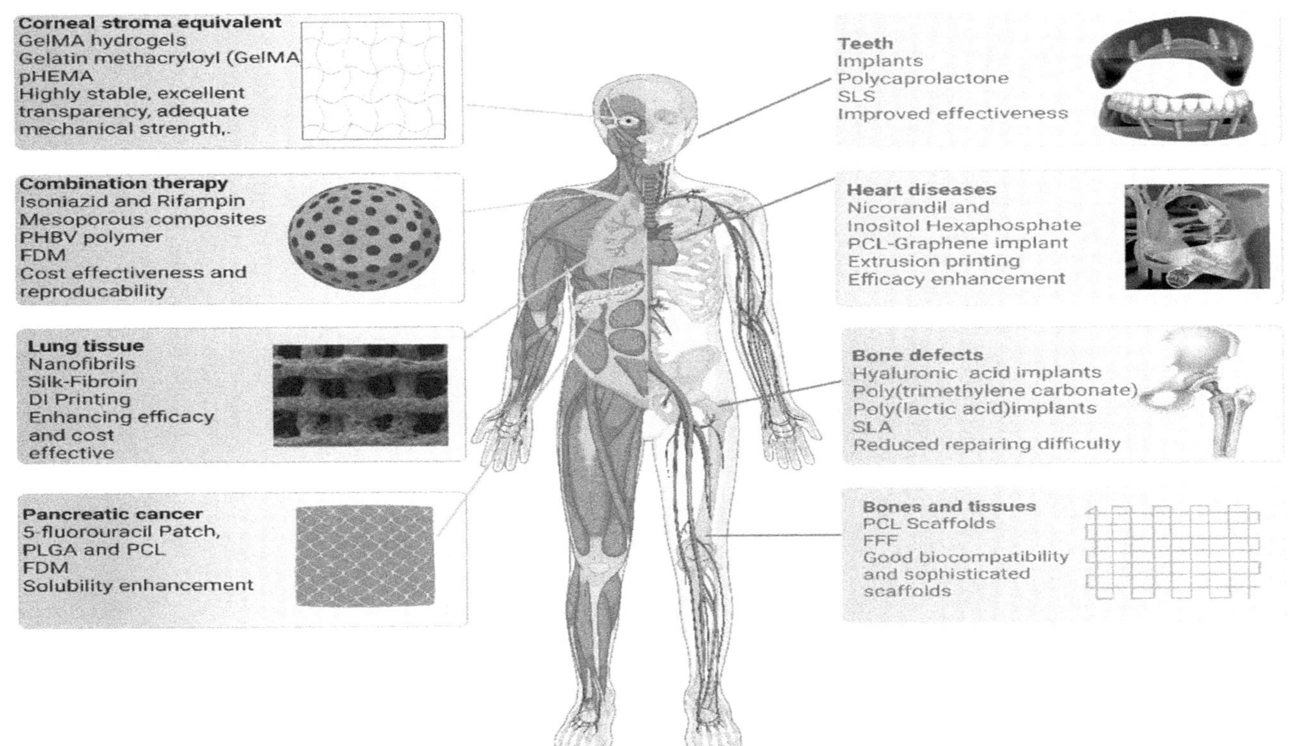

FIGURE 9.2 A visualization of various implants.

medicine. Furthermore, upgradation of this current technology to 5D printing, where is the print head and the printable object have five degrees of freedom is the future of the approach and is yet to be explored.

REFERENCES

Ahmadi, F., Oveisi, Z., Samani, S. M., & Amoozgar, Z. (2015). Chitosan based hydrogels: Characteristics and pharmaceutical applications. *Res Pharm Sci*, *10*(1), 1–16.

Ali, M., Batay, S., & Dastan, S. (2019). 3D printing: A critical review of current development and future prospects. *Rapid Prototyp J*, ahead-of-print. https://doi.org/10.1108/RPJ-11-2018-0293

Alonzo, M., AnilKumar, S., Roman, B., Tasnim, N., & Joddar, B (2019). 3D Bioprinting of cardiac tissue and cardiac stem cell therapy. *Transl Res*, *211*, 64–83 [1878–1810 (Electronic)].

Ambrosi, A., & Pumera, M. (2016). 3D-printing technologies for electrochemical applications [10.1039/C5CS00714C]. *Chem Soc Rev*, *45*(10), 2740–2755. https://doi.org/10.1039/C5CS00714C

Arif, Z. U., Khalid, M. Y., Noroozi, R., Hossain, M., Shi, H. H., Tariq, A., Ramakrishna, S., & Umer, R. (2023). Additive manufacturing of sustainable biomaterials for biomedical applications. *Asian J Pharm Sci*, *18*(3), 100812. https://doi.org/10.1016/j.ajps.2023.100812

Avila, J. D., Stenberg, K., Bose, S., & Bandyopadhyay, A. (2021). Hydroxyapatite reinforced Ti6Al4V composites for load-bearing implants. *Acta Biomater*, *123*, 379–392. https://doi.org/10.1016/j.actbio.2020.12.060

Aydın, L., Kucuk, S., & Kenar, H. (2020). A universal self-eroding sacrificial bioink that enables bioprinting at room temperature. *Polym Adv Technol*, *31*. https://doi.org/10.1002/pat.4892

Bertassoni, L. E., Cecconi, M., Manoharan, V., Nikkhah, M., Hjortnaes, J., Cristino, A. L., Barabaschi, G., Demarchi, D., Dokmeci, M. R., Yang, Y., & Khademhosseini, A. (2014). Hydrogel bioprinted microchannel networks for vascularization of tissue engineering constructs [10.1039/C4LC00030G]. *Lab Chip*, *14*(13), 2202–2211. https://doi.org/10.1039/C4LC00030G

Boetker, J., Water, J. J., Aho, J., Arnfast, L., Bohr, A., & Rantanen, J. (2016). Modifying release characteristics from 3D printed drug-eluting products. *Eur J Pharm Sci*, *90*, 47–52. https://doi.org/10.1016/j.ejps.2016.03.013

Boniatti, J., Januskaite, P., Fonseca, L. B. D., Viçosa, A. L., Amendoeira, F. C., Tuleu, C., Basit, A. W., Goyanes, A., & Ré, M. I. (2021). Direct powder extrusion 3D printing of praziquantel to overcome neglected disease formulation challenges in paediatric populations. *Pharmaceutics*, *13*(8). https://doi.org/10.3390/pharmaceutics13081114

Bouhadir, K. H., Lee, K. Y., Alsberg, E., Damm, K. L., Anderson, K. W., & Mooney, D. J. (2001). Degradation of partially oxidized alginate and its potential application for tissue engineering. *Biotechnol Prog*, *17*(5), 945–950. https://doi.org/10.1021/bp010070p

Brassard, J. A., Nikolaev, M., Hübscher, T., Hofer, M., & Lutolf, M. P. (2021). Recapitulating macro-scale tissue self-organization through organoid bioprinting. *Nat Mater*, *20*(1), 22–29. https://doi.org/10.1038/s41563-020-00803-5

Bukkapatnam, S. T. S. (2023). Autonomous materials discovery and manufacturing (AMDM): A review and perspectives. *IISE Trans*, *55*(1), 75–93. https://doi.org/10.1080/24725854.2022.2089785

Casalini, T., Rossi, F., Castrovinci, A., & Perale, G. (2019). A perspective on polylactic acid-based polymers use for nanoparticles synthesis and applications [review]. *Front Bioeng Biotechnol*, 7. https://www.frontiersin.org/articles/10.3389/fbioe.2019.00259

Chen, Z., Li, Z., Li, J., Liu, C., Lao, C., Fu, Y., Liu, C., Li, Y., Wang, P., & He, Y. (2019). 3D printing of ceramics: A review. *J Eur Ceram Soc*, *39*(4), 661–687. https://doi.org/https://doi.org/10.1016/j.jeurceramsoc.2018.11.013

Chew, S. L., Modica de Mohac, L., & Tolulope Raimi-Abraham, B. (2019). 3D-printed solid dispersion drug products. *Pharmaceutics*, *11*(12).

Courtney, T., Sacks, M. S., Stankus, J., Guan, J., & Wagner, W. R. (2006). Design and analysis of tissue engineering scaffolds that mimic soft tissue mechanical anisotropy. *Biomaterials*, *27*, 3631–3638 [0142–9612 (Print)].

Cowman, M. K., Schmidt, T. A., Raghavan, P., & Stecco, A. (2015). Viscoelastic properties of hyaluronan in physiological conditions. *F1000Res*, *4*, 622. https://doi.org/10.12688/f1000research.6885.1

Daly, A. C., Critchley, S. E., Rencsok, E. M., & Kelly, D. J. (2016). A comparison of different bioinks for 3D bioprinting of fibrocartilage and hyaline cartilage. *Biofabrication*, *8*(4), 045002. https://doi.org/10.1088/1758-5090/8/4/045002

De la Vega, L., A. Rosas Gómez, D., Abelseth, E., Abelseth, L., Allisson da Silva, V., & Willerth, S. M. (2018). 3D bioprinting human induced pluripotent stem cell-derived neural tissues using a novel lab-on-a-printer technology. *Appl Sci*, *8*(12).

de Melo, B. A. G., Jodat, Y. A., Cruz, E. M., Benincasa, J. C., Shin, S. R., & Porcionatto, M. A. (2020). Strategies to use fibrinogen as bioink for 3D bioprinting fibrin-based soft and hard tissues. *Acta Biomater*, *117*, 60–76. https://doi.org/10.1016/j.actbio.2020.09.024

Deshmukh, K., Sankaran, S., Ahamed, B., Pasha, S., Sadasivuni, K. K., Ponnamma, D., AlMa'adeed, M., & Chidambaram, K. (2017). Studies on the electrical properties of graphene oxide oxide-reinforced poly (4-styrene sulfonic acid) and polyvinyl alcohol blend composites. *Int J Nanosci*, *17*. https://doi.org/10.1142/S0219581X17600055

Dominic, P., Leahy, D., & Willis, M. (2010). GPTIPS: An open source genetic programming toolbox for multigene symbolic regression. *Lect Notes Eng Comput Sci*, *2180*.

Ellul, J., & Debono, C. (2022). TinkercadNetConnector: Connecting emulated IoT devices to the outside world. *SoftwareX*, *20*. https://doi.org/10.1016/j.softx.2022.101218

Goh, B. T., Teh, L. Y., Tan, D. B., Zhang, Z., & Teoh, S. H. (2015). Novel 3D polycaprolactone scaffold for ridge preservation – A pilot randomised controlled clinical trial. *Clin Oral Implants Res*, *26*(3), 271–277. https://doi.org/10.1111/clr.12486

Goyanes, A., Det-Amornrat, U., Wang, J., Basit, A. W., & Gaisford, S. (2016). 3D scanning and 3D printing as innovative technologies for fabricating personalized topical drug delivery systems. *J Control Release*, *234*, 41–48. https://doi.org/10.1016/j.jconrel.2016.05.034

Gregor, A., Filová, E., Novák, M., Kronek, J., Chlup, H., Buzgo, M., Blahnová, V., Lukášová, V., Bartoš, M., Nečas, A., & Hošek, J. (2017). Designing of PLA scaffolds for bone tissue replacement fabricated by ordinary commercial 3D printer. *J Bio Eng*, *11*(1), 31. https://doi.org/10.1186/s13036-017-0074-3

Gungor-Ozkerim, P. S., Inci, I., Zhang, Y. S., Khademhosseini, A., & Dokmeci, M. R. (2018). Bioinks for 3D bioprinting: An overview. *Biomater Sci*, *6*(5), 915–946. https://doi.org/10.1039/c7bm00765e

Guo, N., & Leu, M. (2013). Additive manufacturing: Technology, applications and research needs. *Front Mechan Eng*, *8*. https://doi.org/10.1007/s11465-013-0248-8

Haaf, F., Sanner, A., & Straub, F. (1985). Polymers of N-vinylpyrrolidone: Synthesis, characterization and uses. *Polym J*, *17*, 143–152.

Hamidi, Y., & Altan, M. (2017). Process induced defects in liquid molding processes of composites. *Int Polym Process*, *32*. https://doi.org/10.3139/217.3444

Hata, K., Ikeda, H., Nagamatsu, Y., Masaki, C., Hosokawa, R., & Shimizu, H. (2021). Development of dental poly(methyl methacrylate)-based resin for stereolithography additive manufacturing. *Polymers, 13*(24).

He, Y., Derakhshanfar, S., Zhong, W., Li, B., Lu, F., Xing, M., & Li, X. (2020). Characterization and application of carboxymethyl chitosan-based bioink in cartilage tissue engineering. *Journal of Nanomaterials.*

Huang, L., Yuan, W., Hong, Y., Fan, S., Yao, X., Ren, T., Song, L., Yang, G., & Zhang, Y. (2021). 3D printed hydrogels with oxidized cellulose nanofibers and silk fibroin for the proliferation of lung epithelial stem cells. *Cellulose (Lond), 28*(1), 241–257. https://doi. org/10.1007/s10570-020-03526-7

Humphreys, B. D. (2021). Bioprinting better kidney organoids. *Nat Mater, 20*(2), 128–130. https://doi.org/10.1038/s41563-020-00881-5

Ioannou, N., Luo, J., Qin, M., Di Luca, M., Mathew, E., Tagalakis, A. D.,

Izgordu, M. S., Uzgur, E. I., Ulag, S., Sahin, A., Karademir Yilmaz, B., Kilic, B., Ekren, N., Oktar, F. N., & Gunduz, O. (2021). Investigation of 3D-printed polycaprolactone-/polyvinylpyrrolidone-based constructs. *Cartilage, 13*(2_suppl), 626s-635s. https://doi. org/10.1177/1947603519897302

Jain, S., Yassin, M. A., Fuoco, T., Liu, H., Mohamed-Ahmed, S., Mustafa, K., & Finne-Wistrand, A. (2020). Engineering 3D degradable, pliable scaffolds toward adipose tissue regeneration; optimized printability, simulations and surface modification. *J Tissue Eng, 11*, 2041731420954316. https://doi.org/10.1177/2041731420954316

Janarthanan, G., Tran, H. N., Cha, E., Lee, C., Das, D., & Noh, I. (2020). 3D printable and injectable lactoferrin-loaded carboxymethyl cellulose-glycol chitosan hydrogels for tissue engineering applications. *Mater Sci Eng C Mater Biol Appl, 113*, 111008. https://doi.org/10.1016/j.msec.2020.111008

Jiang, Y., Zhou, J., Shi, H., Zhao, G., Zhang, Q., Feng, C., & Xv, X. (2020). Preparation of cellulose nanocrystal/oxidized dextran/gelatin (CNC/OD/GEL) hydrogels and fabrication of a CNC/OD/GEL scaffold by 3D printing. *J Mater Sci, 55*. https://doi.org/10.1007/s10 853-019-04186-0

Karian, H. (2003). *Handbook of Polypropylene and Polypropylene Composites, Revised and Expanded* (2nd Edition). https://doi.org/https://doi.org/10.1201/9780203911808

Khaled, S. A., Burley, J. C., Alexander, M. R., & Roberts, C. J. (2014). Desktop 3D printing of controlled release pharmaceutical bilayer tablets. *Int J Pharm, 461*(1–2), 105–111. https://doi.org/10.1016/j.ijpharm.2013.11.021

Kuebler, S. M., Ananthavel, S., Rumi, M., Marder, S. R., Perry, J. W., Barlow, S., Cumpston, B. H., Dyer, D. L., Ehrlich, J. E., Erskine, L. L., Heikal, A. A., Lee, I. Y. S., McCord-Maughon, D., Qin, J., Röcket, H., & Wu, X.-L. (1999). Two-photon polymerization initiators for efficient three-dimensional optical data storage and microfabrication. OSA Technical Digest. Conference on Lasers and Electro-Optics, 23 May 1999, Baltimore, Maryland.

Lamprou, D. A., & Yu-Wai-Man, C. (2023). 3D-printed long-acting 5-fluorouracil implant to prevent conjunctival fibrosis in glaucoma. *J Pharm Pharmacol, 75*(2), 276–286. https://doi.org/10.1093/jpp/rgac100

Lan, X., Liang, Y., Erkut, E. J. N., Kunze, M., Mulet-Sierra, A., Gong, T., Osswald, M., Ansari, K., Seikaly, H., Boluk, Y., & Adesida, A. B. (2021). Bioprinting of human nasoseptal chondrocytes-laden collagen hydrogel for cartilage tissue engineering. *Faseb J, 35*(3), e21191. https://doi.org/10.1096/fj.202002081R

Lee, A., Hudson, A. R., Shiwarski, D. J., Tashman, J. W., Hinton, T. J., Yerneni, S., Bliley, J. M., Campbell, P. G., & Feinberg, A. W. (2019). 3D bioprinting of collagen to rebuild components of the human heart. *Science, 365*(6452), 482–487. https://doi.org/10.1126/science.aav9051

Lee, K. S., & Cha, C. J. M. R. (2020). Advanced polymer-based bioink technology for printing soft biomaterials. *Macromol Res, 28*, 689–702.

Lee, T. T., García, J. R., Paez, J. I., Singh, A., Phelps, E. A., Weis, S., Shafiq, Z., Shekaran, A., Del Campo, A., & García, A. J. (2015). Light-triggered in vivo activation of adhesive peptides regulates cell adhesion, inflammation and vascularization of biomaterials. *Nat Mater, 14*(3), 352–360. https://doi.org/10.1038/nmat4157

Li, Z., Wang, Q., & Liu, G. (2022). A review of 3D printed bone implants. *Micromachines (Basel), 13*(4). https://doi.org/10.3390/mi13040528

Liaskoni, A., Wildman, R. D., & Roberts, C. J. (2021). 3D printed polymeric drug-eluting implants. *Int J Pharm, 597* [1873–3476 (Electronic)].

Lin, F. S., Lee, J. J., Lee, A. K., Ho, C. C., Liu, Y. T., & Shie, M. Y. (2020). Calcium silicate-activated gelatin methacrylate hydrogel for accelerating human dermal fibroblast proliferation and differentiation. *Polymers (Basel), 13*(1). https://doi.org/10.3390/polym13010070

Liu, W., Feng, Z., Ou-Yang, W., Pan, X., Wang, X., Huang, P., Zhang, C., Kong, D., & Wang, W. (2020). 3D printing of implantable elastic PLCL copolymer scaffolds [10.1039/C9SM02396H]. *Soft Matter, 16*(8), 2141–2148. https://doi.org/10.1039/C9SM02396H

Luffy, S. A., Chou, D. T., Waterman, J., Wearden, P. D., Kumta, P. N., & Gilbert, T. W. (2014). Evaluation of magnesium-yttrium alloy as an extraluminal tracheal stent. *J Biomed Mater Res A, 102*(3), 611–620. https://doi.org/10.1002/jbm.a.34731

Lv, S., Dudek, D. M., Cao, Y., Balamurali, M. M., Gosline, J., & Li, H. (2010). Designed biomaterials to mimic the mechanical properties of muscles. *Nature, 465*, 69–73 [1476–4687 (Electronic)].

Ly, M., Hays, S., Spinelli, S., & Zhu, D. (2022). 3D printing of ceramic biomaterials. *Engineered Regen, 3*. https://doi.org/10.1016/j.engreg.2022.01.006

Martina, M., & Hutmacher, D. (2007). Biodegradable polymers applied in tissue engineering research: A review. *Polym Int, 56*, 145–157. https://doi.org/10.1002/pi.2108

Monslow, J., Govindaraju, P., & Puré, E. (2015). Hyaluronan – A functional and structural sweet spot in the tissue microenvironment [review]. *Front Immunol, 6*. https://www.frontiersin.org/articles/10.3389/fimmu.2015.00231

Müller, M., Öztürk, E., Arlov, Ø., Gatenholm, P., & Zenobi-Wong, M. (2017). Alginate sulfate-nanocellulose bioinks for cartilage bioprinting applications. *Ann Biomed Eng, 45*(1), 210–223. https://doi.org/10.1007/s10439-016-1704-5

Naseri, E., Cartmell, C., Saab, M., Kerr, R. G., & Ahmadi, A. (2020). Development of 3D printed drug-eluting scaffolds for preventing piercing infection. *Pharmaceutics, 12*(9). https://doi.org/10.3390/pharmaceutics12090901

Norotte, C., Marga, F. S., Niklason, L. E., & Forgacs, G. (2009). Scaffold-free vascular tissue engineering using bioprinting. *Biomaterials, 30*(30), 5910–5917. https://doi.org/10.1016/j.biomaterials.2009.06.034

Osidak, E. O., Karalkin, P. A., Osidak, M. S., Parfenov, V. A., Sivogrivov, D. E., Pereira, F., Gryadunova, A. A., Koudan, E. V., Khesuani, Y. D., Kasyanov, V. A., Belousov, S. I., Krasheninnikov, S. V., Grigoriev, T. E., Chvalun, S. N., Bulanova, E. A., Mironov, V. A., & Domogatsky, S. P. (2019). Viscoll collagen solution as a novel bioink for direct 3D bioprinting. *J Mater Sci Mater Med, 30*(3), 31. https://doi.org/10.1007/s10856-019-6233-y

Peeters, P., Bosiers, M., Verbist, J., Deloose, K., & Heublein, B. (2005). Preliminary results after application of absorbable metal stents in patients with critical limb ischemia. *J Endovasc Ther, 12*(1), 1–5. https://doi.org/10.1583/04-1349r.1

Pokala, S., & Samatham, M. (2016). Future of manufacturing technology rapid prototyping technique. *IJMET*, *7*, 2016.

Praveen, S., & Kim, H. S. (2018). High-entropy alloys: Potential candidates for high-temperature applications – An overview. *Adv Eng Mater*, *20*(1), 1700645. https://doi.org/https://doi.org/10.1002/adem.201700645

Robles-Martinez, P., Xu, X., Trenfield, S. J., Awad, A., Goyanes, A., Telford, R., Basit, A. W., & Gaisford, S. (2019). 3D Printing of a multi-layered polypill containing six drugs using a novel stereolithographic method. *Pharmaceutics*, *11*(6). https://doi.org/10.3390/pharmaceutics11060274

Sadasivuni, K. K., Rattan, S., Deshmukh, K., Makhdoomi, A., Ahamed, B., Pasha, S. K., Mazumdar, P., Waseem, S., Grohens, Y., & Kumar, B. (2019). CHAPTER 12: Hybrid Nano-filler for Value Added Rubber Compounds for Recycling; pp. 310–329. https://doi.org/10.1039/9781788013482-00310

Sadia, M., Sośnicka, A., Arafat, B., Isreb, A., Ahmed, W., Kelarakis, A., & Alhnan, M. A. (2016). Adaptation of pharmaceutical excipients to FDM 3D printing for the fabrication of patient-tailored immediate release tablets. *Int J Pharm*, *513*(1–2), 659–668. https://doi.org/10.1016/j.ijpharm.2016.09.050

Saroia, J., Yanen, W., Wei, Q., Zhang, K., Lu, T., & Zhang, B. (2018). A review on biocompatibility nature of hydrogels with 3D printing techniques, tissue engineering application and its future prospective. *Bio-Design Manufactur*, *1*. https://doi.org/10.1007/s42242-018-0029-7

Schuurman, W., Levett, P. A., Pot, M. W., van Weeren, P. R., Dhert, W. J., Hutmacher, D. W., Melchels, F. P., Klein, T. J., & Malda, J. (2013). Gelatin-methacrylamide hydrogels as potential biomaterials for fabrication of tissue-engineered cartilage constructs. *Macromol Biosci*, *13*(5), 551–561. https://doi.org/10.1002/mabi.201200471

Sharma, A., Rawal, P., Tripathi, D. M., Alodiya, D., Sarin, S. K., Kaur, S., & Ghosh, S. (2021). Upgrading hepatic differentiation and functions on 3D printed silk-decellularized liver hybrid scaffolds. *ACS Biomater Sci Eng*, *7*(8), 3861–3873. https://doi.org/10.1021/acsbiomaterials.1c00671

Sharma, R., Smits, I. P. M., De La Vega, L., Lee, C., & Willerth, S. M. (2020). 3D Bioprinting pluripotent stem cell derived neural tissues using a novel fibrin bioink containing drug releasing microspheres [original research]. *Front Bioeng Biotechnol*, *8*. https://www.frontiersin.org/articles/10.3389/fbioe.2020.00057

Tagami, T., Fukushige, K., Ogawa, E., Hayashi, N., & Ozeki, T. (2017). 3D printing factors important for the fabrication of polyvinylalcohol filament-based tablets. *Biol Pharm Bull*, *40*(3), 357–364. https://doi.org/10.1248/bpb.b16-00878

Turner, P. R., Murray, E., McAdam, C. J., McConnell, M. A., & Cabral, J. D. (2020). Peptide chitosan/dextran core/shell vascularized 3D constructs for wound healing. *ACS Appl Mater Interfaces*, *12*(29), 32328–32339. https://doi.org/10.1021/acsami.0c07212

Uddin, M. S., Hall, C., & Murphy, P. (2015). Surface treatments for controlling corrosion rate of biodegradable Mg and Mg-based alloy implants. *Sci Technol Adv Mater*, *16*(5), 053501. https://doi.org/10.1088/1468-6996/16/5/053501

Ulery, B. D., Nair, L. S., & Laurencin, C. T. (2011). Biomedical applications of biodegradable polymers. *J Polym Sci B Polym Phys*, *49*(12), 832–864 [0887–6266 (Print)].

Wei, X., Li, D., Jiang, W., Gu, Z., Wang, X., Zhang, Z., & Sun, Z. (2015). 3D Printable graphene composite. *Sci Rep*, *5*(1), 11181. https://doi.org/10.1038/srep11181

Wong, K. (2012). K.V. Wong, A.Hernandez, "A Review of Additive Manufacturing," ISRN Mechanical Engineering, Vol 2012 (2012), Article ID 208760, 10 pages. *ISRN Mechanical Engineering*, *2012*. https://doi.org/10.5402/2012/208760

Xin, S., Chimene, D., Garza, J. E., Gaharwar, A. K., & Alge, D. L. (2019). Clickable PEG hydrogel microspheres as building blocks for 3D bioprinting [10.1039/C8BM01286E]. *Biomater Sci, 7*(3), 1179–1187. https://doi.org/10.1039/C8BM01286E

Yang, X., Lu, Z., Wu, H., Li, W., Zheng, L., & Zhao, J. (2018). Collagen-alginate as bioink for three-dimensional (3D) cell printing based cartilage tissue engineering. *Mater Sci Eng C Mater Biol Appl, 83*, 195–201. https://doi.org/10.1016/j.msec.2017.09.002

Zanini, N., Carneiro, E., Menezes, L., Barud, H., & Mulinari, D. (2021). Palm fibers residues from agro-industries as reinforcement in biopolymer filaments for 3D-printed scaffolds. *Fiber Polym, 22*. https://doi.org/10.1007/s12221-021-0936-7

Zhang, F., Li, S., Shen, Z., Cheng, X., Xue, Z., Zhang, H., Song, H., Bai, K., Yan, D., Wang, H., Zhang, Y., & Huang, Y. (2021). Rapidly deployable and morphable 3D mesostructures with applications in multimodal biomedical devices. *118*(11), e2026414118. https://doi.org/doi:10.1073/pnas.2026414118

Zhu, J., & Marchant, R. E. (2011). Design properties of hydrogel tissue-engineering scaffolds. *Expert Rev Med Devices, 8*(5), 607–626. https://doi.org/10.1586/erd.11.27

Section VII

Social, Economic, Environmental, Quality, and Regulatory Aspects

10 Social, Economic, and Environmental Justifications for 3D Printing of Pharmaceutical Products

*Himanshu Sharma, Siddhant Jai Tyagi,
Neha Pathak, Adarsh Keshari, Prakhar Varshney,
and Rashmi Pathak*

10.1 INTRODUCTION

Layers of material are deposited on top of one another during the three-dimensional (3D) printing process to produce 3D things from digital models. Prototyping, production, art, education, and medicine are a few examples of the uses of 3D printing. In comparison to conventional fabrication techniques, 3D printing has several benefits, including speed, flexibility, customizability, and less waste (Özeren *et al.*, 2023). The drawbacks of 3D printing include technical restrictions, moral dilemmas, and environmental effects. Future developments in the realm of 3D printing technology might have a profound impact on a wide range of sectors and businesses (Kapadia *et al.*, 2020). By building layers of materials on top of one another, 3D printing technology turns computer models into real objects (Rachmawati *et al.*, 2023). The production of customized medications based on each patient's dosage, shape, color, flavor, and release profile, as well as the development of innovative drug delivery systems like implants, patches, inhalers, and microneedles that can improve the efficacy and safety of currently available medications, are just a few of the many potential uses for 3D printing in the pharmaceutical industry (Ullah *et al.*, 2023). The pharmaceutical industry stands to benefit from 3D printing in several ways, including enhanced patient-centricity and personalized medicine, improved drug product quality and consistency, decreased risk of errors, contamination, and counterfeiting, increased innovation and creativity in drug design and discovery, and the ability to look into new directions and solutions (Chakka & Chede, 2023). Assuring the safety, quality, and efficacy of 3D-printed drugs requires stringent testing and validation methods and standards. Addressing the ethical, legal, and social implications of 3D printing, such as intellectual property rights, data privacy, patient consent, and access to healthcare, as well as overcoming technical and financial obstacles, are other challenges and limitations that 3D printing poses for the pharmaceutical industry (Parry, 2023). The pharmaceutical sector could change because of the revolutionary technology known as 3D printing. To ensure its safe and responsible usage, it also needs careful consideration and regulation. 3D printing is a technology that allows actual objects to be produced from digital models by building complex structures out of multiple layers of material (Priyadarshini *et al.*, 2023). 3D printing has been used by many businesses, including the pharmaceutical sector because it offers advantages like customization, personalization, and on-demand medicine production. Quality control, regulatory limitations, and ethical conundrums are just a few of the risks and challenges associated with 3D printing (Huanbutta *et al.*, 2023). As a result, it is critical to look at the social, economic, and environmental arguments for implementing 3D printing in the pharmaceutical industry in order to weigh its advantages and disadvantages and to determine the best procedures and regulations for its adoption (Eiamin & Herur Ramesh, 2023). Based on the potential to increase drug availability, cost, and access for various populations and requirements, 3D printing in the pharmaceutical industry is socially justified. Drug manufacturing at the point of care is made possible by 3D printing, which lessens the need for supply chains and distribution systems and improves the ability to respond quickly to crises and outbreaks (Desselle *et al.*, 2023). By employing recyclable or biodegradable materials and just manufacturing the necessary quantity of pharmaceuticals, 3D printing can help reduce the amount of waste produced by drug production and consumption. By minimizing the use of animal testing and substances produced from plants, 3D printing can also help conserve biodiversity and natural resources see Figure 10.1 (Kokare *et al.*, 2023).

To ensure that 3D printing is used responsibly and sustainably in the pharmaceutical industry, it is crucial to perform a thorough and impartial review of the grounds for adoption (Bazli *et al.*, 2023). 3D advantages and disadvantages of the various methods are shown in Table 10.1.

10.2   PRECISE DOSAGE AND FORMULATIONS

The ability to produce individualized dosages and formulations for specific patients thanks to 3D printing has the potential to revolutionize personalized medicine. The ability to develop patient-specific drugs thanks to this ground-breaking technology offers several advantages and advances in the medical industry (Chambers *et al.*, 2023). The following are a few of the most significant effects of 3D printing on personalized medicine, see Figure 10.2.

10.2.1   TAILORED MEDICATIONS FOR SPECIFIC CONDITIONS

Unique formulations that are not frequently found on the market are needed for some medical disorders. Using sustained-release mechanisms, alternative drug-delivery methods, or a combination of these to better meet a patient's individual needs, 3D

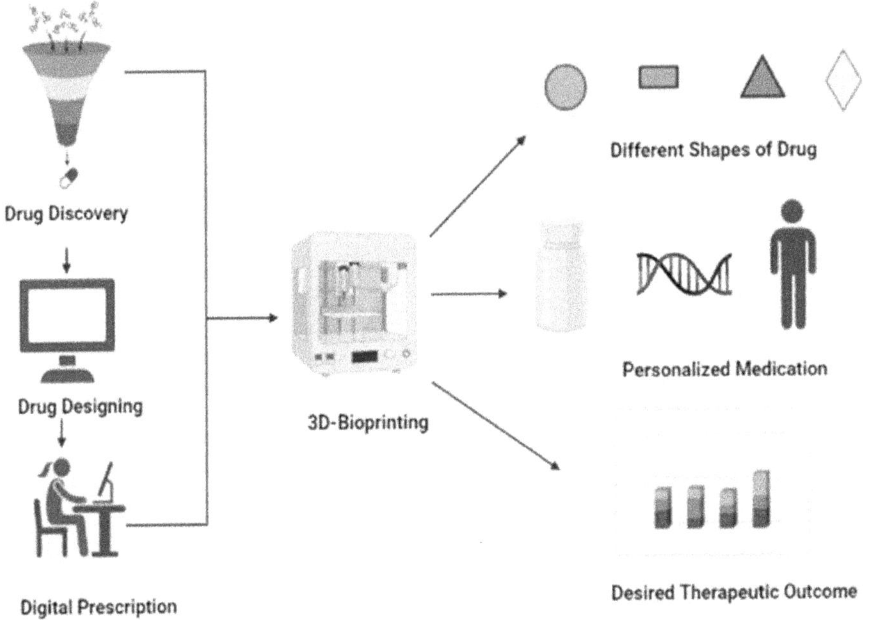

FIGURE 10.1   The process of 3D printing.

TABLE 10.1
Materials Used in Some 3D Printing Methods, Advantages, and Disadvantages of the Various Methods

Methods	Materials	Advantages	Disadvantages
Fused deposition modeling	ABS, PLA, Wax blend, Nylon	High speed, high quality, used for a wide range of material	The porous structure of the binder, and its weak mechanical properties, often required support
Stereolithography	Resin (Acrylate or Epoxy based with proprietary photoinitiator)	Large parts can be built easily, with high accuracy and surface finish	Expensive, not well-defined mechanical properties due to the usage of photopolymers
Selective laser sintering	Metallic powder, polyamide, PVC	High-resolution, high strength	Only metals can be printed, post-processing is required due to its grainy roughness
3D inkjet printing	Photo-resin or hydrogel	Very good accuracy, very high surface finishes	Fragile parts, poor mechanical the properties

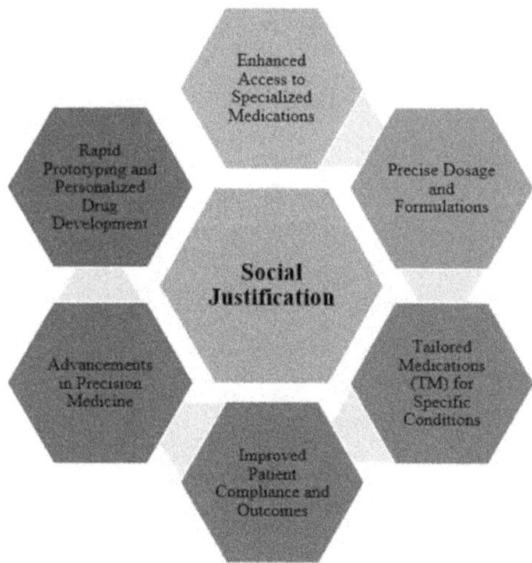

FIGURE 10.2   The role of 3D printing in social justification.

printing enables the development of customized pharmaceuticals. Patients with rare diseases or complex medical conditions particularly benefit from this personalized approach (Shi & McHugh, 2023).

10.2.2 POTENTIAL FOR PATIENT EMPOWERMENT AND ENGAGEMENT IN HEALTHCARE

A revolutionary component of 3D printing technology is its potential to empower and engage patients in healthcare by allowing them to participate in the design and fabrication of their prescription drugs. The usual patient–provider relationship is changed to a more collaborative and patient-centered method by including patients in the process. The following are the main ways that patients' empowerment and involvement might be improved by involving them in the design and manufacture of pharmaceuticals using 3D printing (Sharma *et al.*, 2023).

10.2.3 PERSONALIZATION TREATMENTS

Based on a person's specific medical requirements, 3D printing enables the production of customized pharmaceuticals. Patient input on preferences, tolerances and treatment objectives can be used to actively shape the creation of a patient's drug. As a result, treatment outcomes are better, and patients report feeling more satisfied with their care. This involvement guarantees that the drug is matched to their unique requirements (Handa *et al.*, 2023).

10.2.4 INFORMED DECISION-MAKING

Patients gain a better awareness of their treatment options when they are involved in the design and development of their medications. Patients can choose their healthcare more intelligently as a result of increased patient knowledge about the ingredients, potential adverse effects, and benefits of the prescription. Between patients and healthcare providers, this openness develops a relationship of trust and cooperation (Schroeder *et al.*, 2023).

10.3 ETHICAL CHALLENGES ASSOCIATED WITH THE 3D PRINTING OF PHARMACEUTICAL PRODUCTS

A cautious response is required to the ethical questions and potential difficulties that the 3D printing of medicinal items raises. Even though this cutting-edge technology has many advantages, some complications need to be addressed. Here are some of the main moral issues and difficulties posed by the 3D printing of medicinal products (Manshor *et al.*, 2023).

10.3.1 Quality Control

It is vitally important to guarantee the quality, safety, and efficacy of 3D-printed medicines. The 3D printing method presents difficulty in maintaining dependable and uniform manufacturing standards. For the materials utilized, the precision of the printing process, and the integrity of the finished product to be validated, quality-control methods must be implemented. To ensure that medicines produced by 3D printing adhere to the same high standards as those applied to pharmaceuticals produced traditionally, rigorous testing and regulatory control are required (Wang *et al.*, 2023).

10.3.2 Intellectual Property Issues

Concerns concerning intellectual property rights are raised by how simple it is to reproduce designs and make drugs using 3D printing. Patient safety could be jeopardized and innovation hampered by unauthorized drug reproduction or counterfeiting. It is critical to strike a balance between safeguarding intellectual property and promoting developments in 3D printing technology. In the case of 3D-printed drugs, it is crucial to create proper legal frameworks and enforcement procedures to protect IP rights (Signé, 2023).

10.3.3 Regulatory Frameworks

Drugs produced by 3D printing are subject to a changing regulatory environment. Because of the distinctive features of 3D printing, such as decentralized manufacturing and personalization, regulatory bodies must adjust and create standards that are particular to this technology. A vital component of the regulatory system is ensuring patient safety, quality control, and compliance with current laws. To create thorough and current laws, regulatory agencies must work in conjunction with pharmaceutical businesses and 3D printing industry professionals (Mladenovska *et al.*, 2023).

10.3.4 Accessibility and Equity

While 3D printing makes it easier to get prescription drugs, it is also important to address any accessibility and equality issues that might develop. Not all localities or areas have access to 3D printing facilities or the necessary materials. For disadvantaged groups to stop becoming further marginalized, it is essential to ensure an equitable distribution of 3D printing skills and related training. To prevent adding new obstacles to the accessibility of 3D-printed medicines, economic issues should also be carefully managed (Akinola & Telukdarie, 2023).

10.4 FACTORS IMPACTING THE COST-EFFECTIVENESS OF 3D PRINTING

Some conventional manufacturing processes, like the demand for intricate molds, tooling, and assembly lines, can be eliminated or greatly simplified by 3D printing. By streamlining production and lowering the need for labor and equipment, the number of manufacturing steps can be reduced and thus result in cost savings (Cabibihan *et al.*, 2023). Materials can be wasted far less since 3D printing enables precise and on-demand manufacturing. In contrast to conventional manufacturing techniques, which include subtractive operations (cutting, molding, etc.), 3D printing is an additive manufacturing approach in which materials are deposited layer by layer. With careful planning, waste can be reduced and money can be saved (Wu *et al.*, 2023). By using 3D printing to make customized pharmaceuticals, it is possible to improve patient outcomes and cut expenses associated with inefficient therapies. The effectiveness of a treatment can be increased by adjusting pharmaceutical dosages and prescriptions to the unique needs of each patient, which also lowers the risk of side effects and reduces the need for additional medications or treatments (Uchida & Bruschi, 2023). Traditional pharmaceutical supply chains typically entail several middlemen, shipping, and storage, all of which add to the cost inefficiencies. Pharmaceutical product production can be localized with 3D printing, allowing for on-site or near-to-the-point-of-care manufacturing of drugs. By decentralizing the supply chain, it can reduce its complexity and related expenses, such as those for inventory control and transportation (Uchida & Bruschi, 2023). Comparatively speaking, 3D printing provides more manufacturing flexibility and agility. Production schedules can be optimized, and manufacturers can more quickly adapt to changing demand and better serve the market. Due to a reduced chance of resource overproduction or under-utilization, this agility might result in cost savings (Salim & Sakhri, 2023).

10.5 COST-EFFECTIVENESS OF 3D PRINTING IN THE PHARMACEUTICAL INDUSTRY, CONSIDERING FACTORS LIKE DISTRIBUTION COSTS

The pharmaceutical business can use 3D printing to reduce costs in a variety of ways, including distribution expenses in addition to manufacturing costs. Several benefits that come with 3D printing technology can help reduce costs and increase effectiveness throughout the distribution stage. Let us examine whether 3D printing is economical for the distribution of medicines (Pattanshetti *et al.*,2018). The capacity to manufacture pharmaceuticals locally or more closely to the point of care is one of the major benefits of 3D printing. The requirement for long-distance transportation can be reduced or eliminated as a result of this localized production, which will also lower associated logistical challenges and transportation costs. Decentralized production is made possible by it, facilitating timely medication delivery in far-off places or in times of crisis and possibly lowering distribution costs (Arji *et al.*, 2023). Traditional pharmaceutical distribution frequently entails keeping sizable stockpiles at various points throughout the supply chain to guarantee product availability. With the use of 3D printing, large inventories of drugs can be generated on demand. By lowering the costs of maintaining inventory, such as handling, storage, and the possibility of product expiration, significant cost reductions can be realized (Kocsis *et al.*, 2023). Several intermediaries, such as wholesalers, distributors, and retailers, are a part of the complicated traditional pharmaceutical supply chain. Through the elimination of intermediaries, 3D printing can streamline the supply chain. By eliminating middlemen and their markups, the distribution process can be made more efficient by directly producing drugs at the point of service or through regional production facilities (Perano *et al.*, 2023). Due to the ability of 3D printing, additional packaging and labeling stages are not required when producing pharmaceuticals in their final dosage form. Drugs are frequently packaged and labeled several times before they are delivered to the consumer in the traditional pharmaceutical distribution model. Reduced costs for labor, equipment, and secondary packaging materials are possible by incorporating packaging and labeling into the 3D printing process (Sushir *et al.*, 2023). The adaptability of 3D printing technology allows for a quick reaction to shifts in demand and market dynamics. To lessen the chance of overstocking or understocking, pharmaceutical producers can instantly modify production levels and product offerings. Improved cost-effectiveness, improved distribution routes, and better inventory management are all made possible by this flexibility (Dakić, 2023).

10.6 BENEFITS OF LOCALIZED PRODUCTION, ALLOWING FOR THE CREATION OF SMALL-SCALE MANUFACTURING

The economic benefits of localized production in small-scale manufacturing hubs through 3D printing in the pharmaceutical industry are significant. This approach offers various advantages that can positively impact regional economies and foster sustainable development. Let us explore the economic benefits of localized production through small-scale manufacturing hubs (Nascimento *et al.*, 2019). Establishing small-scale manufacturing hubs for localized 3D printing production creates new employment opportunities. These hubs require skilled technicians, engineers, designers, and operators to manage the production process, quality control, and equipment maintenance. The growth of these local job markets contributes to economic development, reduces unemployment rates, and enhances the overall livelihood of the community (Sanicola *et al.*, 2020). Localized production hubs enable the development of local value chains, fostering economic interdependencies within the region. Supporting industries and services, such as raw material suppliers, equipment maintenance providers, logistics companies, and regulatory consultants, can emerge to support the functioning of the manufacturing hubs. This localization of value chains enhances regional economic resilience and reduces dependence on distant suppliers or intermediaries (Gallaud & Laperche, 2016). By producing medications locally, transportation costs can be significantly reduced. The conventional pharmaceutical manufacturing process involves a lot of long-distance transportation of parts, raw materials, and finished items. Regional manufacturing hubs save money on fuel, shipping, and associated infrastructure by reducing or eliminating the need for extensive transportation networks. The pharmaceutical industry they become more competitive and economically efficient as a result of these cost savings (Wyatt III, 2008). Localized manufacturing facilities increase economic resilience by reducing dependency on external pharmaceutical suppliers. In the event of emergencies, such as disease outbreaks, natural disasters, or disruptions to international supply chains, local manufacturing can offer a reliable supply of essential medications. This resilience maintains access to healthcare, mitigates the financial impact of disruptions, and fosters general economic stability in the area (Golan *et al.*, 2020). The establishment of small-scale manufacturing hubs encourages technology and knowledge transfer. Collaboration between local manufacturers, research institutions, and academic organizations can promote innovation, research, and development. The exchange of expertise and best practices leads to skill enhancement, knowledge creation, and the development of a skilled workforce. This, in turn, drives technological advancement and enhances the region's overall competitiveness in the pharmaceutical industry (Arthur-Holmes *et al.*, 2023).

Localized production hubs create opportunities for entrepreneurial ventures. Small businesses and startups can emerge to serve specific niche markets, develop innovative pharmaceutical products, or provide specialized services related to 3D printing. These entrepreneurial activities foster a dynamic business ecosystem, attract investments, and stimulate economic growth in the region (Audretsch *et al.*, 2023). Localized production hubs equipped with 3D printing technology have the potential to produce high-quality pharmaceutical products for domestic consumption and export. The ability to customize medications, produce rare or orphan drugs, and cater to niche markets can open up new export opportunities. This export potential enhances foreign exchange earnings, strengthens the balance of trade, and contributes to overall economic prosperity (Betz *et al.*, 2023). It is important to note that establishing small-scale manufacturing hubs for localized production requires supportive policies, infrastructure development, and investments in research and development. Additionally, addressing regulatory compliance and quality-control standards is essential to ensure the safety and efficacy of 3D-printed pharmaceutical products. However, with the right ecosystem and enabling environment, the economic benefits of localized production through small-scale manufacturing hubs can be substantial, fostering regional economic growth and sustainable development (Azizfan & Heamatzai, 2023).

10.7 IMPLICATIONS FOR INTELLECTUAL PROPERTY AND PATENT ISSUES

The rise of 3D printing in the pharmaceutical industry has significant implications for patent and intellectual property (IP) issues since it is upending long-standing business frameworks. The ability to digitally copy and create physical goods, including pharmaceutical treatments, offers a variety of challenges to the current framework of intellectual property protection. Let us now examine how patent and intellectual property issues are impacted by 3D printing (Stanko & Rindfleisch, 2023). Using 3D printing increases the likelihood of unlawful duplication and counterfeiting of pharmaceutical products protected by copyright. The ease with which 3D designs can be shared and copied online raises questions about the security of patented drugs. The ability of 3D printing technology to copy patented pharmaceuticals might lead to infringement of intellectual property rights, so jeopardizing the competitive advantage and financial prosperity of pharmaceutical companies (Simon, 2023). Since 3D printing is a distributed and decentralized technology, it could be challenging to identify infringement in this situation. Since 3D printing can happen anywhere, it is harder to find cases of IP infringement than with traditional manufacturing methods, which can be closely watched within restricted spaces. Because of this, it is very challenging to protect intellectual rights and stop unauthorized duplication (Roy & Dheeba, 2023). With the introduction of 3D printing, the laws and regulations pertaining to intellectual property need to be reviewed. The complexities of 3D printing technology and its implications for intellectual property protection could not be adequately covered by the current legal framework. Legislators and regulators have to consider adjusting intellectual property laws to take into account the unique challenges posed by 3D printing, striking a balance between encouraging innovation and defending the rights of patent holders (Rayna & West, 2023). Due to the disruptive nature of 3D printing, open-source projects and collaborative innovation are becoming more and more popular. A number of stakeholders encourage the sharing of 3D printable designs and technologies in order to foster innovation and maximize the benefits of 3D printing. This shift threatens traditional business models that rely on patent exclusivity and exclusive ownership of medicinal products (Rapitsenyane *et al.*, 2023). As 3D printing advances to adjust to the changing environment, new models for royalties and licencing could emerge. Pharmaceutical companies should consider licencing agreements that permit third parties to use their copyrighted designs for 3D printing, subject to specified limitations and fees. Employing this tactic might assist companies in realizing the potential of 3D printing while preserving the security of their intellectual property (Heim, 2023).

10.8 3D PRINTING IN PHARMACEUTICAL PRODUCTION COMPARED TO TRADITIONAL MANUFACTURING PROCESSES

Although 3D printing has the potential to ease some environmental pressures, it also brings with it new difficulties (Elbadawi *et al.*, 2023). Comparing 3D printing in pharmaceutical production to conventional manufacturing, the following analysis looks at the environmental impact see in Figure 10.3.

Mass manufacture of medications employing substantial raw material amounts is a common practice in traditional pharmaceutical manufacturing procedures. By contrast, additive manufacturing, which is more precise and resource-effective,

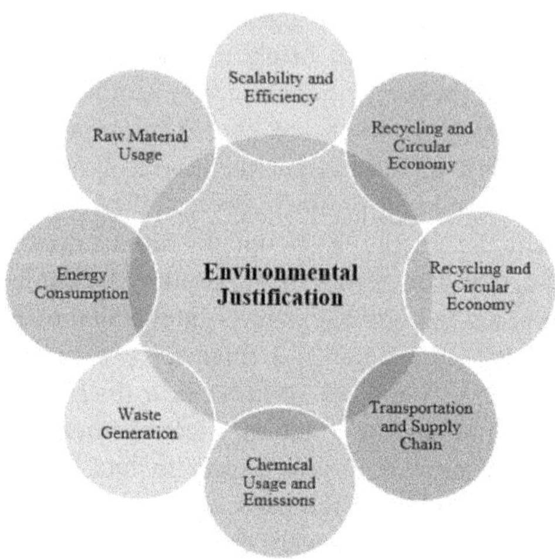

FIGURE 10.3   The role of 3D printing in environmental justification.

is used in 3D printing. By utilizing the necessary amount of material to produce the intended pharmaceutical output, 3D printing can minimize waste, potentially lowering the total environmental impact (Awad *et al.*, 2023). Traditional manufacturing methods typically use more energy than 3D printing. Traditional pharmaceutical production techniques frequently entail energy-intensive procedures including high-temperature reactions and substantial apparatus. In contrast, 3D printing often uses less energy, particularly in small-scale localized manufacturing settings, which could result in energy savings and lower greenhouse gas emissions (Xin *et al.*, 2023). Large amounts of waste, such as rejected goods, extra packaging, and unused raw materials, can be produced during traditional pharmaceutical manufacturing. It is possible that 3D printing is an alternative that is more environmentally friendly because of its exact material consumption, which can reduce waste formation. It is crucial to keep in mind, though, that waste produced by 3D printing might take several forms, depending on the particular 3D printing method being utilized, such as support materials and unsuccessful prints (Caldwell, 2023). Traditional pharmaceutical production employs dangerous chemicals and produces pollutants that could be bad for the environment and people's health. Depending on the materials used, 3D printing can also require the usage of chemicals and the discharge of emissions. As technology develops, attempts are being made to create more environmentally friendly materials and enhance 3D printing processes' emission controls (Kabir *et al.*, 2023). Using 3D printing versus conventional pharmaceutical manufacture can affect how the environment is affected by transportation and supply chain logistics. Transportation of completed goods and raw materials over vast distances can be necessary for traditional manufacturing, which adds to air pollution and carbon emissions. The ability for localized production, on the other hand, is a benefit of 3D printing that lessens the environmental effects of connected long-distance transportation (Besklubova *et al.*, 2023).

10.9 LOCALIZED PRODUCTION AND REDUCED TRANSPORTATION NEEDS

The potential reduction in carbon emissions resulting from localized production and reduced transportation needs is a significant advantage of 3D printing in the pharmaceutical industry. By shifting from centralized mass production to localized production hubs, 3D printing can contribute to lowering carbon emissions in the following ways (Bayram & Çetiner, 2023). Traditional pharmaceutical manufacturing often involves long-distance transportation of raw materials, intermediates, and finished products. This transportation contributes to carbon emissions from vehicles, such as trucks, ships, or planes. With localized production enabled by 3D printing, the need for long-distance transportation is reduced. Raw materials can be sourced locally, and medications can be produced closer to the point of consumption, minimizing transportation distances and associated carbon emissions (Sales & Scholte, 2023). Large-scale pharmaceutical manufacturing typically relies on complex, multi-tiered supply chains that include a large number of vendors, distributors, and intermediaries. Every step in the supply chain requires transportation, which raises carbon emissions. The integration of 3D printing technology with locally produced goods facilitates the optimization and streamlining of the supply chain. Large-scale supply chains and transportation networks are no longer necessary since pharmaceuticals can be produced at or near the site of treatment, which reduces the associated carbon emissions (Abdallah & Nizamuddin, 2023). Energy-intensive processes, large amounts of equipment, and infrastructure can be required for conventional pharmaceutical production methods. However, 3D printing could use less energy, especially in situations where manufacturing is localized. 3D printers consume less energy than traditional production equipment, which can help reduce carbon emissions associated with energy consumption (Tavares *et al.*, 2023).

Large-scale medication production is a frequent practise in conventional manufacturing to achieve economies of scale. This might lead to overproduction, which would increase waste, surplus inventories, and carbon emissions throughout the whole supply chain. 3D printing enables on-demand production, allowing for the optimization of production numbers (Roberts *et al.*, 2023). Medication made on demand, which reduces the possibility of overproduction and the carbon emissions that come from wasted resources (Onyeaka *et al.*, 2023). In localized production, 3D printing might help cut down on packaging waste. Traditionally, pharmaceutical products are packed for long-distance delivery and distribution. As a result, boxes, bubble wrap, and plastic containers are often utilized excessively for packing purposes. By producing medication closer to the point of use, it is possible to reduce the need for large, bulky packaging as well as the carbon emissions associated with the production and disposal of packaging materials (Kazemi *et al.*, 2023). In the pharmaceutical industry, there is a growing interest in and investigation of the sustainability of 3D printing. Reduced waste production and the use of recyclable or biodegradable materials are two strategies to enhance sustainability with 3D printing. Below is a study of these sustainability aspects (Guggenbiller *et al.*, 2023). As environmental concerns gain traction, there is a growing demand for sustainable products and practices. Consumer demand can drive companies to prioritize eco-friendly initiatives, including the

TABLE 10.2
The Use of 3D Printing in the Social, Economic, and Environmental Spheres can be Communicated Aesthetically

Aspect	Social	Economic	Environmental	Aesthetic Communication
Social impact	Enhancing individual lives	Growing the 3D printing industry	Reducing waste and emissions	Visuals of people benefiting from personalized 3D-printed prosthetics
Economic impact	Affordable prototyping	Economical production processes	Recycling materials	Charts illustrating cost savings through 3D printing
Environmental impact	Eco-friendly filaments	Minimizing material waste	Reducing energy consumption	Illustrations with eco-friendly color palettes and nature motifs

Source: Abdur Rahman *et al*. (2023).

adoption of environmentally friendly materials in 3D printing (Pishro, 2023). In conclusion, while challenges exist in implementing environmentally friendly practices in 3D printing, the industry has opportunities to innovate and drive sustainability. By investing in material research, collaborating with various stakeholders, integrating circular economy principles, and raising awareness, the 3D printing sector can move toward more eco-friendly and responsible practices for a more sustainable future see Table 10.2 (Abdur Rahman *et al.*, 2023).

10.10 CONCLUSION

The adoption of 3D printing in the pharmaceutical business has strong social, economic, and environmental arguments. In terms of society, personalized medicine is made possible by 3D printing, allowing for specially formulated medications and dosages that are suited to each patient. This encourages better participation and adherence to pharmaceutical regimens while empowering patients by involving them in their healthcare. To help them feel more in control of and accountable for their health outcomes, patients can also contribute to the development of their medications. 3D printing offers affordable solutions in terms of the economy.

ACKNOWLEDGEMENTS

The authors are thankful to the Principal, Department of Pharmacy, Teerthanker Mahaveer University, Moradabad for providing the necessary facilities.

REFERENCES

Abdallah, S., & Nizamuddin, N. (2023). Blockchain-based solution for pharma supply chain industry. *Computers & Industrial Engineering, 177*, 108997.

Abdur Rahman, M., Haque, S., Athikesavan, M. M., & Kamaludeen, M. B. (2023). A review of environmental friendly green composites: Production methods, current progresses, and challenges. *Environmental Science and Pollution Research, 30*(7), 16905–16929.

Akinola, S., & Telukdarie, A. (2023). Sustainable digital transformation in healthcare: Advancing a digital vascular health innovation solution. *Sustainability, 15*(13), 10417.

Arji, G., Ahmadi, H., Avazpoor, P., & Hemmat, M. (2023). Identifying resilience strategies for disruption management in the healthcare supply chain during COVID-19 by digital innovations: A systematic literature review. *Informatics in Medicine Unlocked*, 101199.

Arthur-Holmes, F., Yeboah, T., Cobbinah, I. J., & Busia, K. A. (2023). Youth in artisanal and small-scale mining (ASM) and higher education nexus: Diffusion of innovations and knowledge transfer. *Futures*, 103201.

Audretsch, D. B., Lehmann, E. E., Otto, J. M., Weiße, L., & Wirsching, K. (2023). The strategic management of places: Applying a framework to analyze local economies. In *The Strategic Management of Place at Work: Why, What, How and Where* (pp. 1–36). Springer.

Awad, A., Goyanes, A., Basit, A. W., Zidan, A. S., Xu, C., Li, W., Narayan, R. J., & Chen, R. K. (2023). A review of state-of-the-art on enabling additive manufacturing processes for precision medicine. *Journal of Manufacturing Science and Engineering, 145*(1), 10802.

Azizfan, S. M. S., & Heamatzai, M. N. (2023). A blueprint for sustainable poverty alleviation and unemployment mitigation: Synthesizing socioeconomic transformation in Afghanistan. *Available at SSRN* https://ssrn.com/abstract=4466714 or http://dx.doi.org/10.2139/ssrn.4466714.

Bayram, G., & Çetiner, B. G. (2023). The disruptive nature of 3D printing technology on mass customization and supply chain in the context of environment and economy. *International Journal of Advances in Engineering and Pure Sciences, 35*(1), 54–65.

Bazli, M., Ashrafi, H., Rajabipour, A., & Kutay, C. (2023). 3D printing for remote housing: Benefits and challenges. *Automation in Construction, 148*, 104772.

Besklubova, S., Tan, B. Q., Zhong, R. Y., & Spicek, N. (2023). Logistic cost analysis for 3D printing construction projects using a multi-stage network-based approach. *Automation in Construction, 151*, 104863.

Betz, U. A. K., Arora, L., Assal, R. A., Azevedo, H., Baldwin, J., Becker, M. S., Bostock, S., Cheng, V., Egle, T., & Ferrari, N. (2023). Game changers in science and technology-now and beyond. *Technological Forecasting and Social Change, 193*, 122588.

Cabibihan, J.-J., Gaballa, A., Fadli, F., Irshidat, M., Mahdi, E., Biloria, N., Mansour, Z., & Abdulrazak, H. (2023). A guided approach for utilizing concrete robotic 3D printing for the architecture, engineering, and construction industry. *Construction Robotics, 7*, 265–278.

Caldwell, D. G. (2023). Automation in food manufacturing and processing. In *Springer Handbook of Automation* (pp. 949–971). Springer.

Chakka, L. R. J., & Chede, S. (2023). 3D printing of pharmaceuticals for disease treatment. *Frontiers in Medical Technology, 4*, 1040052.

Chambers, B. E., Weaver, N. E., & Wingert, R. A. (2023). The "3Ds" of growing kidney organoids: Advances in nephron development, disease modeling, and drug screening. *Cells, 12*(4), 549.

Dakić, M. (2023). Technology use cases. In *Mobile App Development for Businesses: Create a Product Roadmap and Digitize Your Operations* (pp. 295–376). Springer.

Desselle, M. R., Wagels, M., Chamorro-Koc, M., & Caldwell, G. A. (2023). How is point-of-care 3D printing influencing medical device innovation? A survey on an Australian public healthcare precinct. *Journal of 3D Printing in Medicine, 7*(1), 3DP005.

Eiamin, M. A., & Herur Ramesh, S. J. (2023). *3D Printing-Process Optimization for Biocomposites*.

Elbadawi, M., Basit, A. W., & Gaisford, S. (2023). Energy consumption and carbon footprint of 3D printing in pharmaceutical manufacture. *International Journal of Pharmaceutics, 639*, 122926.

Gallaud, D., & Laperche, B. (2016). *Circular Economy, Industrial Ecology and Short Supply Chain* (Vol. 4). John Wiley & Sons.

Golan, M. S., Jernegan, L. H., & Linkov, I. (2020). Trends and applications of resilience analytics in supply chain modeling: Systematic literature review in the context of the COVID-19 pandemic. *Environment Systems and Decisions, 40*(2), 222–243.

Guggenbiller, G., Brooks, S., King, O., Constant, E., Merckle, D., & Weems, A. C. (2023). 3D Printing of green and renewable polymeric materials: Toward greener additive manufacturing. *ACS Applied Polymer Materials, 5*(5), 3201–3229.

Handa, M., Afzal, O., Beg, S., SanapNasik, S., Kaundal, R. K., Verma, R. K., & Shukla, R. (2023). Harnessing personalized tailored medicines to digital-based data-enriched edible pharmaceuticals. *Drug Discovery Today*, 103555.

Heim, I. (2023). *Intellectual Property Management: Interdisciplinary Knowledge for Business Decision-Making*. Springer Nature.

Huanbutta, K., Burapapadh, K., Sriamornsak, P., & Sangnim, T. (2023). Practical application of 3D printing for pharmaceuticals in hospitals and pharmacies. *Pharmaceutics, 15*(7), 1877.

Kabir, Z., Emon, S. Z., & Karim, S. M. A. (2023). Green pharmaceutical production and its benefits for sustainability. In *Microbiology for Cleaner Production and Environmental Sustainability* (pp. 115–140). CRC Press.

Kapadia, S., Kanase, V., Kadam, S., Gupta, P., & Yadav, V. (2020). Chronopharmacology: The biological clock. *International Journal of Pharmaceutical Sciences and Research, 11*(5), 2018–2026. https://doi.org/10.13040/IJPSR.0975-8232.11(5).2018-26

Kazemi, Z., Rask, J. K., Gomes, C., Yildiz, E., & Larsen, P. G. (2023). Movable factory – A systematic literature review of concepts, requirements, applications, and gaps. *Journal of Manufacturing Systems, 69*, 189–207.

Kocsis, S. W., Dialynas, C., & Perkins, R. (2023). *Envisioning the Future of the Pharmaceutical Supply Chain to Advance Public Health in the United States*. Milken Institute, Center for Public Health.

Kokare, S., Oliveira, J. P., & Godina, R. (2023). Life cycle assessment of additive manufacturing processes: A review. *Journal of Manufacturing Systems, 68*, 536–559.

Manshor, M. R., Alli, Y. A., Anuar, H., Ejeromedoghene, O., Omotola, E. O., & Suhr, J. (2023). 4D Printing: Historical evolution, computational insights and emerging applications. *Materials Science and Engineering: B, 295*, 116567.

Mladenovska, T., Choong, P. F., Wallace, G. G., & O'Connell, C. D. (2023). The regulatory challenge of 3D bioprinting. *Regenerative Medicine, 18*.

Nascimento, D. L. M., Alencastro, V., Quelhas, O. L. G., Caiado, R. G. G., Garza-Reyes, J. A., Rocha-Lona, L., & Tortorella, G. (2019). Exploring Industry 4.0 technologies to enable circular economy practices in a manufacturing context: A business model proposal. *Journal of Manufacturing Technology Management, 30*(3), 607–627.

Onyeaka, H., Tamasiga, P., Nwauzoma, U. M., Miri, T., Juliet, U. C., Nwaiwu, O., & Akinsemolu, A. A. (2023). Using artificial intelligence to tackle food waste and enhance the circular economy: Maximising resource efficiency and minimising environmental impact: A review. *Sustainability, 15*(13), 10482.

Özeren, Ö., Özeren, E. B., Top, S. M., & Qurraie, B. S. (2023). Learning-by-doing using 3D printers: Digital fabrication studio experience in architectural education. *Journal of Engineering Research*, 100135.

Parry, E. J. (2023). *A Study Assessing the Viability of Using Fused Filament Fabrication (FFF) Additive Manufacturing (AM) Technology to Manufacture Customised Class I Medical Devices*. Manchester Metropolitan University.

Pattanshetti, S. S., Babar, V., & Patil, B. (2018). *3D Printing Methods for Pharmaceutical Manufacturing: Opportunities and Challenges*. Curr Pharm Des. 24(42):4949–4956. doi: 10.2174/1381612825666181206121701. PMID: 30520367.

Perano, M., Cammarano, A., Varriale, V., Del Regno, C., Michelino, F., & Caputo, M. (2023). Embracing supply chain digitalization and unphysicalization to enhance supply chain performance: A conceptual framework. *International Journal of Physical Distribution & Logistics Management*.

Pishro, A. (2023). *Experimental Research on 3D Printing Recycled Polymer/Aluminum Fraction of Beverage Cartons by Fused Granular Fabrication Method*. Thesis.

Priyadarshini, J., Singh, R. K., Mishra, R., & Dora, M. (2023). Application of additive manufacturing for a sustainable healthcare sector: Mapping current research and establishing future research agenda. *Technological Forecasting and Social Change, 194*, 122686.

Rachmawati, S. M., Putra, M. A. P., Lee, J. M., & Kim, D. S. (2023). Digital twin-enabled 3D printer fault detection for smart additive manufacturing. *Engineering Applications of Artificial Intelligence, 124*, 106430.

Rapitsenyane, Y., Erick, P., Sealetsa, O. J., & Moalosi, R. (2023). The impact of organizational ergonomics on teaching rapid prototyping. In *Intelligent Manufacturing Management Systems: Operational Applications of Evolutionary Digital Technologies in Mechanical and Industrial Engineering* (pp. 319–348). Wiley.

Rayna, T., & West, J. (2023). Where digital meets physical innovation: Reverse salients and the unrealized dreams of 3D printing. *Journal of Product Innovation Management*.

Roberts, H., Milios, L., Mont, O., & Dalhammar, C. (2023). Product destruction: Exploring unsustainable production-consumption systems and appropriate policy responses. *Sustainable Production and Consumption, 35*, 300–312.

Roy, R., & Dheeba, J. (2023). Survey on methodological model of IoT in digital forensic. *2023 International Conference on Intelligent Systems, Advanced Computing and Communication (ISACC)*, pp. 1–6.

Sales, M., & Scholte, S. (2023). *Air Cargo Management: Air Freight and the Global Supply Chain*. Taylor & Francis.

Salim, M., & Sakhri, A. (2023). Revolutionizing supply chain management: Emerging trends and strategies for the future. *Available at SSRN* https://ssrn.com/abstract=4379343 or http://dx.doi.org/10.2139/ssrn.4379343.

Sanicola, H. W., Stewart, C. E., Mueller, M., Ahmadi, F., Wang, D., Powell, S. K., Sarkar, K., Cutbush, K., Woodruff, M. A., & Brafman, D. A. (2020). Guidelines for establishing a 3-D printing biofabrication laboratory. *Biotechnology Advances, 45*, 107652.

Schroeder, T., Seaman, K., Nguyen, A., Gewald, H., & Georgiou, A. (2023). Enablers and inhibitors to the adoption of mHealth apps by patients – A qualitative analysis of German doctors' perspectives. *Patient Education and Counseling*, 107865.

Sharma, D., Patel, P., & Shah, M. (2023). A comprehensive study on Industry 4.0 in the pharmaceutical industry for sustainable development. *Environmental Science and Pollution Research*, 1–11.

Shi, M., & McHugh, K. J. (2023). Strategies for overcoming protein and peptide instability in biodegradable drug delivery systems. *Advanced Drug Delivery Reviews*, 114904.

Signé, L. (2023). *Africa's Fourth Industrial Revolution*. Cambridge University Press.

Simon, C. T. (2023). *Alternative Resources for Theatre: 3D Printing, Woolen Felt and Gelatin Adapted to Produce the Kiss of Blood: Developing Alternate Techniques to Implement Renewable, Biodegradable, and Local Resources to Decrease the Carbon Footprint.* University of Lethbridge.

Stanko, M. A., & Rindfleisch, A. (2023). Digital manufacturing and innovation. *Journal of Product Innovation Management*, 40(4), 407–432. Wiley Online Library.

Sushir, C., Kilor, V., & Rewatkar, A. (2023). Pediatric drug development process: A review. *Asian Journal of Pediatric Research*, 12(2), 23–34.

Tavares, T. M., Ganga, G. M. D., Godinho Filho, M., & Rodrigues, V. P. (2023). The benefits and barriers of additive manufacturing for circular economy: A framework proposal. *Sustainable Production and Consumption*, *37*, 369–388.

Uchida, D. T., & Bruschi, M. L. (2023). 3D Printing as a technological strategy for the personalized treatment of wound healing. *AAPS PharmSciTech*, 24(1), 41.

Ullah, M., Wahab, A., Khan, S. U., Naeem, M., ur Rehman, K., Ali, H., Ullah, A., Khan, A., Khan, N. R., & Rizg, W. Y. (2023). 3D Printing technology: A new approach for the fabrication of personalized and customized pharmaceuticals. *European Polymer Journal*, 112240.

Wang, Y.-C., Chen, T.-C. T., & Lin, Y.-C. (2023). 3D Printer selection for aircraft component manufacturing using a nonlinear FGM and dependency-considered fuzzy VIKOR approach. *Aerospace*, 10(7), 591.

Wu, S., Zeng, J., Li, H., Han, C., Wu, W., Zeng, W., & Tang, L. (2023). A review on the full chain application of 3D printing technology in precision medicine. *Processes*, *11*(6), 1736.

Wyatt III, L. T. (2008). *The Industrial Revolution*. ABC-CLIO.

Xin, C., Li, Z., Hao, L., & Li, Y. (2023). A comprehensive review on additive manufacturing of glass: Recent progress and future outlook. *Materials & Design*, 111736.

11 Quality Control Methods for Three-Dimensional Printed Pharmaceuticals

*Tulja Rani Gampa, Prakash Katakam,
Shanta Kumari Adiki, Nagarajan Sriram, and
Sowmyaranjan Satapathy*

11.1 INTRODUCTION

Clinical pharmacy practice and the pharmaceutical industry are undergoing an ideological shift due to three-dimensional printing (3DP), which is moving away from conventional mass production towards customized therapeutic products. Since the concept allows the on-demand design and manufacture of customizable formulations with adjustable doses, sizes, drug release, and multi-drug combinations, it may benefit patients, pharmacists, and the pharmaceutical industry. Regardless of the technology employed or the number of finished products, quality control (QC) is one of the most essential aspects in the manufacturing process. Recent research has demonstrated the applications of process analytical technologies (PAT) and non-destructive technique (NDT) as an alternative method for conventional end-product testing to evaluate 3DP products (Jorgensen *et al.*, 2023). Similar to conventional dosage forms, 3DP solid oral dose forms (SODF) that are produced in excess can be analyzed using conventional techniques, and finally, the results obtained are compared with the specifications outlined in *Pharmacopoeia* (Brambilla *et al.*, 2021). On the other hand, small-scale, on-demand pharmaceutical 3DP for tailored dosage forms does not have extra finished products or time to conduct quality-control testing by traditional methods, which are intrinsically destructive and time-consuming nature. In situations where NDTs are unavailable or unsuitable, an excessive number of products may be manufactured, in which case destructive QC methods may be applied to the products produced in excess (Okafor-Muo *et al.*, 2020).

11.1.1 IMPORTANCE OF QC IN 3DP PHARMACEUTICALS

The most important topic to consider is how to control the quality of 3DP medication forms. QC includes not only inspecting the finished product but also assessing each stage of the production process, from the receiving of raw materials and testing to the packaging and documentation of the finished product. Continuous improvement helps to achieve higher levels of customer satisfaction, competitiveness, and innovation

DOI: 10.1201/9781003439509-18

with 3DP. This includes validation of the printing equipment and technical processes, quality of materials used, control of critical processes, checking the prepared process data, carrying out visual product control, as well as online monitoring of the accuracy of dimension and shape (Parhi, 2021). Enhancing 3DP quality is essential because poor-quality products may discourage buyers from purchasing them. In addition to chemical tests, microbial tests must be done to check for contamination, which is the key element for any pharmaceutical product.

11.2 FUNDAMENTALS OF QC IN 3DP

The different stages of the 3DP technical process must be carefully verified to ensure consistency, accuracy, and reproducibility of the 3D CAD models. The classic QC process, which includes specific pharmacopoeial tests like content uniformity, homogeneity of mass, hardness, friability, and dissolution, are used to assess conventional solid oral dosage forms. Non-destructive PAT is an alternative approach to the conventional end-product QC process that supports the application of point-of-care manufacturing (Deidda *et al.*, 2019).

11.2.1 Key Parameters Influencing Pharmaceutical 3DP

The primary factors that impact the quality of 3D products depend on the 3DP method used for printouts, for instance, the FDM method, which is an ideal option for small-volume fabrication, has several challenges to overcome, such as the material used, operation, and different specific parameters. The material-specific parameters are related to the physicochemical qualities of the filament, such as its mechanical, thermal, and rheological properties. The physical characteristics of 3D tablets depend on several printing factors, in addition to excipients. Operation-specific factors include the printing processing requirements, such as infill density and printing temperature, which impact the final product quality, the drug-release profile, and the product design. Finally, printer equipment is a machine-specific parameter; improving the equipment's performance and the printing process.

11.2.2 Role of Material Properties in QC

The physical properties and drug-release profiles of 3DP prints depend on the type of materials and technique used for production. Different printing techniques require distinct physicochemical qualities of the excipient and active pharmaceutical ingredient (API). To ensure the quality of 3DP products, the first step is to characterize the printing material. The raw materials used in 3DP such as powders, resins, or filaments have a significant effect on the product quality. In order to find out whether the ingredient is suitable for use in pharmaceutical applications, it is essential to examine its mechanical, chemical, and physical qualities. Melting point analysis and mechanical testing to gauge the material's flexibility and strength are two possible tests. The chemical composition and physical properties of the compound are studied employing tools like Fourier transform infrared spectroscopy (FTIR) and inductively coupled plasma optical emission spectrometry (ICP-OES) (Castro-Sastre *et al.*, 2018). The thermal characteristics of the material are examined utilizing differential scanning calorimetry (DSC) and the structure of the crystal is examined by x-ray diffraction (XRD). The selection of raw materials for 3DP is akin to other pharmaceutical manufacturing processes, where chemicals listed as generally recognized as safe (GRAS) or inactive ingredient database (IID) must be chosen. The chosen material should not generate any hazardous substances either during or after the production process. Additionally, it must be compatible for the API, biodegradable, and suitable for fabrication of 3DP formulations.

11.2.3 Design Considerations for Ensuring Quality in 3DP Pharmaceuticals

The traditional end products are analyzed using chromatographic and spectroscopic methods specified in the official pharmacopoeia, also known as quality by testing (QBT), which are labor-intensive, time-consuming, and destructive methods, whereas x-ray powder diffraction (XRPD) is an NDT (Beccaria and Cabooter, 2020). The pharmaceutical industry is constantly searching for new methods to ensure and enhance the efficacy, quality, and safety of the products. Implementing the new QC techniques for 3DP is challenging due to hardware, software, and regulatory issues. The International Council for Harmonization (Yu *et al.*, 2014) has released general guidelines on pharmaceutical manufacturing that present a systematic approach called quality by design (QbD), which has grown significantly over the last ten years. It was initially designed for manufacturing operations and then applied to analytical chemistry due to its advantages. Even the regulatory organizations place greater emphasis on the implementation of QbD, a science-based approach that enhances process knowledge by reducing process variance and permitting process control measures (Gandhi and Roy 2016) and also focuses on its importance to comprehend the relationship between materials and processes to attain the required level of quality. Critical quality attributes (CQAs) are determined by applying QbD to every unit operation in the process stream (Grangeia *et al.*, 2020). These CQAs are then considered as functions of the critical material attributes (CMAs) and critical process parameters (CPPs). A monograph of every pharmaceutical product is included in *Pharmacopoeia/National Formularies*, which contains its CQA, CPP, and standards for evaluation of finished-product. However, every 3DP product is distinct; it is impractical to establish a monograph for each one of them. Hence, a chapter in *Pharmacopoeia* that is solely dedicated to 3DP may be added that provides general CQAs for every product type in addition to technology-specific CPPs for each 3DP technology.

11.3 NON-DESTRUCTIVE TESTING (NDT) METHODS

PAT and NDT's have gained significant attention in recent years and applied to continuously monitor and assess the specified CQAs and CPPs, thus offering control over the entire production process (Pauli *et al.*, 2019). Non-destructive QC methods must be applied to fully utilize the conceivable benefits of this cutting-edge technology (Dimitrov, 2006). In order to have control over the ongoing 3DP process, the Food and Drug Administration (FDA) introduced PAT in 2004 and also specified the use of simultaneous data analysis tools in conjunction with at-line, in-line, or on-line

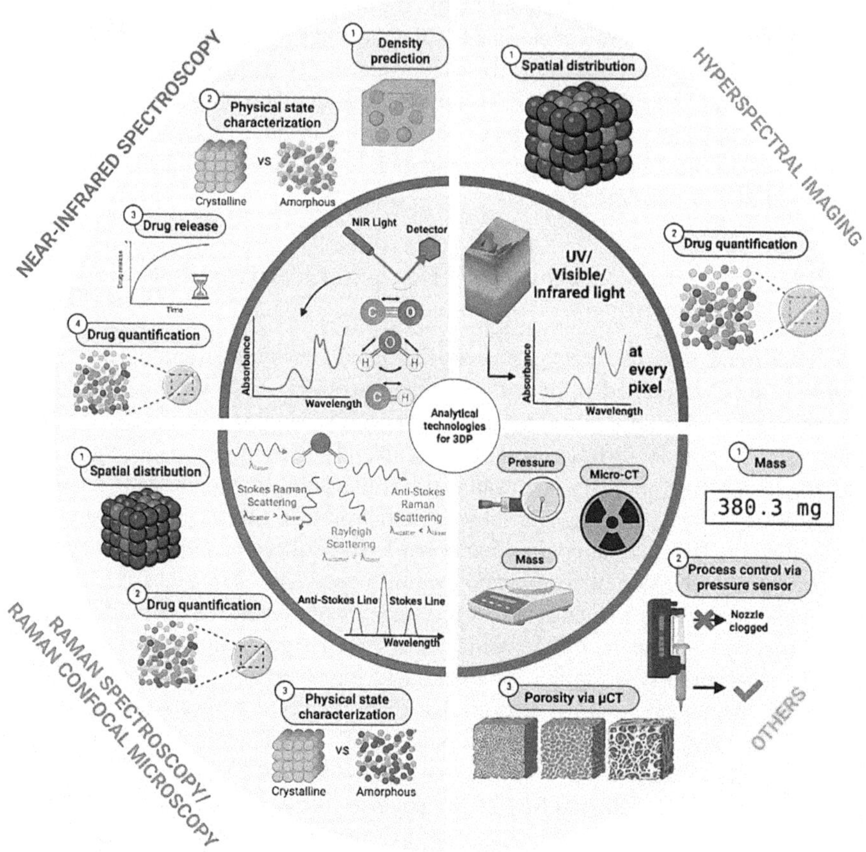

FIGURE 11.1 Various ND methods applied to 3D pharmaceutical product analysis. (Jorgensen, *et al.*, 2023.)

application of non-destructive testing procedures (Edinger *et al.*, 2018). PAT is useful for identifying flaws in 3DP models during the printing process and helps us to identify at which stage the 3DP method has failed. Several NDTs, such as computer vision, laser line Scanner Visual Testing (VT), computer vision, radiographic testing (RT), thermography, electromagnetic testing (ET) (Sheppard, 2020), infrared thermography, and shearography testing, have been used both during and after the process. NDTs and combinations of these techniques with hyperspectral imaging techniques (HSI) are commonly employed to assess individual components in the sample matrix are shown in Figure 11.1.

11.3.1 Visual Inspection and Microscopy Techniques

Visual inspection, the most basic type of NDT, is extensively employed since it can completely eliminate the need for extra testing, saving both money and time. Even though there are some intrinsic disadvantages to this method, visual examination is commonly employed due to its advantages, like its speed, low cost, and lack of equipment requirements. Online monitoring of the production process also helps in anticipating how the operation is performed and identifying any faults in advance. Damage to the model is typically regarded as non-compliant if it is obvious to the "naked eye", and the printing process is stopped and restarted after the errors are examined and rectified. Microscopic examination can be done to verify defects such as voids and inclusions. High-resolution optical technologies, which are non-destructive and low-cost, are used for monitoring 3D operations (Nuchitprasitchai *et al.*, 2017). Optical microscopy is beneficial for a rapid visual assessment, even though it is restricted to surface inspection. Measurement tools, gauges, manual and automatic scanners, tomography, or coordinate computing techniques are used for additional quality-control tests when no evidence of defect is found.

11.3.2 X-ray and CT Scanning for Internal Structure Analysis

NDT techniques are used to identify interior and exterior defects in a product's structure without destroying the individual components (Gholizadeh, 2016). X-ray computed tomography (x-ray CT) is a non-destructive 3D imaging approach that can be applied to view the internal and external geometry of 3D goods saving experimental costs associated with destructive procedures. When it comes to product development and troubleshooting, x-ray CT images (Withers *et al.*, 2021; Khosravani and Reinicke 2020) can provide insights into the potential basic causes of pharmaceutical products' stagnation. It can be used for imaging degradation, analyzing coating thickness, delamination, examining tablet cracks and voids, analyzing aggregates, and analyzing crystalline and amorphous phases. This method is specifically used to determine the density, shape, size, and spatial placement of the interior pores in three dimensions. The mechanical and, ultimately, elastic properties of the 3DP material can be anticipated as a function of porosity, which is related to the microscopic features of the pores determined by x-ray CT.

11.3.3 Ultrasound and Acoustic Methods for Defect Detection

Even 3DP encounters the risk of internal problems such as print errors, residual tension accumulation, or hostile cyber-attacks. One of the most important aspects of the final print evaluation is defect detection, which is crucial for product control in the 3DP sector. Powerful and valuable methods like ultrasonic and acousto-ultrasonic are specifically used in the detection of damage and defects in 3DP products, to ascertain the level of internal defects and in homogeneity in the composite materials and also gives information about the root cause of the failure. The meticulous removal of subpar units with internal flaws such as delamination gaps, cracks, or air bubble entrapment is crucial to achieve reliable manufacturing processes and to reduce the cost of the process.

11.4 PHYSICAL AND MECHANICAL TESTING

In order to ensure that the finished product complies with all standards, mechanical strength, and durability, dissolution tests of the final product must be carried out. The mechanical characteristics of 3DP products are altered by a number of factors, such as 3DP technology, the type of material employed, infill percentage, printing orientation, layer height, cross-sectional area, and the geometric accuracy of the physically produced model. In-fill density should be chosen carefully since it has a significant influence on the weight of the prints, mechanical strength, and drug release (Thakkar *et al.*, 2020). The fill percentage range on 3D printers is set to 0 to 100; 0% produces a hollow print, and 100% produces a fully solid print. Even the temperature variations throughout the FDM process were measured using an extended-range infrared camera (Dinwiddie *et al.*, 2013) and observed its impact on the mechanical qualities of components. A newly developed and established technique for assessing the mechanical strength of 3DP objects is the texture analyzer, also called an instron tensile tester, which examines a number of different properties, including fracture strain, hardness, and Young's modulus.

11.4.1 Tensile, Compression, and Flexural Strength Evaluations

Tensile testing is more appropriate to determine the strength and elasticity of 3DP medicines since it takes tablet geometry into account. If the tensile strength is more than 1.7 MPa, the tablet retains its structural stability throughout commercial production and shipment. For small-scale production of tablets that are not exposed to large mechanical stress, a tensile strength of up to 1 MPa could be adequate (Pitt and Heasley, 2013). Three-dimensional digital image correlation (3D-DIC) technology is useful to assess the specimen's compression testing strain.

11.4.2 Hardness and Friability Testing

The two essential QC tests of solid oral dose forms (SODF) are friability and disintegration, irrespective of the procedure used to fabricate them. Hardness is a valuable and relevant measure for quality assurance and in-process control, despite being an empirical feature (Jarosz and Parrott, 1982). The hardness tester used for conventional tablets is not suitable for 3DP products due to their low or high mechanical strength, and the process used for 3DP production is different from the conventional method. Currently, these are replaced with sophisticated hardness testers that are accurate and can measure hardness, thickness, diameter, and length all at once, making them more user-friendly (Erweka.com). Moreover, the results are presented on the LED screen in the preferred unit, and the user can also adjust the tester's measurement speed. Friability values may vary with the method employed to produce the 3DP prints; for example, tablets produced by the binder-jetting technique are very fragile and usually will not meet the USP friability specifications. There are no specific recommendations for evaluating the friability and hardness of 3DP SODF, so the conventional tablet guidelines must be followed. Thus, it is necessary to create new regulatory frameworks to ensure that the 3DP meets quality standards.

11.4.3 Porosity and Density Measurements

The internal structure of 3DP depends on pre-established design in addition to printing parameters, which vary with the method used for 3DP. The porosity, density, and mechanical strength are interrelated and influence the disintegration, dissolution, and bioavailability of the API. The degree of porosity can be ascertained with different techniques, such as helium pycnometer, mercury porosimetry, nuclear magnetic resonance (NMR), terahertz time-domain spectroscopy (THz-TDS), and x-ray microcomputed tomography (μX-CT) (Markl et al., 2018).

11.5 CHEMICAL AND DRUG-RELEASE ANALYSIS

Printing process requirements, infill density, printing temperature and physical properties of material must be carefully monitored as these factors influence the drug-release profile of 3DP products. After production, the 3DP pharmaceutical products quality must be verified to ensure the safety and therapeutic efficacy of the patient (Beer et al., 2023). So, NDTs of PAT have been used to monitor tablet CQAs, namely drug content (Wartewig and Neubert, 2005), hardness, drug distribution (Eksi-Kocak et al., 2018), solid-state characteristics (Netchacovitch et al., 2017), and characterization by NDT's is due to their quickness, non-destructiveness, and cost-effectiveness (Luypaert et al., 2007).

11.5.1 SPECTROSCOPIC TECHNIQUES (FTIR, UV-VIS) FOR CHEMICAL CHARACTERIZATION

Different types of spectroscopic techniques, like FTIR spectroscopy and XRD, are used for the characterization of materials. To check the impurities in raw materials and the existence of other phases of the powder and to characterize 3DP SOD forms, a scanning electron microscope (SEM) provided with an energy-dispersive x-ray detecting system (ED-XRS), ICP-OES, and micro-optical coherence tomography (μ-OCT) are used.

11.5.2 DRUG CONTENT UNIFORMITY ASSESSMENT

Both content and uniformity are always regarded as the main quality attributes (CQAs) for pharmaceutical products due to their potential to affect both patient safety and efficacy. NIR or NDT are applied to monitor drug content during the fabrication.

11.5.3 IN VITRO DISINTEGRATION AND DISSOLUTION TESTING

The polymer and other components, process variables, and the 3DP technique used for prints have a great influence on the disintegration and release profiles. Depending on the patient's needs, the printing pattern, shell thickness, and filling percentage can all be changed to alter the mechanical strength and finally medication release profile. As per the USP specifications, the disintegration times for different types of conventional solid dosage forms of tablets are different, and even the tablets obtained by the 3DP procedure, more specifically the product from binder-jetting due to its porous structure, show relatively low disintegration times. The other tools, like texture analyzer, can be utilized to calculate the disintegration time.

11.5.4 Quantitative Analysis

The current QC methods available for traditional dosage forms are not suitable for the point-of-care real-time release of printed pharmaceuticals due to their inherent destructiveness, and furthermore, assessments have been carried out offline. In contrast, effective 3DP production can be achieved by evaluating all products in each batch using in-line technologies included in the manufacturing workflow (Sacré *et al.*, 2021; Harms *et al.*, 2019). Near infra-red (NIR), Raman spectroscopy (RS), and terahertz spectroscopy are used for the study of 3DP products (Trenfield, 2021), in which real-time release testing of printlets of 3DP is done at the point of care and need not be removed from the process stream. NIRS and RS aid in obtaining qualitative and quantitative sample information. NIR is used for the QC of 3DP pharmaceutical products due to rapid analysis and thorough physicochemical insights (Talwar *et al.*, 2022; Trenfield, *et al.*, 2023). It proves to be a worthy method for evaluating the amount of drug in 2D and 3DP medicines (Edinger, *et al.*, 2017; Pollard *et al.*, 2023) and is also used for characterization of a single drug (paracetamol) in a point-and-shoot manner (Trenfield, *et al.*, 2018). RS scattering signals for API are frequently higher compared to those for excipients, and the fingerprint is precisely proportionate to the analyte concentration. Additionally, with little or no sample preparation, transmittance NIRS (tNIRS) and reflectance NIRS (rNIRS) are appropriate for the quantitative and qualitative analysis of samples (Jorgensen *et al.*, 2023).

11.6 SURFACE CHARACTERIZATION TECHNIQUES

If the real-time monitoring of the 3DP process is omitted due to a lack of specialized mechanisms for tracing and checking the printing process's progress, then many 3D printers will proceed to print all the layers with dimensional anomalies in the printlets. On the other hand, *in situ* visual inspections and monitoring assists in identifying errors at various stages during the 3DP process and helps to minimize the printing of defective components, which in turn reduces the waste of material resources and production time. Automatic process monitoring becomes crucial when manufactured in huge quantities utilizing hundreds of 3D printers. To detect problems in real time, sophisticated technology must be applied to develop fully functional monitoring systems. A variety of techniques were developed to monitor and evaluate the quality of the 3DP product, such as a multi-camera system consisting of five supervising features, each with a Raspberry Pi camera; rotating the camera around the printed item; a 3D reconstruction approach (Malik *et al.*, 2019), image-sensing device; a three-dimensional digital image correlation system (3D-DIC) (Holzmond *et al.*, 2017); artificial intelligence (AI) algorithms and machine learning (Farhan Khan *et al.*, 2020); and texture analysis utilizing the gray-level co-occurrence matrix (GLCM) and particular Haralick features as online measurement methods.

11.6.1 Scanning Electron Microscopy for Surface Morphology

An electron microscope is employed to evaluate the morphological features of the powder particles. SEM is an essential imaging tool used for surface characterization, and its micrographs provide information regarding the layering pattern on the surfaces of the 3D-printed tablets. The other one is transmission electron microscope (TEM), which is often used to examine the internal structure of samples. NDT offers the advantage of not causing damage to the unit being evaluated when compared to destructive techniques, such as TEM and SEM (Goldstein *et al.*, 2018).

11.6.2 ROUGHNESS ANALYSIS AND SURFACE PROFILOMETRY

The layer-by-layer construction of the components in 3DP technology introduces some characteristics that affect their quality, release rates, and performance. Dimensional accuracy, porosity, surface roughness, and necessary borders are critical quality indicators that can be attained by modifying the 3DP operation-specific factors. Work has been done to examine the impact of many factors, including orientation, layer thickness, building style, printing speed, dimensional accuracy of 3DP forms and temperature of the nozzle, platform, and chamber, on the surface roughness (Wang *et al.*, 2016). Due to the continuous invention of new substances and processes, it is usually a challenging task for QC to find reliable methods to appropriately test the material surfaces. The most commonly used methods to determine surface roughness of the printed objects include vision, microscopy like optical microscopy, and laser profilometry, optical profilometry, pin profilometry, micro x-ray CT, optical scanning, CT scanning (Hartcher-O'Brien *et al.*, 2019), and Nanovea's 3D non-contact profilometer are used (Ramirez, Nanovea.com).

11.6.3 CONTACT ANGLE MEASUREMENTS FOR WETTABILITY STUDIES

The wettability of the solid surface depends on the angle formed by the selected liquid on the specific solid surface. There are some indirect methods like liquid penetration (both thin-film wicking and column), the sessile drop technique, and the Wilhelm plate in which the penetration rate or pressure is correlated to contact angles (Alghunaim *et al.*, 2016). The sessile drop method, which involves placing a drop of liquid on a surface and measuring the angle of contact at the three-phase (liquid, solid, or vapor) contact line of the drop, is most widely used for checking the contact angle of flat and non-porous surfaces but cannot be used for porous and rough surfaces.

11.7 REGULATORY CONSIDERATIONS AND COMPLIANCE

Regulating standards, however, demand that the quality, purity, and product in every batch must meet certain specifications. The regulatory frameworks that govern the production, shipment, and compounding of on-demand and commercial 3DP products vary from nation to nation. Furthermore, there are no clear guidelines that manufacturers need to abide by in order to get permission for the commercialization of their devices and pharmaceutical products. The United States Food and Drug administration (USFDA), Healthcare Products Regulatory Agency (MHRA) and UK's Medicines, have released the documents endorsing the use of 3DP for point-of-care (PoC) manufacture, along with regulatory challenges.

11.7.1 Current Regulatory Landscape for 3DP Pharmaceuticals

The FDA approval of a 3DP pharmaceutical product (Spritam®) in 2015 is a turning point in the history of 3DP technology in the pharmaceutical field. Even though all regulatory agencies place a top priority on the quality of pharmaceutical substances to ensure the patients' safety, no proper guidelines have been issued till now for the production of 3DP products (Cui *et al.*, 2021). In addition, it is not clear that regulatory permission is required only for the finished product or at all phases of product design, including during manufacture. Even the safety precautions and standard operating procedures are to be considered in the 3DP process because toxic substances may be released at different steps of the 3DP process, like fusion, extrusion, or heating, that affect the skin or respiratory organs (Gioumouxouzis *et al.*, 2019).

11.7.2 Good Manufacturing Practices (GMP) in 3D Printing

3DP has shown considerable potential in the pharmaceutical market and has the capability to revolutionize personalized medicine production and drug discovery in the pharmaceutical industry. Various regulatory practices, such as good manufacturing techniques (GMPs), good documentation practices (GDPs), and good laboratory practices (GLPs), are applied to maintain the manufacturing standards of pharmaceutical products. Therefore, it is also necessary to develop suitable regulations for the production and marketing of 3DP pharmaceutical formulations, like GMP accreditation, which is required for premises that produce and distribute 3DP pharmaceutical formulations (Acosta-Velez, 2016).

11.7.3 Quality Assurance and Documentation Requirements

QbD is an alternative strategy to pharmaceutical product quality assurance that has recently gained popularity. Proper documentation and traceability are also necessary for QC in 3DP to ensure that all manufacturing and QC processes are accurately recorded, managed, and verifiable. Recording the materials utilized, the settings of the 3DP process, and the findings of the inspection are all part of this. By providing this documentation, it is possible to trace the final product's origin and ensure its traceability. Document management and storage may require the use of electronic document management.

11.8 CASE STUDIES AND REAL-WORLD APPLICATIONS

Several aspects of a 3DP product, including its mechanical qualities, dimensional accuracy, surface quality, and compliance with specifications are considered and assessed to establish the quality of the product by NDTs. It was reported that the NIRS was employed for in-line process control of different layers of UV-curable printing inks (Mirschel *et al.*, 2014), evaluation of 3DP pharmaceuticals (films and tablets), and near-infrared chemical imaging to study inkjet-printed pharmaceuticals (Vakili *et al.*, 2015). Raman confocal spectroscopy finds its use in examining the

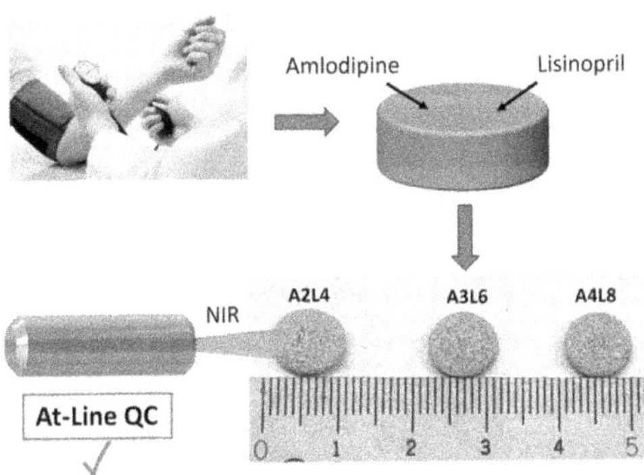

FIGURE 11.2 Determining the dosage content in polyprintlets using a portable NIR device. (Trenfield *et al.*, 2020.)

distribution of the medication and polymer within the 3DP tablet. *In situ* sensors and cameras are used to acquire process data for quality analysis and real-time monitoring of the 3DP techniques. A thermal camera is utilized to collect facts regarding the potential degradation processes (Aho *et al.*, 2019), which aids in chemical mapping of the drug and excipients and also to observe the variations in the solid forms of the finished product.

According to Figure 11.2, a study was carried out to determine the dose content of the polyprintlets containing two different medications (lisinopril and amlodipine) placed into cylindrical polyprintlets and 3D-printed films, with drug concentration ranges from 1–20% w/w and 1–3% w/w, respectively, by a portable NIR spectrometer non-destructively, and calibration models were also established (Trenfield *et al.*, 2020) and compared with HPLC output.

A quality management system, "certify-as-you-build", can watch a printlet throughout the printing process and identify print flaws in real time by comparing the created geometry with the computational model and 3D-DIC can be used to capture the structure and record the real-time flaws in 3DP product (Holzmond and Li, 2017). Figure 11.3 represents the real-time fault detection of specific and general defects by 3D-DIC.

11.8.1 Exemplary QC Strategies in 3DP Drug Formulations

Non-destructive testing is frequently used to provide efficient QC and preventive or predictive maintenance without altering the properties or original state of the material. One of the main purposes of the adaptation of QbD and PAT is to facilitate real-time release testing (RTRT), ensuring the quality of the medicinal product without damaging end-products. Taguchi's strategy is to complement approaches to conventional experimental design methods because it combines engineering and management approaches with statistical ones to produce improved-quality products and reduce costs quickly.

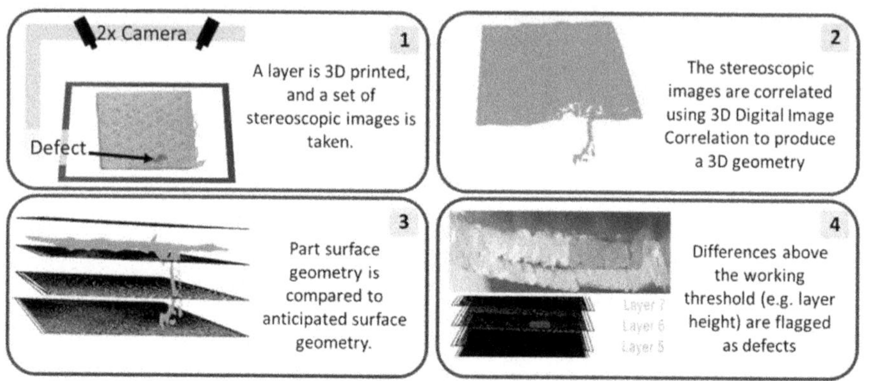

FIGURE 11.3 Real-time fault detection of both specific and general defects by using 3D-DIC. (Holzmond, *et al.*, 2017.)

11.8.2 Lessons Learned from Successful Implementation of QC Methods

Several factors, such as production process, the material being used, and the existence of contaminants, influence the selection and application of a non-destructive testing technique as each approach has its own guiding principles. Even the regulatory measures need to place a lot of emphasis on the quality assurance and management steps that lead to product formation by using new approaches to ensure quality throughout the production process.

11.8.3 Future Trends and Advancements in QC for Pharmaceutical 3D Printing

3DP is a breakthrough innovation; it provides novel approaches for both patients and the pharmaceutical industry that have a significant impact on the pharmaceutical sector. The QC methods that are employed for traditional pharmaceutical products are not suitable for 3DP products so NDTs are adopted for the characterization of 3DP pharmaceuticals. Spectroscopic techniques like NIRS, Fourier transform NIRS, HSI coupled with NIRS and RS, or Raman confocal microscopy can be installed offline, at-line, or in-line, and they can yield both quantitative and qualitative data. Another method, using an advanced algorithm, has been developed by ZoomlabTM (Tracy *et al.*, 2023), which helps to select the optimal excipients for a given API. This method minimizes costs by reducing the requirement for several laboratory tests, reducing wastage of expensive excipients, and checking the compatibility of various excipient–API combinations virtually. The numerous technological and legal challenges and the availability of online non-destructive quality-control procedures that 3D printing technology is currently confronting will be resolved in the near future.

11.9 CONCLUSION

3DP has received significant attention from the pharmaceutical industry over the past ten years owing to its rapid production, affordable price, and versatility in pharmaceutical formulations, thus enabling patients to obtain more effective and safer medication. In the pharmaceutical sector, quality control is a fundamental and crucial activity that ensures high-quality pharmaceutical products. The primary objective is to ensure that the product is safe, efficient, consistent, and reproducible throughout the entire manufacturing procedure. So it is critical to improve 3D printing quality since low standards could discourage consumers from buying 3D-printed products. Conventional QC techniques that have become prevalent in large-scale manufacturing represent the end-product testing paradigm; such approaches are generally destructive and inappropriate for the 3DP. This demands the development of a non-destructive PAT that requires little to no sample preparation and retains the integrity of the finished product. PAT is currently gaining recognition in research as a QC technique that allows the monitoring of the production process by offering real-time evaluation and management of critical process parameters and previously established CQA. Non-destructive techniques like 3D-DIC, photogrammetry techniques, NIR, RS, and hyper imaging are employed to reduce manufacturing oversights, material waste, variations, and imperfections in the 3DP process, as well as to enhance product quality during the manufacturing process. QC techniques and regulatory strategies like GMP at every stage of manufacture are crucial in enhancing the quality of 3DP formulations.

ACKNOWLEDGEMENTS

The authors are thankful to the management of Malla Reddy Pharmacy College for their unwavering support.

REFERENCES

Acosta-Velez, G. 3D pharming: direct printing of personalized pharmaceutical tablets. Polym Sci [Internet]. 2016 [cited Oct 28, 2023];2(1). Available from: www.primescholars. com/articles/3d-pharming-direct-printing-of-personalized-pharmaceutical-tablets-99603.html

Aho J, Bøtker JP, Genina N, Edinger M, Arnfast L, Rantanen J. Roadmap to 3D-printed oral pharmaceutical dosage forms: feedstock filament properties and characterization for fused deposition modeling. J Pharm Sci. 2019;108(1):26–35. doi: 10.1016/j.xphs.2018.11.012, PMID 30445005.

Alghunaim A, Kirdponpattara S, Newby B-MZ. Techniques for determining contact angle and wettability of powders. Powder Technol. 2016;287:201–15. doi: 10.1016/j.powtec.2015.10.002

Beccaria M, Cabooter D. Current developments in LC-MS for pharmaceutical analysis. Analyst. 2020;145(4):1129–57. doi: 10.1039/c9an02145k, PMID 31971527.

Beer N, Kaae S, Genina N, Sporrong SK, Alves TL, Hoebert J, et al. Magistral compounding with 3D printing: a promising way to achieve personalized medicine. Ther Innov Regul Sci. 2023;57(1):26–36. doi: 10.1007/s43441-022-00436-7, PMID 35943712.

Brambilla CRM, Okafor-Muo OL, Hassanin H, ElShaer A. 3DP printing of oral solid formulations: a systematic review. Pharmaceutics. 2021;13(3):358. doi: 10.3390/pharmaceutics13030358, PMID 33803163.

Castro-Sastre A, Fernández-Abia AI, Rodriguez-Gonzalez P, Martínez-Pellitero S, Barreiro J. Characterization of materials used in 3D-printing technology with different analysis techniques. In: International Vienna DAAAM, Proceedings of the 29th International DAAAM Symposium; 2018, pp. 947–54. doi: 10.2507/29th.daaam.proceedings.136

Cui M, Pan H, Su Y, Fang D, Qiao S, Ding P, Pan W. Opportunities and challenges of three-dimensional printing technology in pharmaceutical formulation development. Acta Pharmaceut Sin B. 2021; *11*(8):2488–504. https://doi.org/10.1016/j.apsb.2021.03.015

Deidda R, Sacre P-Y, Clavaud M, Coïc L, Avohou H, Hubert P, et al. Vibrational spectroscopy in analysis of pharmaceuticals: critical review of innovative portable and handheld NIR and Raman spectrophotometers. TrAC Trends Anal Chem. 2019;114:251–9. doi: 10.1016/j.trac.2019.02.035

Dimitrov D, Schreve K, de Beer N. Advances in three dimensional printing – state of the art and future perspectives. Rapid Prototyp J. 2006;12(3):136–47. doi: 10.1108/13552540610670717

Dinwiddie RB, Love LJ, Rowe JCM, Vogeler F, Coppens K. Realtime process monitoring and temperature mapping of a 3D polymer printing process. In: Proceedings of the SPIE, The International Society for Optical Engineering Faes; 2013.

Edinger M, Bar-Shalom D, Rantanen J, Genina N. Visualization and non-destructive quantification of inkjet-printed pharmaceuticals on different substrates using Ramanspectroscopy and Raman chemical imaging. Pharm Res. 2017;34(5):1023–36. doi: 10.1007/s11095-017-2126-2, PMID 28251424.

Edinger M, Jacobsen J, Bar-Shalom D, Rantanen J, Genina N. Analytical aspects of printed oral dosage forms. Int J Pharm. 2018;553(1–2):97–108. doi: 10.1016/j.ijpharm.2018.10.030, PMID 30316794.

Eksi-Kocak H, Tamer S, Yilmaz S, Eryilmaz M, Boyaci IH. Tamer quantification and spatial distribution of salicylic acid in film tablets using FT-Raman mapping with multivariate curve resolution. Asian J Pharm Sci. 2018;13:155–62.

Erweka.com [cited Oct 2, 2023]. Tablet hardness testers [Internet]. Available from: www.erweka.com/tablet-hardness-testers.html

Evans J. PAT minimises regulatory concerns around 3D-printed medicines [Internet]. synTQ. 2021 [cited Oct 28, 2023]. Available from: www.syntq.com/pat-minimises-regulatory-concerns-around-3d-printed-medicines-2/

Farhan Khan M, Alam A, Ateeb Siddiqui M, Saad Alam M, Rafat Y, Salik N, Al-Saidan I. Real-time defect detection in 3D printing using machine learning. Mater Today: Proceed. 2021;*42*:521–28. https://doi.org/10.1016/j.matpr.2020.10.482

Gandhi A, Roy C; Quality by Design (QbD) in pharmaceutical industry: tools, perspectives and challenges. PharmaTutor. 2016;4(11):12–20.

Gholizadeh S. A review of non-destructive testing methods of composite materials. Procedia Struct Integr. 2016;1:50–7. doi: 10.1016/j.prostr.2016.02.008

Gioumouxouzis CI, Karavasili C, Fatouros DG. Recent advances in pharmaceutical dosage forms and devices using additive manufacturing technologies. Drug Discov Today. 2019;24(2):636–43. doi: 10.1016/j.drudis.2018.11.019, PMID 30503803.

Goldstein J I, Newbury DE, Michael JR, Ritchie NWM, Scott JHJ, Joy DC. Scanning electronmicroscopy and X-raymicroanalysis. Microscopy Microanal. 2018;24(6):768. Springer, 550 pp. ISBN:978-1-4939-6674-5. https://doi.org/10.1017/S1431927618015271

Grangeia HB, Silva C, Simões SP, Reis MS. Quality by design in pharmaceutical manufacturing: a systematic review of current status, challenges and future perspectives. Eur J Pharm Biopharm. 2020;147:19–37. doi: 10.1016/j.ejpb.2019.12.007, PMID 31862299.

Harms ZD, Shi Z, Kulkarni RA, Myers DP. Characterization of near-infrared and Raman spectroscopy for in-line monitoring of a low-drug load formulation in a continuous manufacturing process. Anal Chem. 2019;91(13):8045–53. doi: 10.1021/acs.analchem.8b05002, PMID 31140783.

Hartcher-O'Brien J, Evers J, Tempelman E. Surface roughness of 3DP materials: comparing physical measurements and human perception. Mater Today Commun. 2019;19:300–5. doi: 10.1016/j.mtcomm.2019.01.008

Holzmond O, Li X. In situ real time defect detection of 3D printed parts. Addit Manufactur. 2017;*17*:135–42. https://doi.org/10.1016/j.addma.2017.08.003

Jarosz PJ, Parrott EL. Tensile strengths and hardness of tablets. J Pharm Sci. 1982;71(6):705–7. doi: 10.1002/jps.2600710625, PMID 7097540.

Jorgensen AK, Ong JJ, Parhizkar M, Goyanes A, Basit AW. Advancing non-destructive analysis of 3D printed medicines. Trends Pharmacol Sci. 2023;*44*(6): 379–93. https://doi.org/10.1016/j.tips.2023.03.006

Khosravani MR, Reinicke T. On the use of X-ray computed tomography in assessment of 3D-printed components. J Nondestr Evaluat. 2020;*39*(4). https://doi.org/10.1007/s10921-020-00721-1

Luypaert J, Massart DL, Vander Heyden Y. Near-infrared spectroscopy applications in pharmaceutical analysis. Talanta. 2007;72(3):865–83. doi: 10.1016/j.talanta.2006.12.023. PMID 19071701.

Malik A, Lhachemi H, Ploennigs J, Ba A, Shorten R. An application of 3D model reconstruction and augmented reality for real-time monitoring of additive manufacturing. Procedia CIRP. 2019;81:346–51. doi: 10.1016/j.procir.2019.03.060

Markl D, Strobel A, Schlossnikl R, Bøtker J, Bawuah P, Ridgway C, et al. Characterisation of pore structures of pharmaceutical tablets: a review. Int J Pharm. 2018;538(1–2):188–214. doi: 10.1016/j.ijpharm.2018.01.017, PMID 29341913.

Mirschel G, Daikos O, Heymann K, Decker U, Scherzer T, Sommerer C, et al. In-line monitoring of printing processes in an offset printing press by NIR spectroscopy: correlation between the conversion and the content of extractable acrylate in UV-cured printing inks. Prog Org Coat. 2014;77(11):1682–7. doi: 10.1016/j.porgcoat.2014.05.012

Netchacovitch L, Dumont E, Cailletaud J, Thiry J, De Bleye C, Sacré PY, et al. Development of an analytical method for crystalline content determination in amorphous solid dispersions produced by hot-melt extrusion using transmission Raman spectroscopy: a feasibility study. Int J Pharm. 2017;530(1–2):249–55. doi: 10.1016/j.ijpharm.2017.07.052, PMID 28746834.

Nuchitprasitchai S, Roggemann M, Pearce JM. Factors effecting real-time optical monitoring of fused filament 3D printing. Prog Addit Manufactur. 2017;2(3):133–49. doi: 10.1007/s40964-017-0027-x

Okafor-Muo OL, Hassanin H, Kayyali R, ElShaer A. 3DP of solid oral dosage forms: numerous challenges with unique opportunities. J Pharm Sci. 2020;109(12):3535–50. doi: 10.1016/j.xphs.2020.08.029, PMID 32976900.

Parhi R. A review of three-dimensional printing for pharmaceutical applications: quality control, risk assessment and future perspectives. J Drug Deliv Sci Technol. 2021;64:102571. doi: 10.1016/j.jddst.2021.102571

Pauli V, Roggo Y, Pellegatti L, Nguyen Trung NQ, Elbaz F, Ensslin S. Process analytical technology for continuous manufacturing tableting processing: a case study. J Pharm Biomed Anal. 2019;162:101–11. doi: 10.1016/j.jpba.2018.09.016, PMID 30227355.

Pitt KG, Heasley MG. Determination of the tensile strength of elongated tablets. Powder Technol. 2013;238:169–75. doi: 10.1016/j.powtec.2011.12.060

Pollard TD, Seoane-Viaño I, Ong JJ, Januskaite P, Awwad S, Orlu M, et al. Inkjet drug printing onto contact lenses: deposition optimisation and non-invasive dose verification. Int J Pharm X. 2023;5:100150. doi: 10.1016/j.ijpx.2022.100150, PMID 36593987.

Ramirez J. Surface roughness statistical analysis using 3d profilometry [Internet]. Nanovea. com [cited Oct 29, 2023]. Available from: https://nanovea.com/App-Notes/roughness-statistical-analysis.pdf

Sacré P-Y, De Bleye C, Hubert P, Ziemons E. PAT applications of NIR spectroscopy in the pharmaceutical industry. In: Portable Spectroscopy and Spectrometry; 2021, pp. 67–88. Wiley.

Sciencedirectassets.com [cited Sep 30, 2023].

Sheppard CJR. Scanning optical microscopy. Adv Imag Electron Phys. 2020;213:227–325.

Talwar S, Pawar P, Wu H, Sowrirajan K, Wu S, Igne B, et al. NIR spectroscopy as an online PAT tool for a narrow therapeutic index drug: toward a platform approach across lab and pilot scales for development of a powder blending monitoring method and endpoint determination. AAPS J. 2022;24(6):103. doi: 10.1208/s12248-022-00748-4, PMID 36171513.

Thakkar R, Pillai AR, Zhang J, Zhang Y, Kulkarni V, Maniruzzaman M. Novel on-demand 3-dimensional (3-D) printed tablets using fill density as an effective release-controlling tool. Polymers (Basel). 2020;12(9):1872. doi: 10.3390/polym12091872, PMID 32825229.

Tracy T, Wu L, Liu X, Cheng S, Li X. 3D printing: innovative solutions for patients and pharmaceutical industry. Int J Pharm. 2023;631:122480. doi: 10.1016/j.ijpharm.2022.122480, PMID 36509225.

Trenfield SJ. Quality Control of 3DP Pharmaceuticals Using Process Analytical Technologies; 2021. UCL (University College London).

Trenfield SJ, Goyanes A, Telford R, Wilsdon D, Rowland M, Gaisford S, Basit AW. 3D printed drug products: non-destructive dose verification using a rapid point-and-shoot approach. Int J Pharmaceut. 2018;549(1–2):283–92. https://doi.org/10.1016/j.ijpharm.2018.08.002

Trenfield SJ, Tan HX, Goyanes A, Wilsdon D, Rowland M, Gaisford S, Basit, AW. Non-destructive dose verification of two drugs within 3D printed polyprintlets. Int J Pharmaceut. 2020;577:119066. https://doi.org/10.1016/j.ijpharm.2020.119066

Trenfield SJ, Xu X, Goyanes A, Rowland M, Wilsdon D, Gaisford S, et al. Releasing fast and slow: non-destructive prediction of density and drug release from SLS3DPtablets using NIR spectroscopy. Int J Pharm X. 2023;5:100148. doi: 10.1016/j.ijpx.2022.100148, PMID 36590827.

Vakili H, Kolakovic R, Genina N, Marmion M, Salo H, Ihalainen P, et al. Hyperspectral imaging in quality control of inkjet printed personalised dosage forms. Int J Pharm. 2015;483(1–2):244–9. doi: 10.1016/j.ijpharm.2014.12.034, PMID 25527212.

Wang WM, Zanni C, Kobbelt L. Improved surface quality in 3D printing by optimizing the printing direction. Comput Graph Forum. 2016;35(2):59–70. doi: 10.1111/cgf.12811

Wartewig S, Neubert RH. Pharmaceutical applications of mid-IR and Raman spectroscopy. Adv Drug Deliv Rev. 2005;57(8):1144–70. doi: 10.1016/j.addr.2005.01.022, PMID 15885850.

Withers PJ, Bouman C, Carmignato S, Cnudde V, Grimaldi D, Hagen CK, et al. X-ray computed tomography. Nat Rev Methods Primers. 2021;1(1):1–21.

Yu LX, Amidon G, Khan MA, Hoag SW, Polli J, Raju GK, et al. Understanding pharmaceutical quality by design. AAPS J. 2014;16(4):771–83. doi: 10.1208/s12248-014-9598-3, PMID 24854893.

12 3D-Printed Pharmaceuticals
Current Regulatory Scenario

Raja Rajeswari Kamisetti, Ajmeer Ramkishan, Prakash Katakam, and Subhas Sahoo

12.1 INTRODUCTION

3D printing (3DP), an expository advancing technology in versatile fabrication systems including pharmaceuticals, bio-medicine, aviation and automobiles and so on with its ubiquitous utilization with an expectation to grow significantly to \$42.9 billion by 2025 (CAGR Markets press release, Tracy *et al.*, 2023). However, despite its potential and focus on digital savings, there is no systematic plan for 3DP. While compliance with rules is generally lacking in nations like India, certain countries have specific regulations focused on certain areas such as medical equipment.

These innovations are contemporary with multiple edges to the pharmaceutical industry, during early stages of drug development by their less time and expenditure. The timelines in the developmental stages was marked during the COVID-19 pandemic requiring rapid drug development and repurposing trials. In the course of pre-clinical and clinical formulation development, this technology is a prototype tool to rapidly evaluate intermittent batches of dissimilar drug product replications with a jolt on critical quality imputes.

3DP is a viable alternative to traditional manufacturing processes in the pharmaceutical business for producing personalized medications, offering cost savings compared to conventional procedures. However, these formulas have significance in improving medicinal effects. Formulations can be customized to individual patient requirements using 3DP under controlled conditions, a procedure already employed in the healthcare sector. Many manufacturers use this technology for the mass production of personalized hearing aids.

Industries worldwide must proactively adjust and shape the direction of technology, while governments should prioritize 3DP. In recent times, major nations such as China, the United States (US), and the European Union (EU). China has been actively developing its 3DP business and implementing policies to regulate these technologies. In 2017, an action plan called the "Additive Manufacturing Industry Development Action Plan (2017–2020)" was created (www.gov.cn/xinwen/2017-12/14/content_5246754.htm).

DOI: 10.1201/9781003439509-19

In 2018, "Centre of Medical Devices Evolution" of China issued suggestions for the management and directive of 3DP medical equipment that are specifically custom-built additive-manufactured medical devices (www.cmde.org.cn/CL0063/6954.html). In 2020, technical guidelines were adhered to permit the production of 3DP replacement vertebrae www.cmde.org.cn/CL0112/21043.html) and an acetabular cup (www.cmde.org.cn/CL0112/21042.html).

In 2017, the Federal government made a significant shift when the Foods and Drugs Administration of USA (FDA) issued recommendations aimed at additive produced medical devices (Martin *et al.*, 2017). The agency authorized the production of 3D-printed parts for commercial engines (www.ge.com/news/reports/the-faa-cleared-the-first-3d-printed-part-to-fly-2).

The Federal government has attempted to regulate the misuse of 3DP of firearms by introducing multiple laws in Congress (H.R.7115 2015). Despite being obscured by darkness, regulatory rules have been developed based on important recommendations.

12.1.1   Key Regulatory Considerations for 3DP Pharmaceuticals

Design and development: the design and development of 3D-printed pharmaceuticals must be carefully controlled to ensure the safety and efficacy with regard to the products. This includes material choices and design of the dosage form, and the printing process.

Manufacturing: the manufacturing of 3DP pharmaceuticals must be done in conformity with good manufacturing processes (GMP). This ensures that the products are produced consistently and reliably, and that they meet the required quality standards.

Quality control: 3DP pharmaceuticals must be subject to rigorous quality-control testing to ensure their safety and efficacy. This testing should include the tests to determine the identification, pureness, strength, effectiveness, and stability of the pharmaceuticals.

Labeling: the labeling of 3DP pharmaceuticals must be accurate and complete, and it must comply with all applicable regulations. The labeling should include information about the ingredients, the dosage, the route of administration, and the storage conditions.

The regulatory landscape for 3DP pharmaceuticals is still sprouting, but it is apparent that these products will be subject to austere regulations to warrant the safety and efficacy of these products, which have the potential to revolutionize the way to deliver medicines.

12.2   US FOOD & DRUG ADMINISTRATION (USFDA)

The regulating body is responsible for ensuring the safety and efficacy for the medical supplies such as medicines, biological products, and medical-devices, including 3D-printed medical products. The USFDA does not have strict monitoring in place for 3D printers, but it does closely oversee the automated processes and production of these 3D printers if the resulting product are medical devices that meet quality standards.

3DP devices must adhere to regulatory regulations, like all other devices. Premarket requirements relate to medical devices before they are launched, whereas post-market essentials use on medical products after they are sold.

There are three groups of medical equipment: Class I, Class II, and Class III. As you move from Class I to Class III, regulatory control grows.

The futuristic 3D printing technology and FDA's policy relates to the following:

(a) the fabrication, labeling, marketing, manufacturing, and analysis of regulated products, *(b)* the dispensation, at ease, for assessment or endorsement of regulatory submissions and *(c)* scrutiny and implementation of guidelines.

But the authority also states that a substitutional determine if it meets the criteria of the relevant laws. Hence, this outlined guidance is predominantly organized into two specific sections:

12.2.1 DESIGN AND MANUFACTURING CONSIDERATIONS

This involves addressing technical factors to comply with Quality Systems (QS) standards for a device based on its governing category or applicable legislation. The guidelines cover manufacturing issues and thoroughly address all regulatory criteria needed to develop a quality system for device manufacturing (U.S. Food and Drug administration, 2017).

12.2.2 DEVICE TESTING CONTEMPLATIONS

The section 510(k) of the guidance describes how to submit premarket notification submissions, related to applications of premarket approval (PMA), humanitarian device exemption (HDE), investigational device exemption (IDE) and *de novo* requests for 3D-printed devices.

The device categorization system defines the statutory prerequisites for general device types. Mostly devices belonging to Class I are exempted from section 510 (k), however the rules are mandatory for the devices belonging to Class II and Class III devices (www.gov.cn/xinwen/2017-12/14/content_5246754.htm).

Based on their inventiveness, 3DP has versatile medical applications, medical devices are regulated by the Center for Devices & Radiological Health (CDRH). The Center for Biologics Evaluation and Research (CBER) regulates biologics and the drugs are regulated by the Center for Drug Evaluation and Research (CDER).

Whilst the general 3DP devices are controlled by CDRH, the CBER oversees the regulatory oversight of all applications of additive manufacturing that use biological, cellular, or tissue-based materials. The CDER oversees medication applications involving 3DP, while the Office of the Combination Products (OCP) supervises goods with components typically overseen by multiple FDA Centres.

The FDA has not yet established a definitive policy regarding 3D-printed pharmaceuticals, but it has affirmed that they would be regulated as drugs or medical devices, depending on the specific product. The Foods, Drugs, and Cosmetics

(US-FDC) Act regulates drugs, whereas the Medical Device Amendments of 1976 (MDA) governs medical devices.

12.2.3 Recommendations: Quality System (QS) Regulation Amendments

The FDA published a guidance document (Feb 23/2022), appealing for public comment on device cGMP necessities as guided by Part-820 of 21 CFR to comprise the global standards meant for medical device QMS defined by ISO 13485:2016 standards.

12.2.4 Flexibility of the Quality Systems (QS)

Despite the fact that the current QS regulations provide ample and effectual requirements for the setting up of a QMS with worldwide accepted regulations of 13485 of ISO for medical devices that are followed by various regulatory agencies.

12.2.5 Applicability

This system encourages firms to create a distinct quality system that adheres to and is suitable for their particular products and operations, as outlined in 21 CFR 820.5. The rules of QS requires device producers to commercialize their finished products. US authorities classify items like tubings for blood and x-ray machines for diagnostic purposes as complete devices since these items are considered accessory items of finished-devices. Therefore, all accessory manufacturers must comply with QS regulations.

12.2.6 GMP Exclusions

The USFDA decided that some medical devices exempted from the requirement of GMP and are specified in 862 to 892 of 21 CFR and mentioned in the Federal Register. The GMP requirements' indemnity does not preclude maintaining complaint files (820.198 of 21 CFR) or common record-keeping specifications (820.180 of 21 CFR).

Medical devices made under an experimental device exemption (IDE) are excluded from design control criteria outlined in 21 CFR 820.30 of the QS regulation.

The Device Manual containing the operating setting as shown in Figure 12.1 ought to contain the following:

    i.   Recognize particulars from the device
    ii. Expound the details and make resolutions
    iii. Operate and control the device, its components.

It is also vital that devices

    iv. Collect input from the user and
    v. Respond to provided feedback.

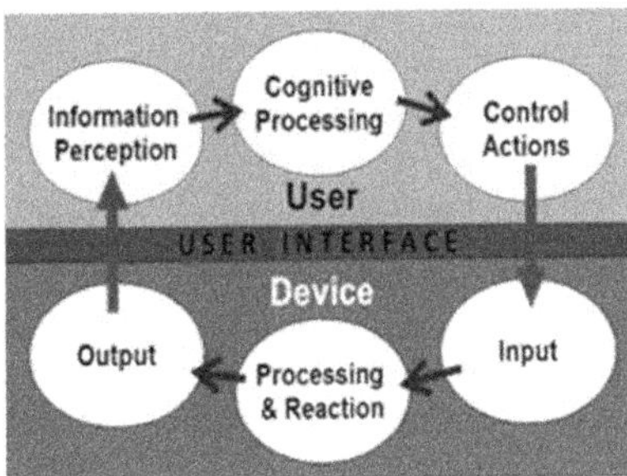

FIGURE 12.1   The user interface of medical equipment in an operating setting. (From www. fda.gov/media/80481/download)

12.2.7   Significance of Human Factors-Medical Devices

The user-device interface is designed with human factors and ergonomics in mind, encompassing all aspects of the device from unboxing, setup, calibration, usage, to maintenance tasks like cleaning, battery replacement, and repairs.

The practice of designing for human factors and usability aims to minimize risks associated with use and dangers while ensuring safety, efficiency, and effectiveness. The beneficial results of implementing in medical devices, human factors and usability engineering comprise

i.   More secure components and attachments, such as power wires, leads, tubing, and cartridges.
ii.   Effective controls and display interaction.
iii.   Proper user comprehension of the condition and functioning of the device.
iv.   Enhanced user comprehension of a user's present clinical status.
v.   Efficiently managing warning signal system.
vi.   Simplified gadget upkeep/restoration.
vii.   Decreased dependence on instruction manuals.
viii.   Reduced necessity for user instruction and reeducation.
ix.   Decreased user vulnerability and mistakes.
x.   Minimal likelihood of negative incidents and minimal likelihood of product withdrawals.

Commercial development of 3DP is highly sought after and is under the CDER. In 2015, the bureau authorized its initial 3DP medicine, an anti-epileptic medication tailored for persons with dysphagia (Aprecia Pharmaceuticals LLC 2015). CDER has not issued official recommendations on 3DP pharmaceuticals but is increasing its research in collaboration with interested producers through its Emerging Technology Programme   (www.fda.gov/drugs/news-events-human-drugs/cder-researchers-expl ore-promise-and-potential-3d-printed-pharmaceuticals).

TABLE 12.1
FDA's Approaches on 3D Printing Technologies

Models of Anatomy	Prosthetic Models	Implantable Devices
During clinical trials and innovation at the Veterans Health Administration as anatomical models for treatment procedures and patient consultation.	In the manufacture of customized orthotics and prosthetic devices tailored to the specific needs of each patient (VHA Innovation Ecosystem, 2022).	ProMade Point-of-care Centre for Complex Orthopaedic Solutions in New York, established by the Hospital for Special Surgery (HSS) and Lima Corporate SPA, offers customized 3DP solutions for replacing joints in individual patients (ProMade, 2022).

12.2.8　FDA: Emerging Approaches

3DP's uniqueness lies in its ability to enable personalized, on-demand, and decentralized production of medications using patient-specific imaging data (Morey 2020). Table 12.1 describesFDAs approaches on 3D printing technologies. Table 12.2 and 12.3 showcases the framework of FDA towards the development and approvals of 3DP technologies.

12.2.9　FDA Framework

(a)　Former version

TABLE 12.2
FDA's Former Version on 3D Printing Approvals

Condition	Summary
A	Low-risk 3D printing carried out by medical experts
B	Devices purposefully created by the maker under authorized procedures such as a fully integrated system
C	Devices created by a producer through a verified procedure: extra qualifications needed for healthcare professionals
D	At the point-of-care is where the manufacturer is situated
E	Medical proficiency

Source:　Zidan *et al.* (2018).

(b) Updated version

TABLE 12.3
FDA's Updated Version on 3D Printing Approvals

Scenario	Description	Entity Responsible for Designing and Developing the Gadget	Entity Utilizing a 3D Printing Machine to Manufacture Devices	Entity Accountable for Adhering to Relevant Regulatory Mandates
1	Healthcare institution utilizing a medical device manufacturing system (MDPS)	Conventional manufacturer	Healthcare facility	Conventional manufacturer
2	Conventional manufacturing located on or near the healthcare institution premises	Conventional manufacturer	Conventional manufacturing, including contractual process	Conventional manufacturing, including any prospective contract manufacturer
3	Healthcare facility taking up all conventional manufacturer duties	Medical facility	Medical facility	Medical facility

12.2.10 FDA-Approved 3D-Printed Medical Devices and Drug Products in Various Categories

List of approved products and devices are shown in Tables 12.4, 12.5, and 12.6, respectively.

12.2.11 USFDA-Approved Drug Products and Devices

Table 12.7 summarizes the legal and regulatory requirements mandatory for the Medical Device manufacturers. The overview of the regulations statuatory for 3DP in US, EU, and Australia are shown in Table 12.7.

12.2.12 Advocacy for the Prospects

i. *Counsel.* Guidance on device risk and regulations should be clear and specific for all categories of devices. The manufacturers should mention the manuals with all specifications and also the risks, technical errors, rectifications and the required statuatory framework guidelines are to be specified by the agency.

TABLE 12.4

3DP Medical Devices and Drug Products Approved by FDA

Category	Device	Applications
Orthopedics	3D-printed implants, such as knee and hip replacements	Customized design fit for each patient's anatomy
Craniofacial surgery	3D-printed models of the skull and facial bones	Surgeries and craft custom implants
Dental	3D-printed crowns, bridges, and inlays	Match a patient's natural dental alignment
Otolaryngology	Hearing aids and implants	Tailorable with robustness for each patient's ear canal
Urology	Stents and other implants	to treat urinary infections and ailments
Vascular surgery	3DP models of blood vessels	To plan surgeries and create custom grafts
Oncology	3D-P models of tumors	To plan radiation therapy and surgery
Drug delivery	3D-printed tablets and capsules	designed to release drugs at a controlled/modified pattern

TABLE 12.5

List of 3D Printing Drug Products and Devices

3DP tool	Formulation	Active Pharmaceutical Ingredient
Semi-solid extrusion	Bilayer tablet (polypill)	Guaifenesin (Roberts *et al.*, 2015)
	Multiple active tablets (polypill)	Nifedipine, Captopril, Glipizide (Martinez *et al.*, 2017)
Stereo-lithography	Hydrogel	Ibuprofen (Alvaro Goyanes and Usanee Det-Amornrat, 2016)
	Face mask	Salicylic acid (Fina, 2017)
	Tablet	Paracetamol (Salmoria GV and LA Zepon KM., 2013)
	Solid dosage form	Progesterone (Goyanes A *et al.*, 2016)
Fused Deposition Modeling	Caplet	Caffeine (Jamróz W *et al.*, 2017)
	Tablet	Hydrochlorothiazide (Scoutaris *et al.*, 2011)
	Oral film	Aripiprazole (Wu BM *et al.*, 1996)
Binder jetting	Tabular device	Methylene blue and alizarin yellow (Wang *et al.*, 2016)
Binder jetting	Cubic tabular device	Pseudoephedrine (Katstra WE *et al.*, 2000)
	Tablet	Chlorpheniramine maleate and fluorescein
	Oro-dispersible tablet	Levetiracetam (Jacob et al., 2017)
Inkjet	Implant	Levofloxacin (Huang W *et al.*, 2007)
	Nano-suspension	Folic acid (Wu W, 2009 and B. J, 2013).
	Nanoparticle	Rifampicin (Sandler N, 2011)
3D printing	Multidrug implant	Rifampicin and isoniazid (Wu W, 2009 and Pardeike J *et al.*, 2011)
Thermal Inkjet	Solution	Salbutamol sulfate (Buanz and Basit AW, 2011).

TABLE 12.6
USFDA-Approved Drug Products and Devices

Product	Applications	Manufactured by
Spritam® (levetiracetam), approved in 2015	Anti-epileptic designed to disintegrate quickly in the mouth, prepared by Zipdose technology enabling a single high-dose delivery (up to 1000 mg) in a highly absorbent composition that quickly disintegrates upon contact with a small amount of liquid (Wang *et al.*, 2016).	Aprecia Pharmaceuticals, USA
OsteoFab®	Orthodontic implant is the only polymeric medical device additive manufacturing platform with properties that include osseointegration, antibacterial and antiviral performance, bone-like mechanics, perfect fit, and radiolucency.	Oxford Performance Materials Inc, USA
Unite 3D™	The Bridge Fix mechanism incorporates an innovative foot and ankle joint fusion system that enhances stability using 3DP and OsseoTi® porous metal technology, eliminating the need for conventional surgical plates, screws, and staples (Dodziuk, 2016).	Zimmer Biomet Holdings, USA

TABLE 12.7
Summary of Legal and Regulatory Needs for Producers of Medical Devices

Description	Relevance to Device Makers
Registration of company and entry of devices	For the requirements of registration by the owner/operator for Commercial distribution: FDCA 510, 21 USC360; 21 CFR part 807; For manufacturing: 21 CFR 80720 (a)
Applicability to device manufacturing	PMN to be submitted by the manufacturer: 21 CFR-80781 (a) and 21 CFR § 80720 To market new device 510 (k), at least 90 days in advance FDCA 510 (k), 21 USC-360 (k); 21 CFR part 807, subpart E
(GMPs) /Quality System Regulation (QSR)	GMP/QSR requirements: 21 CFR § 8201 (a) (1) Facilities and Control: FDCA-520 (f) (1), 21 USC- 360j (f) (1); 21 CFR part 820

ii. *Legitimate.* The regulatory agencies must frame guidances for 3DP products and all are critically controlled, for their safety and efficiency.

iii. *Well-timed and extended oversight.* There is an urgent need for the agencies to issue official guidances and enforce the same during premarket review, post-market surveillance, and subsequent inspections. The gaps identified must be considered and thoroughly studied collaborating with professional medical associations and hospital accrediting organizations and certification standards for 3DP products and devices further to broaden the scope of oversight.

iv. *Oversight.* Sophistication and digitalization of technologies should be adopted by the agency and all stakeholders for future development of measures that guarantee patient safety while promoting an environment conducive to revolutionary advancements. This systematic action, might harmonize the quality management system requirements for global regulations.

12.2.13 Summary of USFDA Regulations on 3DP Technologies

3DP is geared up to entail the patients of a particular category like multiple doses in single dosage form. Their manufacture is exempted from sections 501(a)(2)(B), 502(f)(1) and 505 of the FD&C Act is more concerned about the accurate dose, efficiency, safety, stability, and biopharmaceutical aspects.

12.3 EUROPEAN MEDICINES AGENCY (EMA)

EMA suggests the statutory bodies must inculcate optimal tools to keep pace with scientific and technological drift and thus ensure the sound assessment of trial-blazing and complexive therapies. Specific EU product harmonization legislation describes 3D printing products as "Harmonized products" as per the Machinery Directive (Guide to application of the Machinery Directive 2006/42/EC - Edition 2.2).

3D printers that are complied with the Machinery Directive 2006/42/EC with respect to design and manufacture can be distributed in domestic marketplace without any additional or differing requirements imposed by Member States regarding manufacture and positioning in the market. 3DP devices are covered by EU guidelines under 93/42/EEC of Medical Devices Directive (Wang *et al.*, 2016). EU legal framework is technologically balanced without any specific mandatory technical aspects for their development.

12.3.1 Legal Framework for 3D Printers

Laser-operated 3D printers for metal product manufacturing should follow the relevant harmonized standards "Machinery Directives 4" as cited in the *Official Journal of the European Union* (earlier known as OJEC – the Official Journal of the European Community) are as follows:

i. EN ISO 12100 pertains to the machine safety and provides common principles for designing, assessment, and reduction of the risk.

ii. EN 60204-1 pertains to the safety standards for electric instruments used in machinery.

iii. EN 13849-1 pertains to the machine safety, specifically focusing on safety of of control system spare parts.

iv. EN 13850 pertains to the machine safety and specifically focuses on the design principles for emergency stop functions.

v. EN ISO 11553-1 pertains to machines that process laser equipment.

vi. EN 1127-1 pertains to explosion environments and methods for preventing and protecting against explosions.

vii. EN ISO 19353 pertains to the safety of machinery, specifically focusing on preventive maintenance and protection from fire.

For printing plastic objects, fire and explosion also relevant.

Additionally, considered for few non-harmonized standards for laser based production and safety;

viii. EN 60825-1 pertains to the safety standards for laser goods, specifically focusing on equipment categorization and requirements.

ix. EN 60825-4 pertains to the safety standards for laser-based product, specifically focusing on laser guards.

12.3.2   EU Legal Framework for 3DP Products

3DP are qualified for the approvals according to the definitions prescribed in the legislation. Medical device accessories must comply with medical device laws in order to be considered devices, as stated in Directive 93/42/EEC34[34]. Even if a medical device's component does not comply with the Medical Devices Directive 93/42/EEC's regulatory status, it is still anticipated that the component meet all of the device's safety requirements.

EN ISO 13485:2016 offers guidelines for QMS of Medical Devices and regulatory strategies outlined in ISO 13485:2016 and EN ISO 13485:2016/AC:2018. It emphasizes the importance of having a validated manufacture procedure, as detailed in Sec. 7.5.6 under EN ISO 13485:2016, which includes equipment qualification.

12.3.3   Harmonized Benchmarks for Accessories and Similar Tools for Medical Devices

i. Despite of the lack of harmonized standards specifically applicable to tooling and other accessories, in the medical devices' sector, still the manufacturers may be instructed to follow all measures of standards.

ii. Existing safety standards can be updated in specification to the manufacture processes to all types of products produced by 3D technology.

iii. There is an urgent need to upgrade the necessary guidance for the choice of safe and efficient materials like the components included in the case of ventilator valves, etc.

iv. Proper recommendations are required to be applied for suitable post-processing, such as cleaning, sterilization, biocompatibility of the devices manufactured to make sure for the nonappearance of free solid particles and other possibly dangerous materials.

v. The EU regulation on medical devices includes obligations related to high safety and quality standards, manufacturer-supplied information, and medical electrical equipment.

vi. Specifications for device design and related modules may be proposed by reaching a contract with the manufacturer or by contacting a national competent body, in addition to harmonized standards (https://health.ec.europa.eu/medical-devices-sector/new-regulations/contacts_en).

vii. The body recommends issuing a declaration of compliance for device qualifications.

12.3.4 Contemporary Published List of Harmonized Top-Notch Guidelines under the Medical Devices and Related Components

i. EN ISO 17510-1:2009 Sleep apnea breathing therapy - Part 1: Devices (ISO 17510-1:2007) and Part 2: Masks and accessories (ISO 17510-2:2007)

ii. EN 12342:1998+A1:2009 Respiratory tubings employed in apparatus for anaethesia and in ventilators are specified in the EN ISO 8835-3:2009 standard. Part 3 of the ISO 8835-3:2007 standard covers the systems for the conveyance and reception of active anesthetic gas scavenging systems used in inhalational anaesthesia. The document reference is EN ISO 8835-3:2009/A1:201

iii. The standard code is EN ISO 5366-1:2009. Tracheostomy tubes for adults (ISO 5366-1:2000) - Part 1: Tubes and connectors

iv. EN ISO 7376:2009 Equipment for anesthesia and respiration: laryngoscopes used for intubation of trachea

v. EN 13544-1:2007+A1:2009 Equipment for respiration therapy - Nebulizing systems (Part 1)

vi. EN 13544-2:2002 with Amendment 1:2009 Equipment for respiration therapy - Part 2: Intubation and associated components

12.3.5 3DP Products: Design Parameters

I. The details of the specifications will describe the scientific designs and needs for the product. Identify and confirm the necessary qualifications for the relevant 3D printer (3DP) and the procedures and parameters for the mass manufacturing of 3D items (https://health.ec.europa.eu/medical-devices-sector/new-regulations/contacts_en).

Further, the EMA strictly adheres to and signifies the issues related to the material used in 3D-printed products to be safe and performability are assessed for the purpose of the products. Examples include thermal, mechanical, chemical, and resistance to sterilization.

12.4   REGULATORY SCENARIO: AUSTRALIA

Australia: Australia updated its medical device regulatory framework prior to conducting clinical trials on 3DP medical devices. Current regulatory framework describes and specifically recommends the use of 3DP technologies. And to be followed for the mass production of similar 3DP devices.

12.5   PERSONALIZED MEDICAL DEVICES

Personalized medical devices are categorized as custom devices tailored to individual patients' anatomy or physiology, such as orthotics, dental crowns, or prosthetic limb sockets, are ideal for clinical use. These cater to unique and uncommon needs that cannot be met by mass-produced medical devices.

12.5.1   A PRODUCER MUST

a. Submit a device declarations' certificate outlining the main concepts related to the device's planned performance and design production. Evaluate the industrial process outcomes to ensure the device meets its intended functionality and design specifications.
b. Inform the relevant secretary about potential adverse reactions or recalls of the marketed device.

12.5.2   REGULATORY PERSPECTIVE

A 3DP medical device is mandated to fulfill the given below:

c. Custom-made gadgets, as per the EU MDR (Medical Device Regulation) definition, are not produced in large quantities.
d. Exemptions for specially designed equipment to be included in the Australian Register of Therapeutic Goods (ARTG).
e. ARTG inclusivity for reimbursement through normal health technology assessment (HTA) procedures, including the following:
   i. Customized medical devices.
   ii. Mass manufacture is done using standardized device templates that match a patient's anatomy and physiological parameters.
   iii. Reimbursement qualifications for patient-specific medical devices are required if they are incorporated in Australian Register for Therapeutic Goods (ARTG).
   iv. MTAA (Medical Technology Association of Australia) supports the idea that cutting-edge standards applicable to medical devices in common can also apply to 3DP equipment for medical purposes. Showing adherence to the Essential Principles of performance and safety.

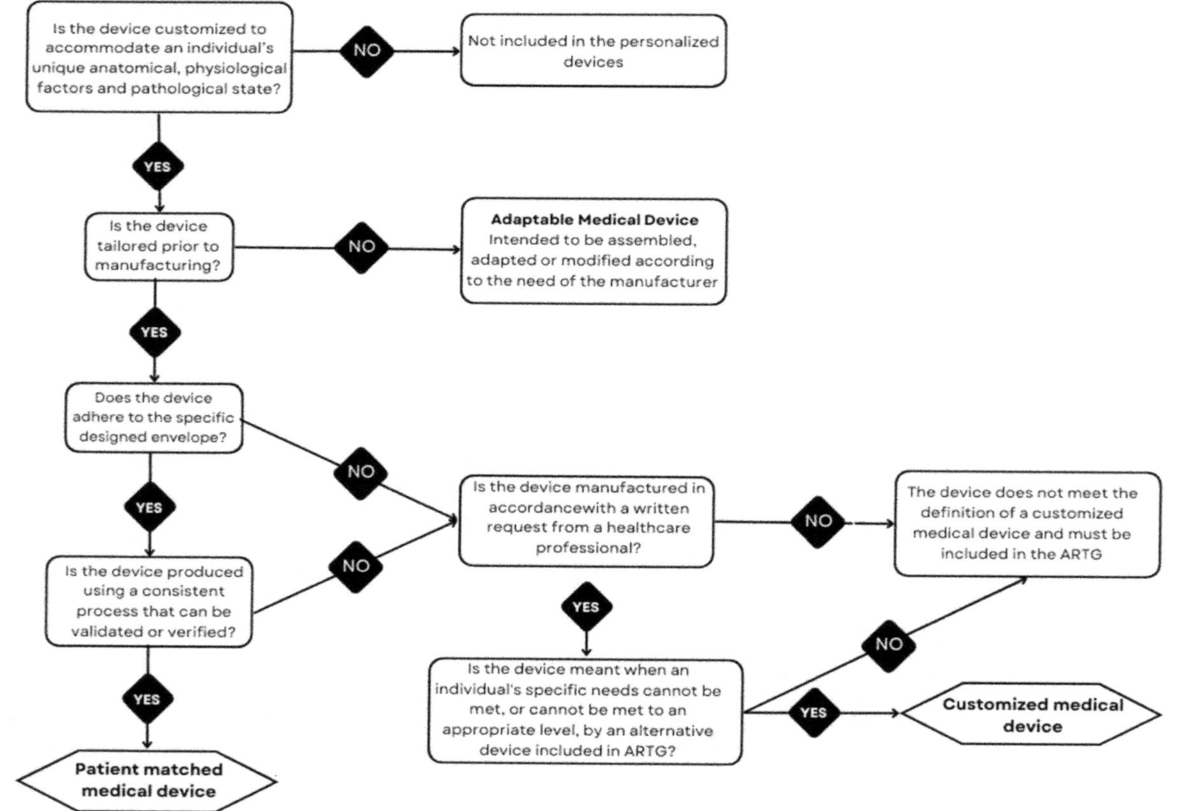

FIGURE 12.2 Personalized medical devices' decision tree regulatory overview. (Personalized medical devices including 3D Printing TGA V5. 1. August 2022.)

TABLE 12.8
Regulatory Overview of 3D Printing in US, EU, and Australia

	US	EU	Australia
Regulatory Agency	CDER (USFDA)	EMA	TGA
Classification	Class III	Class III	Class III
Law/directive	Included under Additive Manufactured Medical Devices	3DP Report on crucial technology-based products	Personalized and 3DP devices
Design input	Patient matched device designed using patient medical image	Esthetical preferences of the patients	Patient-customized device
Functional requirements	Operative qualification	Operational qualification (as per the FDA)	Realistic anatomical Geometries
Performance requirements	Additive Manufacturing and Hot Isostatic Process	Additive manufacturing	Safety
Design process and output	Standard development with documentation	Not applicable	Not applicable
Authentication and validation	non-disruptive assessments/Quality	Non-destructive evaluations/Quality	Safety, performance and Clarification/Quality management System
Regulatory perspective	Intellectual Property, bureaucratic distribution, premarket restrictions and control	Protecting human health and safety	Regulated according to biological framework
Regularity	ISO/ASTM 52915	ISO/ASTM TC 261 - ASTM F42 - CEN/TC 438Digital Single Market ECCommunications, 201	ISO 31485
Acceptance	QMS certification	CE marking	QMS certification

Sources: Dodziuk et al. (2016a, b) and Wang et al. (2016).

Medical device production systems (MDPS) are a novel statutory concepts exclusively meant for healthcare for customized production of patient-matched devices. An overview of a decision tree by the regulatory authority for personalized medical devices is represented in Figure 12.2.

12.6 CONCLUSION

At this present moment, 3DP devices are regularized similarly to the ones designed by conventional strategies. This statuatory substructure should be applicable despite the fact that 3DP devices are employed immediately after production, without allowing for extended quality-control procedures. The FDA has amended the guidance documents on 3DP. The Australian agency has already paved the way for superior regulations, and the guidelines within the EU need to be brought up to date. The investigations and laws of 3DP is to be fostered in the mere future. The laws on intellectual property need to be specified and regulated to withhold offences and mistreatments for not-for-profit applications. The potential of 3DP for creating customized pharmaceuticals is undeniable; regardless of how, machine diversifications are basic for proper pharmaceutical use. Furthermore, within-reach fabrication methods are worthwhile for public safety and efficient treatment procedures, and making their path into the commercial market by collaborative actions of regulation and patent authorities should collaborate with businesses.

REFERENCES

Applying Human Factors and Usability Engineering to Medical Devices. Guidance for Industry and Food and Drug Administration Staff, 2016. Available from www.fda.gov/media/80481/download

Aprecia Pharmaceuticals LLC, "FDA Approves the First 3D Printed Drug Product," News release, August 3, 2015, www.aprecia.com/news/fda-approves-the-first-3d-printed-drug-product

Banks J, "Adding value in additive manufacturing: Researchers in the United Kingdom and Europe look to 3D printing for customization," *IEEE Pulse*, vol. 4, pp. 22–26, 2013.

Buanz ABM, Basit AW. Preparation of personalized-dose salbutamol sulphate oral films with thermal ink-jet printing. Pharm. Res., vol. 28, no. 10, pp. 2386–2392, 2011.

Buanz ABM, Gaisford S, Basit AW, "Preparation of personalized-dose salbutamol sulphate oral films with thermal ink-jet printing," *Pharm. Res.*, vol. 28, no. 10, p. 2386, 2011.

Centre for Medical Device Evaluation, National Medical Products Administration, People's Republic of China, "Guidelines for the Technical Review of Custom Additive Manufacturing Medical Device Registration," February 26, 2018. www.cmde.org.cn/CL0063/6954.html

Centre for Medical Device Evaluation, National Medical Products Administration, People's Republic of China, "3D printing artificial vertebrae registration technical review guidelines (No. 36 of 2020)," June 5, 2020. www.cmde.org.cn/CL0112/21043.html

Centre for Medical Device Evaluation, National Medical Products Administration, People's Republic of China, "3D printed acetabular cup product registration technical review guidelines (No. 36 of 2020)," June 5, 2020. www.cmde.org.cn/CL0112/21042.html

Dodziuk H. Applications of 3D printing in healthcare. *Kardiochir Torakochirurgia Pol*, vol. 13, no. 3, pp. 283–293, 2016a. https://doi.org/ 0. 5114/kitp. 2016.62625

Dodziuk H. The Bridge Fix mechanism: An innovative foot and ankle joint fusion system utilizing 3D printing and OsseoTi® porous metal technology. *J. Ortho. Innov.*, vol. 9, no. 3, pp. 123–130, 2016b.

Fina F, Goyanes A, Gaisford S, Basit AW, "Selective laser sintering (SLS) 3D printing of medicines," *Int. J. Pharm.*, vol. 529, pp. 285–293, 2017.

Gallagher MB, "3 Questions: The Risks of Using 3D Printing to Make Personal Protective Equipment," Massachusetts Institute of Technology, March 26, 2020, https://news.mit.edu/2020/3q-risks-using-3d-printing-make-personal-protective-equipment-0326

General Electric, "The FAA cleared the first 3D printed part to fly in a commercial jet engine from GE," April 14, 2015. www.ge.com/news/reports/the-faa-cleared-the-first-3d-printed-part-to-fly-2

Goyanes A, Det-Amornrat U, "3D scanning and 3D printing as innovative technologies for fabricating personalized topical drug delivery systems," *J. Control. Release*, vol. 234, pp. 41–48, 2016.

Goyanes A, Martínez-Pacheco R, Basit AW, "Fused-filament 3D printing of drug products: Microstructure analysis and drug release characteristics of PVA-based caplets," *Int. J. Pharm.*, vol. 234, pp. 290–295, 2016.

Guide to application of the Machinery Directive 2006/42/EC - Edition 2.2. Available from https://osha.europa.eu/en/legislation/guidelines/guide-application-machinery-directive-200642ec

H.R.7115 – 3-D Firearms Prohibitions Act, 115th Congress, 2017–2018, www.congress.gov/bill/115th-congress/house-bill/7115/text?r=1&fbclid=IwAR2ara4EL2d6RHk5M_hNXHOKLaYlPcYmAScl_hBgTIV0unCw_dk5VPPGO4E

Hospital for Special Surgery, "First Surgeries Completed With Patient-Specific 3D Printed Implants Produced at the LimaCorporate ProMade Point-of-care Center at Hospital for Special Surgery," News release, March 8, 2022, https://news.hss.edu/first-surgeries-completed-with-patient-specific-3d-printed-implants-produced-at-the-limacorporate-promade-point-of-care-center-at-hospital-for-special-surgery/.

https://health.ec.europa.eu/medical-devices-sector/new-regulations/contacts_en

Huang W, Zheng Q, Sun W, Yang X, "Levofloxacin implants with predefined microstructure fabricated by three-dimensional printing technique," *Int. J. Pharm.*, vol. 339, pp. 33–38, 2007.

Jacob J, Coyle N, Thomas GW, Donald CM, Henry LS, Nemichand BJ. "Rapid disperse dosage form containing levetiracetam," US9339489B2 (Patent), 2017.

Jamróz W, Kurek M, Szafraniec J, Syrek K, "3D printed orodispersible films with Aripiprazole," *Int. J. Pharm.*, vol. 533, no. 2, pp. 413–420, 2017.

Katstra WE, Teung P, Rowe CW, Giritlioglu B, Cima MJ, "Oral dosage forms fabricated by three-dimensional printing," *J. Control. Release*, pp. 1–9, 2000.

Khaled SA, Burley JC, Alexander MR, Yang J, Roberts CJ, "3D Printing of tablets containing multiple drugs with defined release profiles," *Int. J. Pharm.*, vol. 494, no. 2, pp. 643–650, 2015.

Markets and Markets, "3D Printing Market Worth $42.9 Billion by 2025 With a Growing CAGR of 23.3%." www.marketsandmarkets.com/PressReleases/3d-printing.asp

Martin, N, "FAA Drafts Plan to Regulate Additive Manufacturing of Aerospace Components," October 23, 2017. www.executivegov.com/2017/10/faa-drafts-plan-to-regulate-additive-manufacturing-of-aerospace-components/

Martinez PR, Goyanes A, Basit AW, Gaisford S, "Fabrication of drug-loaded hydrogels with stereolithographic 3D printing," *Int. J. Pharm.*, 2017, doi: 10.1016/j.ijpharm.2017.09.003

Morey B, "Metal 3D Printing Comes to Mayo's Engineering Division," SME, May 20, 2020, www.sme.org/technologies/articles/2020/may/metal-3d-printing-comes-to-mayos-engineering-division/

Pardeike J, Schrödl N, Voura C, Gruber M, Khinast JG, "Nanosuspensions as advanced printing ink for accurate dosing of poorly soluble drugs in personalized medicines," *Int. J. Pharm.*, vol. 420, no. 1, pp. 93–100, 2011.

ProMade Point-of-care Centre for Complex Orthopaedic Solutions in New York. Established by the Hospital for Special Surgery (HSS) and Lima Corporate SPA. 2022.

Salmoria GV, Klauss P, Zepon KM, "The effects of laser energy density and particle size in the selective laser sintering of polycaprolactone/progesterone specimens: Morphology and drug release," *Int. J. Adv. Manuf. Technol.*, vol. 66, pp. 1113–1118, 2013.

Sandler N, Maattanen A, Ihalainen P, Kronberg L, Viitala T, "Inkjet printing of drug substances and use of porous substrates towards individualized dosing," *J. Pharm. Sci.*, vol. 100, pp. 3386–3395, 2011. www.gov.cn/xinwen/2017-12/14/content_5246754.htm

Scoutaris N, Alexander MR, Gellert PR, Roberts CJ, "Inkjet printing as a novel medicine formulation technique," *J. Control. Release*, 2011, doi: 10.1016/j.jconrel.2011.07.033

Tracy T, Wu L, Liu X, Cheng S, Li X, "3D printing: Innovative solutions for patients and pharmaceutical industry," *Int. J. Pharm.*, vol. 631, 2023.

U.S. Food and Drug Administration, "CDER Researchers Explore the Promise and Potential of 3D Printed Pharmaceuticals," 2017, www.fda.gov/drugs/news-events-human-drugs/cder-researchers-explore-promise-and-potential-3d-printed-pharmaceuticals

U.S. Food and Drug Administration, "Statement by FDA Commissioner Scott Gottlieb, M.D., on FDA Ushering in New Era of 3D Printing of Medical Products; Provides Guidance to Manufacturers of Medical Devices," News release, December 4, 2017, www.fda.gov/news-events/press-announcements/statement-fda-commissioner-scott-gottlieb-md-fda-ushering-new-era-3d-printing-medical-products

VHA Innovation Ecosystem, "3D Printing at VHA," 2022, www.va.gov/INNOVATIONECOSYSTEM/assets/images/covid-images/3D-Printing-Overview-HIMSS_v2.pdf

Wang J, Goyanes A, Gaisford S, Basit AW. "Stereolithographic (SLA) 3D printing of oral modified-release dosage forms," *Int. J. Pharm.*, vol. 503, no. 1–2, pp. 207–212, 2016. https:// doi.org/ 10. 1016/j. ijpha rm. 2016. 03. 016

Wu BM, Borland SW, Cima LG, Sachs EM, "Solid free-form fabrication of drug delivery devices," *J. Control. Release*, vol. 40, pp. 77–87, 1996.

Wu W, Zheng Q, Liu Y, Sun J, "A programmed release multi-drug implant fabricated by three-dimensional printing technology for bone tuberculosis therapy," *Biomed. Mater.*, vol. 4, 2009.

Zidan A et al., "Extrudability analysis of drug loaded pastes for 3D printing of modified release tablets," *Int J Pharm*, vol. 554, pp. 292–301, 2019, https://doi.org/10.1016/j.ijpharm.2018.11.025

Zidan A et al., "Development of mechanistic models to identify critical formulation and process variables of pastes for 3D printing of modified release tablets," *Int J Pharm*, vol. 555, pp. 109–123, 2019, https://doi.org/10.1016/j.ijpharm.2018.11.044

Index

For Product Safety Concerns and Information please contact our EU
representative GPSR@taylorandfrancis.com
Taylor & Francis Verlag GmbH, Kaufingerstraße 24, 80331 München, Germany

www.ingramcontent.com/pod-product-compliance
Ingram Content Group UK Ltd.
Pitfield, Milton Keynes, MK11 3LW, UK
UKHW022316100726
473146UK00009B/493